MASSAGE THERAPY

INTEGRATING RESEARCH AND PRACTICE

Trish Dryden, MEd, RMT
Centennial College, Toronto

Christopher A. Moyer, PhD
University of Wisconsin–Stout, Menomonie

Editors

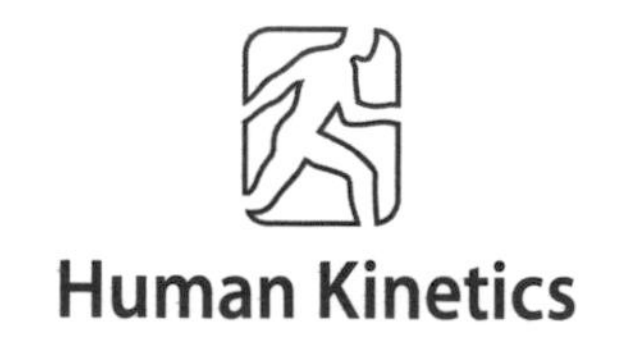

Human Kinetics

Library of Congress Cataloging-in-Publication Data

Massage therapy : integrating research and practice / Trish Dryden, Christopher A. Moyer, editors.
p. ; cm.
Includes bibliographical references and index.
ISBN 978-0-7360-8565-6 (hard cover) -- ISBN 0-7360-8565-3 (hard cover)
I. Dryden, Trish, 1954- II. Moyer, Christopher A., 1970-
[DNLM: 1. Massage. 2. Evidence-Based Practice. WB 537]

615.8'22--dc23

2011047784

ISBN-10: 0-7360-8565-3 (print)
ISBN-13: 978-0-7360-8565-6 (print)

The web addresses cited in this text were current as of November 9, 2011, unless otherwise noted.

Acquisitions Editor: Myles Schrag; **Developmental Editor:** Kevin Matz; **Assistant Editors:** Steven Calderwood, Anne Cole, and Melissa J. Zavala; **Copyeditor:** Joy Wotherspoon; **Indexer:** Michael Ferreira; **Permissions Manager:** Dalene Reeder; **Graphic Designer:** Fred Starbird; **Graphic Artist:** Denise Lowry; **Cover Designer:** Keith Blomberg; **Photographs (interior):** © Human Kinetics, unless otherwise noted; **Photo Asset Manager:** Laura Fitch; **Photo Production Manager:** Jason Allen; **Art Manager:** Kelly Hendren; **Associate Art Manager:** Alan L. Wilborn; **Illustrations:** © Human Kinetics; **Printer:** Thomson-Shore, Inc.

Printed in the United States of America 10 9 8 7 6 5 4 3 2 1

The paper in this book is certified under a sustainable forestry program.

Human Kinetics
Website: www.HumanKinetics.com

United States: Human Kinetics, P.O. Box 5076, Champaign, IL 61825-5076
800-747-4457
e-mail: humank@hkusa.com

Canada: Human Kinetics, 475 Devonshire Road Unit 100, Windsor, ON N8Y 2L5
800-465-7301 (in Canada only)
e-mail: info@hkcanada.com

Europe: Human Kinetics, 107 Bradford Road, Stanningley, Leeds LS28 6AT, United Kingdom
+44 (0) 113 255 5665
e-mail: hk@hkeurope.com

Australia: Human Kinetics, 57A Price Avenue, Lower Mitcham, South Australia 5062
08 8372 0999
e-mail: info@hkaustralia.com

New Zealand: Human Kinetics, P.O. Box 80, Torrens Park, South Australia 5062
0800 222 062
e-mail: info@hknewzealand.com

E4900

Contents

Foreword

The future of the massage therapy profession depends on the ability of massage therapists—not just professional researchers—to understand the importance of high-quality research and to embrace how it can influence their work. This will allow our profession to grow in effectiveness and allow us to create stronger connections with other health care providers. But research has always seemed hopelessly abstract and disconnected from the daily needs of a massage practice. Further, research literacy has never been a standard part of core curriculum in massage therapy education. One reason for this vacuum is that we have lacked resources that demonstrate how to weave research findings and clinical practice together.

Here is a book that begins to fill that vacuum. I believe it has the potential to change our whole profession.

My work with the Massage Therapy Foundation has made me a spokesperson for massage therapy research, but I never hide the fact that my background is not in the sciences. My education in research methodology and statistical analysis has been . . . let's call it haphazard. I reluctantly entered this world only because it became clear that the massage therapy profession would hit an intractable and unpleasant dead end without the ability to communicate in a research-based, evidence-informed context. Slowly, slowly, I have learned to speak this language and to appreciate all that this way of thinking has to offer. For this, I owe a debt of gratitude to many people, several of whom are contributors to this text.

Imagine my delight, then, to be invited to write the foreword for *Massage Therapy: Integrating Research and Practice.* This groundbreaking work would have made my entrance into the world of evidence-informed practice so much easier. The chapters on qualitative and quantitative research alone explained several years' worth of confusions that I have accumulated since I began trying to sort out research language. This is a technical manual that will be useful to those who are comfortable in the research world. The text will also be inviting to people who may be hesitant or nervous about climbing this learning curve.

This book does five crucial things:

1. It makes the compelling case that research literacy is a necessary skill even among entry-level massage therapists.
2. It introduces key concepts in a way that is both simple and accurate. As a teacher of a complex topic, I know how often the tipping point between simplicity and accuracy is narrow indeed.
3. It emphasizes the application of research by giving clear examples of tying published findings to everyday practice scenarios.
4. By emphasizing the practical application of research findings, it acknowledges the importance of the feedback loop that must exist between clinicians and researchers.
5. It lays the groundwork for its own future development as the mass of evidence about massage therapy continues to grow.

I am thrilled to welcome *Massage Therapy: Integrating Research and Practice* to the resources that are available for students and practitioners of massage. And I am jealous of the newest generation of massage therapists who will have this guide into a part of their education that defines the future of our profession.

Ruth Werner, President
Massage Therapy Foundation

Preface

Massage therapy is a rapidly growing profession. The United States Department of Labor (2011) predicts that employment of massage therapists is expected to increase by 19% from 2008 (122,400) to 2018 (145,600), faster than the average for all occupations. Similar growth can be expected in Canada and other nations.

Paralleling this growth is a substantial increase in the number of research studies that examine its value for promoting human health and well-being. Increasingly, health care practitioners, educators, and researchers are faced with a dilemma: How does one keep up? Massage therapy research tends to be scattered across a range of journals in the medical and behavioral sciences, making merely finding the latest articles challenging and time consuming. Once they are found, making sense of those articles—for example, determining which ones are sound and which ones are flawed—usually requires a background in scientific research that may not have been part of a practitioner's training.

Despite these obstacles, every professional therapist working today needs to have some understanding of the research process and knowledge of the latest findings, which confirm (and, occasionally, disconfirm) current practices, promote innovation and progress, and help ensure that therapy is delivered in ways that are optimally safe and effective. The research process is slowly transforming the massage therapy profession from one that has been largely based on tradition to one that is increasingly based on evidence. In the future, the profession's answer to questions that take the form of "Why do massage therapists do X?" will less frequently be "Because that's what we've always done." Increasingly, the answer will need to be "Because we have evidence that X works." This is a profound change.

Massage Therapy: Integrating Research and Practice was produced in recognition of this change and as a tool for advancing the development of evidence-informed practice. With this in mind, our goal was straightforward: to produce the best single source of the latest research with relevance to the practice of massage therapy. By compiling this information in a single book, we present readers with a synthesis of information from diverse fields, including kinesiology, medicine, nursing, physical therapy, and psychology. We strived to do this in a way that is clear and concise, without resorting to oversimplification.

Note that this book does not require you to begin on the first page and end with the last page (though there would be no harm in doing so). Rather, we have organized the book into 23 topic-specific chapters that can be read either individually or in any order, depending on your interests and current needs. Feel free to skip around. Without knowing what order you will choose for yourself, we can confidently say this: The reader who takes in all of these chapters will cover a lot of ground and will learn the most up-to-date information available on these topics. This is because each chapter has been authored by experts carefully selected for their specific knowledge, experience, and ability to synthesize the best evidence with implications for clinical practice and future research. For example, the chapters in part III represent those populations and conditions for which there is now enough substantive evidence to warrant a full discussion in this book. In future editions, it is our intention to not only update and expand those chapters as new evidence becomes available but also to add chapters covering other populations and conditions as scientific examination of massage therapy expands.

We expect this book to be indispensible to both students and current practitioners of massage therapy. For both of these groups, knowledge of the information contained in these pages will ensure that they bring to their practice the most accurate information currently available. It will also allow them to ground their practice in the latest research findings. Just as important, this knowledge also will greatly assist aspiring and practicing massage therapists to work collaboratively with other health care practitioners. This trend toward interprofessionalism is already well underway, and it is likely to become increasingly important as the profession continues to progress. For that reason, we also expect this book to be a valuable resource to other health care practitioners, educators, and researchers who are interested in learning more about massage therapy and the development of patient-centered, evidence-informed, integrative health care.

Whether you are a veteran massage therapist, an aspiring student of massage therapy, or the practitioner of another health modality who wishes to learn more about massage therapy, the following chapters will present you with the best evidence for this safe and effective health intervention.

INSTRUCTOR RESOURCES

Massage Therapy: Integrating Research and Practice includes an ancillary test package as an aid for instructors. The test package includes more than 200 questions, including multiple choice, true or false, and short answer/essay questions. Instructors can access the test package at

www.HumanKinetics.com/MassageTherapy

REFERENCE

United States Department of Labor, Bureau of Labor Statistics. 2011. Occupational Outlook Handbook, 2010-11. www.bls.gov/oco/ocos295.htm.

Acknowledgments

Working with Christopher Moyer is an adventure and joy. Meticulous and caring, Chris is a wonderful colleague and friend and I look forward to our continued work together. I am also hugely indebted to Stacey Shipwright, Research Analyst at Centennial College, for her unwavering faith in the project, administrative support, and also for her wonderful chapter contribution. A huge thank you also goes to our principal editor from Human Kinetics, Kevin Metz, whose careful reading of the text, respectful questions, and helpful additions were invaluable, and to my many colleagues and friends at Centennial College, especially President Ann Buller and the executive team, for their mentorship and support.

I am deeply grateful to the chapter authors for their scholarship and contribution to increasing safe and effective client care and respectful, interprofessional practice. To my many clients over thirty years of practice, whose sharing of their healing journeys teaches me about the true value of compassionate touch and human connection; and to my many students, colleagues, dear friends and mentors who continue to ask the tough questions and challenge the answers.

Finally, and most importantly, I am grateful to my beloved family—my husband Lee, our children Bryn and Jesse, and my sister Diane—for their laughter and their love, and to my parents Betty and George, and my brother Derek—whose many gifts in life and in death—continue to inspire me.

Trish Dryden

There are many folks who supported me in the completion of this project. The love and support of my parents, Jack and Elaine, and my siblings, Stephen and Tatiana, is the foundation that makes any of my projects possible. I never could have completed this project without my friend and colleague Trish Dryden, whose intelligence, wit, and motivation make working with her a pleasure, and I feel lucky that the two of us both arrived at the idea for this book independently. Stacey Shipwright deserves thanks for providing Trish and myself with outstanding organization, planning, and coordination that helped us to make our idea a reality. I also want to thank each of the authors who contributed to this book's individual chapters; there is no way this book could have been created without your tremendous knowledge and dedication. I am also grateful to the Psychology Department at University of Wisconsin-Stout for granting me a course release that made completing this book a little easier, to the Massage Therapy Foundation who have been a terrific resource to me in many ways, and to Rosemary Chunco for being a good friend and an enthusiastic supporter of this book's mission.

Above all, thanks go to my wife, Jessica, who gives me love, support, and motivation. I never would have thought to undertake this project had I not first seen her complete three books of her own, and her advice was invaluable. Finally, I also want to acknowledge all the members, both past and present, of our pet family. Their love and companionship fills our lives with joy and meaning.

Christopher A. Moyer

Contributors

Carla-Krystin Andrade, PhD, PT
University of California

Amanda Baskwill, BEd, RMT
Humber College

Patricia J. Benjamin, PhD

Karen T. Boulanger, MS, CMT
The University of Iowa

Paul Clifford, BSc, RMT
Sir Sandford Fleming College

Trish Dryden, MEd, RMT
Centennial College

Paul Finch, PhD, DpodM
Conestoga College Institute of Technology and Advanced Learning

Andrea D. Furlan, MD, PhD
Institute for Work and Health, University of Toronto, Toronto Rehabilitation Institute

Stuart Galloway, PhD
University of Stirling

Kimberly Goral, MS, NCTMB
Boston University

Michael D. Hamm, LMP CCST
Cortiva Institute at Seattle

Bodhi G. Haraldsson, RMT
Massage Therapists Association of British Columbia

Angus Hunter, PhD
University of Stirling

Marta Imamura, MD, PhD
University of São Paulo School of Medicine

Emma L. Irvin, BA
Institute for Work and Health, University of Toronto, Toronto Rehabilitation Institute

Janet R. Kahn, PhD, LMT
University of Vermont, Integrated Healthcare Integrative Consulting

Ania Kania, BSc, RMT
University of Calgary

Albert Moraska, PhD
University of Colorado at Denver

Christopher A. Moyer, PhD
University of Wisconsin–Stout

Douglas Nelson, LMT, NMT
MMT MidWest, Inc.

Janice E. Post-White, PhD, RN, FAAN
University of Minnesota School of Nursing

Cynthia J. Price, PhD, LMT
University of Washington

Stacey Shipwright, BA, RMT
Centennial College

Diana L. Thompson, LMP
Hands Heal

Marja Verhoef, PhD
University of Calgary

Joan M. Watt, MA, MCSP, MSMA
University of Stirling

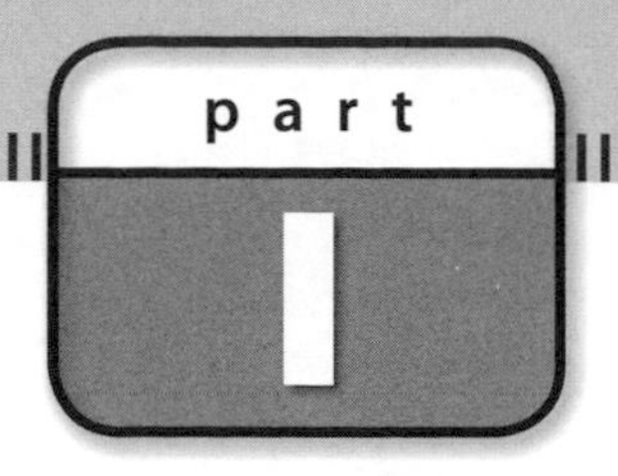

HISTORICAL DEVELOPMENT AND BACKGROUND

To understand the current state of massage therapy research and practice, and where they are headed, we must first put their origins in context. The chapters presented here illustrate the long and interesting history of massage therapy, and connect it with the modern shift toward evidence-based and outcome-based approaches in healthcare.

The chapters in Part I begin with an overview of the history and development of research in massage over the past 150 years and conclude by outlining a step by step clinical decision-making process on integrating research and practice.

Historical Overview

Patricia J. Benjamin, PhD

> Respecting the physiological action of Massage, it is necessary to speak with caution. Here, as is so often the case, practice has preceded theory. The art of Massage has been acquired, but we know little of its mode of action . . . It is easy to theorize, but we want carefully observed facts and accurately recorded experiments.
>
> *(Murrell 1890, 74)*

Massage research has experienced a renaissance in the past 20 years. The number and quality of studies has increased dramatically, and it is becoming easier to access research reports. Research literacy is on the rise among massage therapists (Dryden et al. 2004).

It may surprise some to learn that this is not the first period of interest in research about massage. Over a century ago, there was similar interest in scientific massage, based on anatomy and physiology. Experiments were conducted to determine how it works. In this precursor to the current evidence-based age of health care, empirics were scoffed at and scientific investigation was lauded as the way to gain merit as a respected therapeutic system. Some thought that massage was on its way to becoming "a special branch of the art of medicine" (Graham 1902, 41).

This prediction was vastly overblown, as the history of massage in the 20th century confirms. The use of massage in conventional health care languished for many decades. It is now considered to be complement and alternative to conventional medicine. How did this come to be? What forces dampened the interest in massage in the mid-20th century and what forces have led to this latest revival? The answers to these questions provide insight into why it is important to keep the momentum for massage research going strong in the future.

EMPIRICS

The words *empiric* and *empiricism* have special meaning in the history of medicine. They are not to be confused with the more neutral term *empirical,* which describes knowledge gained through observation using the physical senses. The distinction is particularly important when trying to understand how massage came to be considered alternative to contemporary conventional medicine, since much of its history is actually linked to the medical establishment.

empirical

▸ Concerned with the acquisition of knowledge through observation or experience.

empiric

▸ A historical term for a charlatan, or a dishonest or unqualified practitioner, who was guided solely by experience.

empiricism

▸ The position that knowledge comes largely or entirely from experience. Historically, this was a pejorative term that referred to medical practice that disregarded science in favor of experience.

At the time, *empiric* was a pejorative term akin to *quack* and *charlatan*. It was often applied to what was considered fringe or alternative medicine. In this context, *empiricism* actually suggested practitioners who showed a disregard for scientific methods while relying solely on experience. The terms *empiric* and *empiricism* were often used in a derogatory sense by physicians, especially in the early 20th century, in their attempts to raise standards in the medical profession and to distinguish themselves from quack medicine and from those with competing views of health and healing.

CYCLES OF BOOM AND BUST

The history of massage research can be envisioned as cycles of boom and bust that have a somewhat predictable trajectory. First, champions for massage promoted its therapeutic value to the general public and to other health professionals. Their beliefs are accounted for by rational explanations based on science and clinical observations. Case studies are provided to support their claims.

Next, a call was made to back up empirical data with more rigorous scientific experimentation. This type of request typically involves established health professions, including their professional societies and publications. As long as massage is valued as a therapeutic agent, massage research continues. However, when massage is devalued for some reason, interest wanes and research largely disappears. This cycle occurred in medical circles in the late 19th century and in physical therapy in the 20th century.

A new cycle for massage research has begun, and the latest champions are within the emerging profession of massage therapy. Their efforts are multiplied by concurrent public and government interest in complementary and alternative medicine (CAM), or complementary and integrative health care (CIHC), as it is sometimes now named. Subsequent sections of this chapter outline how an infrastructure is being built to support massage research in the coming years. Although history is best told with a little hindsight, the end of the chapter describes some of the latest developments to bring this chronicle of massage research up to the present time.

This look at the history of massage research is necessarily brief due to space constraints. It is also limited to sources that are available in English. Although it focuses on development of massage research in North America, European influence is noted where relevant. Only major historical developments and players are included here. The many minor but important factors are left to a more extensive account. This chapter serves as an introduction to some of the characters, events, and progress made in the past 150 years that are nudging massage out of the realm of conjecture and onto the more solid footing of science-based knowledge.

EARLY CHAMPIONS OF MASSAGE

For centuries, the writings of ancient Greek and Roman physicians were consulted on the use of frictions, rubbing, and unctions to treat human ailments. These included the works of Hippocrates (460-370 BCE), the father of medicine, who famously observed “the physician must be experienced in many things, but assuredly also in rubbing, for things that have the same name have not the same effects . . . Hard rubbing binds; soft rubbing loosens; much rubbing causes parts to waste; moderate rubbing makes them grow” (Graham 1902, 21).

Centuries later during the Age of Enlightenment, a time in Western society when reason was advocated as the source of legitimacy and authority, physicians began to report their own observations of frictions and rubbing in the treatment of diseases. These cases were published in the journals of fledgling medical societies in Western Europe and in the American colonies in the 1700s. The articles were typically written by individual physicians reporting on interesting cases, with results explained by the prevailing beliefs about human physiology.

Then in the next century, two popular systems of manual therapy would emerge and lay the foundation for massage therapy as we know it today. They built on the accumulated knowledge about medical rubbing and movements, and they gained respect in medical circles as they demonstrated positive clinical results and proposed rational explanations for their methods. These systems were Ling's medical gymnastics (Swedish movement cure) and Mezger's massage.

Ling

Pehr Henrik Ling (1776-1839) of Sweden developed a system of active and passive movements for treating chronic diseases that included soft-tissue manipulation. He based his system on knowledge of anatomy and physiology and "conducted his researches with the most scrupulous exactness, and frequently in the most earnest manner recommended his companions to do the same. He did not acknowledge a new movement to be a good one, until he was able to render to himself an exact account of its effects" (Roth 1851, 10).

With government funding, Ling established the Royal Institute of Gymnastics in Stockholm in 1813, which included a school and clinic. Ling's reputation spread widely. By the mid-1800s, physicians and lay practitioners from Russia, Germany, France, England, and the United States came to the Royal Institute to learn his system.

Mezger

Johann Mezger, MD of Amsterdam (1838-1909), gained renown by curing the chronic joint problem of Denmark's crown prince with his system of soft-tissue techniques. Mezger later emerged as a minor celebrity, and he was sought by other physicians who wanted to learn his system of massage. His technique categories of effleurage, petrissage, friction, tapotement, and the use of French terminology (such as *massage, masseuse, masseur*) characterize classic Western massage to this day.

Mezger's massage was considered far more sophisticated than medical rubbing found elsewhere. The observation was made that "there is as much difference between Mezger's Massage and the so-called English Massage, as there is between champagne and gooseberry. It is oysters and marcobrunner *versus* ginger-beer and whelks" (Murrell 1890, 23). By the early 20th century, massage and the Swedish movements began to appear together, and the two systems were conflated into what was later known variously as Swedish massage and remedial massage.

EARLY MASSAGE STUDIES

By the beginning of the 20th century, a considerable store of practice-based knowledge about the use of massage had been collected by physicians and lay practitioners, particularly in Western Europe and North America. This information was published in medical journals, monographs, and a growing number of textbooks.

A few prominent physicians championed the use of massage in medical circles. Noteworthy among them were J.B. Zabludowski (1851-1906) and Albert Hoffa (1859-1907) of Germany, William Murrell of England (1853-1912), and Douglas Graham of Boston in the United States (1848-1928). The writings of these men, particularly Murrell and Graham, are valuable for the background they provide, especially the descriptions of studies related to massage. These early massage textbooks illustrate research that attempted to put massage in the realm of science.

Authors often cited each other, reporting on cases improved by massage. In many cases, it was simply noted that the condition improved and the patient resumed normal activity. Occasionally, they provided a more detailed description, such as "under [massage's] influence, appetite and digestion improve, and the circulation becomes more rigorous, colour returns, and the quantity of food consumed is sometimes astonishing" (Murrell 1890, 201).

Authors sometimes debated the efficacy of different treatments, such as the treatment of sprains by massage versus immobility in a plaster cast. One early study had a control group that received the standard treatment at the time, which was immobilization, while the others received massage. It was noted that "Muller treated 37 cases of sprains with massage, and found the mean duration of treatment till recovery to be 9 days, against 25.6 days that 42 cases required under immobilization" (Graham 1902, 351).

Sometimes interest centered on the treatment for a particular pathology. For example, Dr. Weir Mitchell promoted his rest cure as treatment for a condition called neurasthenia. Massage was thought to be an important part of treatment because it was believed to improve appetite. In an experiment to test this hypothesis, it was found that after one week of systematic 20-minute daily massage, all participants in the study gained weight. Measurements included appetite, amount of food eaten, weight gained, quantity of nitrogen assimilated, temperature in the axilla, pulse rate, and frequency and depth of breathing (Murrell 1890, 74-75). Although the research design had serious flaws by today's standards, it demonstrates the combination of qualitative and quantitative methods to measure the effects of massage.

Basic research on animals was conducted to explain the therapeutic effects of massage in terms of physiology. Popular topics included the effects of massage on blood and lymph circulation, urine output, and recovery after muscle exertion. In one study by Professor von Mosengeil, a student of Mezger, rabbits were used to measure the effects of massage on the circulatory and lymphatic systems (Murrell 1890, 78-79).

Many massage studies were conducted at universities, particularly in Europe. However, in at least one instance, experiments occurred at a natural healing institution, the Battle Creek sanitarium in Michigan, directed by J. Harvey Kellogg, MD (1852-1943). In his *Art of Massage* (1895), Kellogg mentions experiments conducted in the sanitarium's physiology laboratory, which illustrates that massage was no longer solely informed by clinical experience but also by scientific experiment. Kellogg states the purpose of these investigations to be "verifying the physiological effects obtained by other investigators . . . and determination of the special effects which are characteristic of different procedures of massage . . . which had not previously been fully studied" (Kellogg 1895, vi). See figure 1.1.

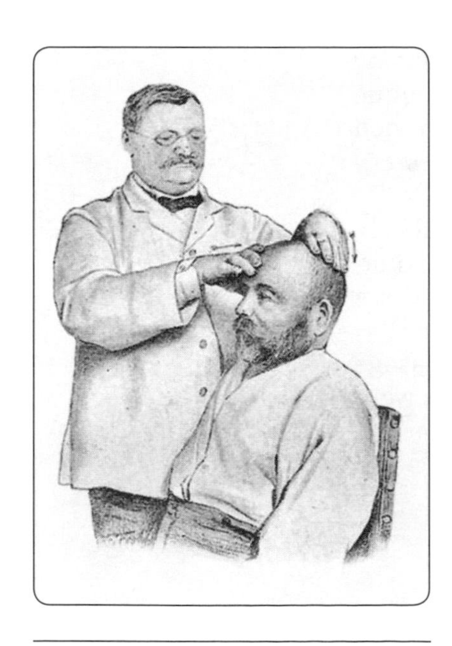

Figure 1.1 Massage of the Head.

From Zabludowski's Technik der Massage by Eiger 1911.

TWO PATHS FOR MASSAGE

A few late 19th century realities are worthy of note. One is that regular medicine at this time was based largely on clinical experience. Medical science linking pathologies and physiology began to gain acceptance in the 1860s, but the main emphasis remained on practice-based knowledge well into the next century (Porter 1997).

Another reality is that in the 19th century in Europe and North America, medical practice was loosely regulated, resulting in the availability of a wide variety of approaches to healing. In addition to regular or conventional medicine (i.e., *allopathic*), unconventional medicine techniques included homeopathy, eclectic medicine, hydropathy, and natural healers. Among the many cures promoted were the rest cure, the water cure, and the Swedish movement cure. Medical gymnasts provided treatment to patients for a variety of pathologies with active and passive movements, including massage. The professions of naturopathic physician, chiropractor, and osteopath were all formed in the 1890s.

Some might say that it was a time of vibrant diversity in options for healing. Others would call it a hotbed of quackery and runaway empiricism. For the most part, medical schools of all types were proprietary, leading to many abuses and unsubstantiated claims for the methods that they promoted. Snake oil hucksters, patent medicine salesmen, and lightning bonesetters peddled cures of dubious efficacy. Massage textbooks often lamented the proliferation of untrained practitioners with crude skills and little knowledge.

The landscape of medicine changed dramatically in the United States after the Food and Drug Act of 1906 and the publication of the Flexner report by the Carnegie Foundation in 1910. The Food and Drug Act demanded that claims for cures be substantiated, while the Flexner report was responsible for causing major changes in allopathic medical training. Scientific research became the basis of medical knowledge and medical training became the responsibility of universities. The amount of training needed to become a physician increased, the number of medical schools declined, and the American Medical Association acquired greater influence over medicine. Nonallopathic healers were largely branded as empirics and quacks.

Physicians now focused almost entirely on the use of drugs and surgery, and massage lost its standing as a branch of medicine.

Subsequently, the practice of massage continued on two different paths. Natural healers, working outside of the medical profession, continued to practice massage in an empirical manner. However, many masseuses and masseurs elected to work in tandem with regular medicine to develop the profession of physiotherapy (i.e., physical therapy). At the same time, massage research continued in the early decades of the 20th century.

PHYSIOTHERAPY AND MASSAGE

Physiotherapy in North America traces its roots to World War I and the treatment of wounded soldiers with massage and Swedish movements. The high demand for skilled therapists produced the first wave of practitioners, who developed the profession known as *physical therapy* in the United States and *physiotherapy* in Canada, the United Kingdom, and other English-speaking countries. (For the purposes of this chapter, physiotherapy will be considered as one profession, albeit with variations in different countries.)

In response to the demand for rehabilitation specialists, a group of Canadian nurses underwent a year's training in rehabilitation massage and exercise prior to working with injured troops in France. On their return to Ontario, they organized the first group of massage therapists in Canada. Subsequently, these practitioners trained in remedial massage and found work treating patients with polio and industrial injuries. The focus of the profession later broadened to include treatment of orthopedic injuries, including sports injuries. The Ontario Board of Regents began regulating the practice of massage in 1919 (Dominion of Canada 1920).

Mennell

James B. Mennell, MD (1880-1957) was an important transitional figure who championed massage from the beginning to the middle of the 20th century. He was a physician, physiotherapist, and lecturer at London's St. Thomas Hospital, and he wrote the textbooks about remedial massage that were used in military rehabilitation centers throughout the United Kingdom during World War I. He influenced both Canada and the United States with his rehabilitation training centers, including the Canadian Medical Service in Toronto and Walter Reed Army Hospital in Washington, DC, which were both established just prior to 1918.

Mennell wrote *Massage: Its Principles and Practice* (1917), which focused primarily on orthopedic treatments. His work was adopted by physiotherapists in both the United States and Canada and was influential through its last edition in 1945. Mennell recounted a familiar story of how he learned about massage:

> The views expressed in these pages are founded on the result of several years of close observation, study, and experiment. It is possible some of my deductions are erroneous, but at least they are capable of being argued and are not merely arbitrary (Mennell 1920, 2).

McMillan, Beard, and Tappan

Mary "Mollie" McMillan (1880-1959) trained in physiotherapy in England and later served as director of Reed College Clinic for Training Reconstruction Aides in Physical Therapy in Portland, Oregon, in 1919. She served as the director of physical therapy at Harvard Medical School from 1921 to 1925 and wrote *Massage and Therapeutic Exercise* (1921), the first comprehensive text on physiotherapy written by an American physical therapist. Although McMillan was clearly aware of prior massage research, her text was almost exclusively a how-to book with few references.

Gertrude Beard (1887-1971) was the first director of the physical therapy program at Northwestern University Medical School in Evanston, Illinois, one of the earliest accredited programs in the United States. She cowrote the textbook *Massage: Principles and Techniques* in 1964, which explained and illustrated the use of massage in physical therapy. The massage techniques described were largely based on clinical observations, but the bibliography shows that some massage research was consulted.

Frances Tappan (1917-1999) was first director of the physical therapy program established in 1950 at the University of Connecticut. Continuing the tradition of wartime training in remedial massage, Tappan was a product of army rehabilitation programs in World War II. Her first book, *Massage Techniques: A Case Method Approach* (1964), made note of research while describing massage developed from clinical experience.

The research cited by Beard and Tappan highlights massage effects related to cases common in physiotherapy. Individual citations included the following: "Effect of massage on metabolism: A survey" (Cuthbertson 1933), "Effects of massage on denervated skeletal muscle" (Suskind, Hajek, and Hines 1946), "The effect of massage upon the skeletal system of the dog" (Kosman, Wood, and Osborn 1948), "The effects of massage on the circulation in normal and paralyzed extremities" (Wakim 1949), and "Effect of various procedures on the flow of lymph" (Elkins et al. 1953). In addition, the number of individual journals that they cited, including *Archives of Physical Medicine, Archives of Physical Therapy, British Journal of Physical Medicine, Journal of the American Physical Therapy Association, Physiotherapy, Physical Therapy Review,* and *Principles and Practice of Physical Therapy*, is evidence of the growth of research in physiotherapy during this period.

Beard specifically noted the decline in the amount of massage prescribed by physicians following WWII. She speculated that this was due to the time, strenuous effort, and manual skill it demanded. She also admits that the basis for prescribing massage had been largely empiric (i.e., practice based) rather than scientific (i.e., evidence based). Within physiotherapy, interest in massage waned after the 1960s, and the quantity of massage research declined.

LATEST CYCLE OF MASSAGE RESEARCH

As a therapeutic practice, massage languished for much of the 20th century, apart from some interest in massage for palliative care within nursing. Then, in the 1980s, the massage therapy profession emerged from the tradition of natural healers, and a new wave of massage research began. The desire to be included in evidence-based integrative health care motivated massage studies for a variety of specific conditions. Today the range of massage topics being researched is very broad, paralleling the interest in massage research that occurred over a century ago.

In the past 20 years, several separate streams have come together to create a positive climate for massage research and to lay the foundation for the future. Interest in massage research has shifted from that of a few isolated health care professionals, gaining institutional and governmental support that it never had before. The following are a few examples of recent institutional developments that support massage research.

Touch Research Institute

A breakthrough study in massage for infants in the 1980s propelled massage into the public consciousness. Tiffany Field's study of massage for preterm infants showed improved weight gain and developmental behaviors (1986). The conclusion that the massage intervention shortened hospital stays and saved the hospital money caught the attention of the health care industry. It also led to a grant from Johnson and Johnson, which Field used to establish the Touch Research Institute (TRI) at the University of Miami's School of Medicine in 1992. Since that time, TRI and its partners have conducted more than 100 studies on the therapeutic effects of touch and massage therapy.

Massage Therapy Foundation

In the early 1990s, the American Massage Therapy Association proposed a strategic plan for professional development of the field that included the establishment of a foundation to promote massage research (AMTA 1990). The AMTA Foundation was incorporated as a nonprofit corporation in 1992, and was later renamed the Massage Therapy Foundation (MTF). The MTF has been a driving force in massage research since its creation.

In 1999, MTF convened a three-day conference to frame a research agenda for the massage therapy field. The Massage Research Agenda Workgroup (MRAW) included physicians, clinical and experimental scientists, social scientists, and massage therapists from the United States, Canada, and Europe. The participation of the massage therapy profession was believed to be essential for generating research that would be relevant and valuable to massage therapists and their clients. This proactive stance was designed to reverse the frequent practice in CAM research of failing to include practitioners in the conceptualization of research.

The resulting *Massage Therapy Research Agenda* (2002) identified five goals for the future. The first was to build a research infrastructure within the massage therapy profession and to establish research as a core competency in massage therapists' education. The other goals focused on funding studies in the following areas: the safety and efficacy of massage therapy, the physiological mechanisms of massage, massage from a wellness paradigm, and the massage therapy profession itself.

The MTF provides grants for massage research. Since 2001, it has maintained a web-based database of massage research studies (www.massagetherapyfoundation.org/researchdb.html). In 2005, the MTF started an annual student case-report competition, adding a contest of practitioner case reports in 2007. In a landmark move, the MTF established the first free, online, peer-reviewed journal for massage research, the *International Journal of Therapeutic Massage and Bodywork: Research, Education, and Practice* (www.ijtmb.org) in 2009.

The National Center for Complementary and Alternative Medicine

In the 1990s, growing public use of alternative medicine coincided with U.S. government attention to CAM therapies, including massage therapy. The Office of Alternative Medicine (OAM) had been established within the U.S. National Institutes of Health (NIH) in 1992 to explore "unconventional medical practices" and to recommend further research on the subject (NIH 2011). Its 1994 report summarized OAM findings related to CAM. OAM was elevated to a center in 1999, when it became the National Center for Complementary and Alternative Medicine (NCCAM). NCCAM has since awarded several research grants for studies of manual therapies, including massage. It has also sponsored several research conferences.

The Holistic Health Research Foundation of Canada

The Holistic Health Research Foundation of Canada (HHRC) was founded in 2003 as a charitable organization to support multidisciplinary research, public awareness, and professional education in complementary and alternative health care. It established a dedicated massage therapy research fund in 2005 in partnership with the College of Massage Therapists of Ontario and with the support of the Canadian Massage Therapy Alliance and the Massage Therapists' Association of British Columbia. It has awarded massage research grants annually since 2007. Refer to the Canadian Interdisciplinary Network for Complementary and Alternative Medicine Research Network (IN-CAM) for current status.

The International Society for Complementary Medicine Research

The International Society for Complementary Medicine Research (ISCMR) was established in 2003 at the 10th Annual Symposium of Complementary Health Care in

London. Its mission is to foster complementary and integrative medicine research and to serve as "a platform for knowledge and information exchange to enhance international communication and collaboration" (ISCMR 2010).

Massage Research Conferences

A natural outgrowth of growing interest in massage therapy has been the advent of massage research conferences and the inclusion of massage in CAM research conferences. These have been sponsored by both government agencies and non-governmental organizations. One of the first was in 1999, when the Massage Therapists' Association of British Columbia sponsored the Touch Research Symposium in Vancouver, Canada. Since that time, a number of conferences have provided a venue for presentations, discussions, and further development of massage research infrastructure. A list of these is presented in table 1.1.

Table 1.1 Major CAM and Massage Research Conferences

Date	Conference, place, and sponsor
1999	In-Touch Research Symposium in Vancouver, Canada
2002	International Symposium on the Science of Touch in Montreal, Canada
2004	2nd International Symposium on the Science of Touch in Montreal
2005	Highlighting Massage Therapy in CAM Research in Albuquerque, New Mexico
	Conference on the Biology of Manual Therapies in Bethesda, Maryland
2006	North American Research Conference on Complimentary and Alternative Medicine in Edmonton, Canada
2007	1st International Fascia Research Conference in Boston, Massachusetts
2009	North American Research Conference on Complementary and Integrative Medicine in Minneapolis, Minnesota
	2nd International Fascia Research Conference in Amsterdam, Netherlands
2010	Highlighting Massage Therapy in CIM Research in Seattle, Washington
	5th International Conference on Complementary Medicine Research in Tromso, Norway
2012	International Research Conference on Integrative Medicine in Portland, Oregon
	3rd International Fascia Research Conference in Vancouver, Canada

MOMENTUM FOR THE FUTURE

Both massage research and the history of massage itself have had their ups and downs through the decades, as noted by Graham (1902, 48):

> From this outline of the history of massage we may conclude that, like many other matters in and out of medicine, it has not been steadily progressive, at times being highly esteemed, at others treated with indifference or even contempt, until the weight of eminent authority or the pressure of popular opinion has again raised it from oblivion.

While the current interest in massage research rides the wave of enthusiasm for CAM therapies, it will hopefully be sustained from within the massage therapy profession and by the infrastructure of organizations that provides its direction and funding. Perhaps the recent explosion in the number of research studies and the promising results demonstrating its efficacy will finally provide the momentum needed to ensure that massage therapy has a place in integrative health care, now and in the future.

SUMMARY

The history of massage therapy research published in English primarily extends over the past 150 years with works such as Ling's medical gymnastics (also known as the Swedish movement cure) and Mezger's massage. Although the earliest references to the use of massage appear in writings as far back as the works of Hippocrates (460-370 BCE), by the beginning of the 20th century, a considerable store of practice-based knowledge about the use of massage had been collected by physicians and lay practitioners. This information was published in medical journals, monographs, and a growing number of Western textbooks. Early massage research was associated with the new science of physiology, and massage was viewed as a medical practice. Over time, interest in massage research waxed and waned, depending on whether massage was associated with conventional or unconventional medicine or was aligned with either science or medical quackery.

In Europe and North America, the middle of the 20th century saw a resurgence of interest in massage for rehabilitation. However, massage research languished during this time. A new wave of massage research began in the 1980s, motivated by increased professionalization and massage practitioners' increased desire to be aligned with evidence-based integrative health care. This shift parallels the massage research cycle that occurred over a century ago.

Critical Thinking Questions

1. What is the importance of the work of Ling and Mezger to the development of massage research in the 19th century?
2. How did massage come to be considered alternative to contemporary conventional medicine, when much of its history is linked to the medical establishment?
3. Why were the terms *empiric* and *empiricism* often used in a derogatory sense by physicians, especially in the early 20th century?
4. When and how did massage practice and research become associated with physiotherapy?
5. Which factors have resulted in the resurgence of interest in massage therapy research over the past 20 years?

REFERENCES

American Massage Therapy Association. 1990. *In touch with the future: Massage therapy in the 1990s, issues of professional development.* Evanston, IL: American Massage Therapy Association.

———. 2002. *Massage therapy research agenda*. Evanston, IL: AMTA Foundation.

Beard, G., and E. Wood. 1964. *Massage: Principles and techniques*. Philadelphia: Saunders.

Cuthbertson, D.P. 1933. Effect of massage on metabolism: A survey. *Glasgow M.J.* 2: 200-213.

Dominion of Canada. 1920. *Sessional papers vol. LVI: Fourth session of the thirteenth Parliament.* Toronto, ON: King's Printer.

Dryden T., H. Boon, M. Verhoef, and S. Mior. 2004. *Research requirement: Literacy among complementary and alternative health care (CAHC) practitioners*. Ottawa, ON: Natural Health Products Directorate.

Elkins, E.C., J.F. Herrick, J.H. Graindlay, F.C. Mann, and R.E. DeForest. 1953. Effects of various procedures on the flow of lymph. *Arch Phys Med* 34: 81-89.

Field, T., S. Schanberg, F. Scafidi, C.R. Bauer, N. Vega Lahr, R. Garcia, J. Nystrom, and C. Kuhn. 1986. Tactile/kinesthetic stimulation effects on preterm neonates. *Pediatrics* 77: 654-658.

Graham, D. 1902. *A treatise on massage*. Philadelphia: Lippincott.International Society for Complementary Medicine Research (ISCMR). 2010. www.iscmr.org.

IN-CAM. www.incamresearch.ca

International Society for Complementary Medicine Research (ISCMR). 2010. www.iscmr.org

Kellogg, J.H. 1895. *The art of massage: Its physiological effects and therapeutic applications.* Battle Creek, MI: Modern Medicine.

Kosman, A.J., E.C. Wood, and S.L. Osborn. 1948. The effect of massage upon the skeletal muscle of the dog. *Arch Phys Med* 29: 489-490.

McMillan, M. 1921. *Massage and therapeutic exercise*. Philadelphia: Saunders.

Mennell, J.B. 1917. *Massage: Its principles and practice.* Philadelphia: Blakiston.

———. 1920. *Physical treatment by movement, manipulation and massage*. 2nd ed. Philadelphia: Blakiston.

———. 1945. *Physical treatment by movement, manipulation and massage*. 5th ed. Philadelphia: Blakiston.

Murrell, W. 1890. *Massotherapeutics or massage as a mode of treatment.* Philadelphia: Blakiston.

NIH. 2011. "Important events in NCCAM history." Last modified May 31. http://www.nih.gov/about/almanac/organization/NCCAM.htm

Porter, R. 1997. *The greatest benefit to mankind: A medical history of humanity*. New York: Norton.

Porter, R. 2003. *Quacks: Fakers and charlatans in medicine*. Stroud, UK: Tempus.

Roth, M. 1851. *The prevention and cure of many chronic diseases by movements*. London: Churchill.

Suskind, M.I., N.A. Hajek, and H.M. Hines. 1946. Effects of massage on denervated skeletal muscle. *Arch Phys Med* 27: 133-135.

Tappan, F. 1964. *Massage techniques: A case method approach*. New York: Macmillan.

United States Government. 1992. *Alternative medicine: Expanding medical horizons. A report to the National Institutes of Health on Alternative Medical Systems and Practices in the United States.* Washington, DC: Government Printing Office.

Wakim, K.G. 1949. The effects of massage on the circulation in normal and paralyzed extremities. *Arch Phys Med* 30: 135.

White House Commission on Complementary and Alternative Medicine Policy. 2002. *Final report.* Washington, DC: Department of Health and Human Services.

chapter

2

Evidence-Based and Outcome-Based Approaches in Massage

Carla-Krystin Andrade, PhD, PT
Paul Clifford, BSc, RMT

Massage therapists now discuss outcomes and evidence for massage more frequently. Yet, many practicing therapists remain unclear about how they can put these concepts into practice when treating their clients. This chapter outlines the general principles of the approaches for evidence-based practice and outcome-based massage. It also uses a *clinical decision-making process* to show therapists how to integrate outcomes and evidence into the development and progression of massage interventions for their clients.

clinical decision-making process

▸ A repeatable, logical series of steps that therapists can use to gather, synthesize, and analyze information on a client's condition. They can then use the results to create and progress treatment regimens.

WHY WE NEED EVIDENCE, OUTCOMES, AND CLINICAL DECISION MAKING

Effective therapists systematically collect and analyze information from their clients throughout the therapeutic encounter. They also cultivate an inquiring attitude toward the use of massage in their clinical practices. Questions that reflect this inquiring attitude include the following: What are this client's main issues? What results is this client seeking? Which treatment techniques should I use? How will I know if the client is improving?

The search for answers to these questions has led massage therapists to identify *evidence* for why some protocols work and others do not. In addition, it has prompted them to look beyond generic guidelines for the treatment of *medical conditions* to specific *outcomes* that are relevant for individual clients. Finally, it has led therapists to create more structured and effective approaches to clinical decision making, such as those included in outcome-based massage and evidence-based practice (see table 2.1).

evidence

▸ Information on clinical care that therapists collect in a systematic manner.

medical conditions

▸ Diseases, illnesses, or injuries that result in pathophysiological changes, impairments, and disability.

outcomes

▸ The therapeutic effect of a treatment that can be established for impairments related to a client's medical condition or a client's wellness goals.

EVIDENCE-BASED PRACTICE

Evidence for massage is information on massage practice that researchers and therapists collect in a systematic manner (Sackett et al. 2000). In the past, therapists relied heavily on their clinical intuition and past experience to guide treatment decisions. In today's health care arena, therapists need evidence in order to provide the best care possible to their clients (Achilles and Dryden 2004; Menard and Piltch 2009; Menard 2008), to identify which practices are useful and safe for their clients, and to educate themselves and their clients about what massage can and cannot do. A solid foundation of evidence also facilitates acceptance of the value of massage and accountability for its increased second-party reimbursement. The use of evidence to guide clinical decision making is *evidence-based practice* (EBP). The transition from an experience-based approach to practice to EBP is not necessarily intuitive; hence, structured methodologies that can provide guidance on these issues are needed.

evidence-based practice

▸ The application of evidence based–medicine principles to other health care professions.

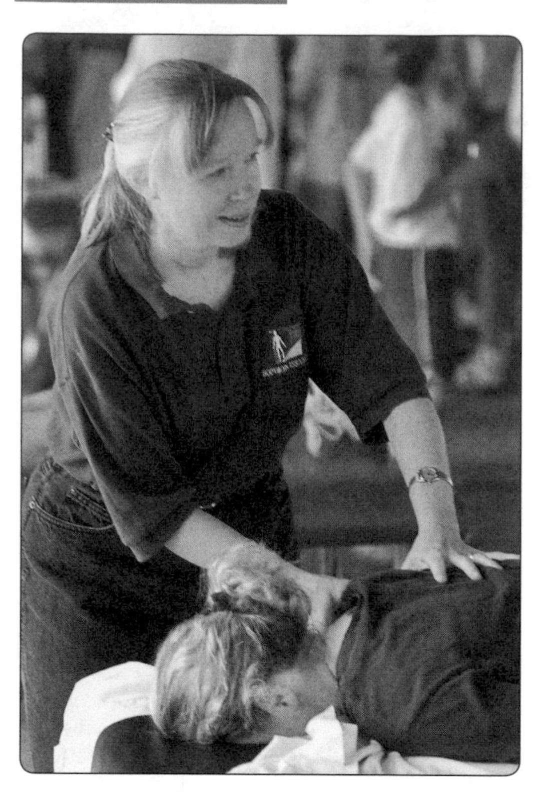

In today's health care arena, therapists need evidence in order to provide the best care possible to their clients and to identify which practices are useful and safe.

Defining Evidence-Based Practice

Sackett and colleagues (2000), who developed the concept of *evidence-based medicine,* define the three components for EBP as best research evidence, clinical expertise, and client values. Best research evidence is the best available clinical, client-centered research that examines the accuracy, safety, and efficacy of assessment tests and therapeutic interventions. Clinical expertise is therapists' ability to use their clinical skills and past experience to identify each client's unique health needs and the potential risks and benefits of interventions. Finally, client values are the unique preferences, goals, and expectations that each client brings to the therapeutic relationship. The integration of these components is the goal of EBP.

Evaluating Evidence

Many therapists, for whom finding the time to locate and read evidence is challenging enough, find the additional step of evaluating evidence daunting. Fortunately, three approaches provide guidance to therapists. First of all, Sackett and others (2000) created a hierarchy of *levels of evidence* that ranks research designs based on the extent to which they provide strong evidence of a cause-and-effect relationship between the treatment and the outcome. In this respect, studies at the top of the hierarchy, such as randomized clinical trials, are considered better evidence than those at the bottom, such as qualitative studies. This hierarchy may raise concerns within the field of massage therapy (MT) because the lower-ranked research designs are considered by some to be optimal for studying complex, holistic, or wellness-oriented aspects of massage (Finch 2007).

evidence-based medicine

▸ An approach developed by Sackett and colleagues (2000) that involves the integration of best research evidence with clinical expertise and client values.

levels of evidence

▸ A hierarchy of research designs created by Sackett and colleagues (2000) that ranks several types of research studies, with studies at the top of the hierarchy providing the strongest evidence of a cause-and-effect relationship between the intervention and the outcome.

Both Jonas and Finch offer alternatives to this hierarchical approach. Jonas (2001) proposes an *evidence house* that includes many kinds of rigorous research methods—different rooms in the house—without ranking the types of research designs. He suggests that including a variety of qualitative and quantitative research methodologies provides a more balanced and complete picture of massage and how it works. Finch (2007) describes how practitioners act like an *evidence funnel* in the sense that they receive evidence from many sources, and then filter it by evaluating its relevance and merits before integrating it with their own expertise and the client's preferences.

In addition to these systems for evaluating evidence, there are several excellent MT-specific handbooks (Hymel 2006; Menard 2009) that therapists can use for assistance in locating and evaluating evidence. In practical terms, it may be more efficient for a therapist who is new to the concepts of evidence-based practice to use preappraised sources, such as practice guidelines, clinical protocols, or plans of care published by professional associations (Grant et al. 2008).

OUTCOME-BASED MASSAGE

Outcome-based massage or OBM (Andrade and Clifford 2008) helps us answer the question: Do we treat two clients with the same medical condition in the same way? Until recently, it was difficult for many therapists to (a) identify detailed differences between two clients with the same medical condition and (b) design different treatment regimens to treat the clinical issues stemming from those differences. Although therapists intuitively knew that two clients with the same medical condition (for example, low back pain) had different presentations and responded differently to the same massage protocol, they lacked a structured approach for identifying those differences and treating them accordingly. OBM provides therapists with a practical method for planning massage treatments that address the client's specific presenting *impairments* or stated *wellness* goals.

Defining Outcome-Based Massage

OBM is the use of a systematic clinical decision-making process for the following processes:

- Identifying the impairments associated with the client's medical condition or wellness goals.
- Specifying desired and relevant outcomes for clients based on their impairments or wellness goals.
- Selecting massage techniques, based on the evidence, that can achieve the desired outcomes.
- Applying those massage techniques using effective psychomotor skills.

Simply put, OBM is massage that therapists plan and perform with the goal of achieving specific therapeutic effects that relate to a client's presenting impairments or wellness goals.

Several basic assumptions underlie OBM. First of all, not all outcomes are relevant for a given client or situation. Second, therapists can use massage to produce a variety of distinct outcomes related to impairments and wellness goals. Third, therapists can structure the massage treatment to produce some outcomes and not others. In addition, therapists can measure the client's progress toward the achievement of the desired outcomes. Finally, outcomes can encompass (a) client-centered outcomes based on the client's physical, psychological, social, and spiritual needs and (b) broader outcomes oriented toward whole systems that consider the therapeutic environment and the therapist–client interaction (Ritenbaugh et al. 2003).

Client-Centered Outcomes for the Treatment of Impairments

An outcome for a client with a medical condition is a desired change in a specific impairment that stems from that client's medical condition (Andrade and Clifford 2008). An impairment is any loss in body function or abnormal body structures that occur as a result of a medical condition. These impairments and their effects are

evidence house

▸ A concept proposed by Jonas (2001) in which various kinds of rigorous research methods, treated as different rooms in a house, are organized nonhierarchically. Instead, each method is considered an equally important contribution to the overall structure.

evidence funnel

▸ A concept proposed by Finch (2007) that describes how practitioners combine, or *funnel*, information from many sources, filter it by evaluating its relevance and merits, and then integrate it with their own expertise and the client's preferences.

outcome-based massage

▸ An approach developed by Andrade and Clifford (2008) that involves the use of a systematic clinical decision-making process for (a) identifying the impairments associated with the client's medical condition or the client's wellness goals; (b) specifying desired and relevant outcomes for the client, based on impairments or wellness goals; (c) selecting massage techniques, based on available evidence, that can achieve the desired outcomes; and (d) applying those massage techniques using effective skills.

impairments

▸ Loss of body function or abnormality of body structures that occurs as a result of a medical condition.

wellness

▸ A state of being that encompasses a balance of body, mind, and spirit, as well as clients' self-perception of well-being that is distinct from their state of health.

usually visible or palpable. Example of impairments include adhesions, elevated muscle resting tension, postural adaptive shortening, edema, anxiety, and depression. Each medical condition has a characteristic set of potential impairments (Goodman, Boissonault, and Fuller 2003). For example, the impairments associated with fibromyalgia may include muscle pain, muscle tenderness, elevated muscle resting tension, tender points, anxiety, disturbed sleep, and altered body image.

Different clients with the same medical condition can, however, present with different combinations of the characteristic impairments. Consequently, they will require different outcomes and different treatment regimens. Recent work on summarizing the effects of massage concluded that reduction of anxiety and musculoskeletal pain, including low back pain, are among the most established outcomes for massage (Moyer, Dryden, and Shipwright 2009). Nevertheless, massage may also have other important outcomes, such as improvements in mood, sleep, and breathing, and reduction of stress, lymphedema, and some cancer-specific impairments, such as nausea and fatigue. Table 2.1 outlines a variety of outcomes for massage that relate to medical conditions.

Table 2.1 Impairments Appropriate for Treatment with Massage and Related Outcomes

Impairment in body structures and functions	Outcomes
MUSCULOSKELETAL	
Adhesions/scarring	• Increased tissue mobility • Decreased scarring
Impaired connective tissue integrity: fascial restrictions, abnormal connective tissue density, tethering of nerve sheathes, and decreased mobility of skin and superficial and deep fascia	• Separation and lengthening of fascia • Promotion of dense connective tissue remodeling • Increased connective tissue mobility
Impaired joint integrity: inflammation of joint capsule or ligaments, restrictions of joint capsule and ligaments	• Decreased signs of inflammation of joint capsule, tendons, or ligaments • Decreased capsular and ligament restrictions • Increased joint mobility • Increased joint integrity
Impaired joint mobility: decreased voluntary range of motion	Increased joint mobility: increased voluntary range of motion
Impaired muscle integrity: decreased muscle extensibility, decreased muscle resiliency, tendinopathies, trigger points, muscle strains and tears	• Increased muscle extensibility • Increased muscle resiliency • Decreased signs of inflammation and promotion of healing of tendons • Decreased trigger-point activity • Increased joint mobility • Decreased signs of inflammation and promotion of healing of muscle
Impaired muscle performance (strength, power, endurance)	• Enhanced muscle performance secondary to the enhancement of muscle extensibility, reduction of pain, reduction of muscle spasm, reduction of resting tension, enhancement of joint mobility, normalization of joint integrity, and reduction of trigger-point activity • Balance of agonist/antagonist muscle function • Increased ease and efficiency of movement

Impairment in body structures and functions	Outcomes
	MUSCULOSKELETAL
Abnormal muscle-resting tension and muscle spasm	• Decreased muscle spasm • Normalized muscle-resting tension • Increased joint mobility • Ease and efficiency of movement
Postural malalignment	• Normalized postural alignment • Increased postural awareness • Lengthening of adaptive shortening
Edema, joint effusion	• Decreased joint effusion • Decreased edema • Increased joint integrity • Increased joint mobility
	MULTISYSTEM
Altered body image	Improved body image and physical self-acceptance
Impaired sensation secondary to entrapment neuropathy or nerve-root compression	Normalized sensation secondary to the reduction of nerve and nerve-root compression due to fascial restrictions, postural malalignment, and trigger points
Pain	• Reduction of pain through primary treatment of dysfunction (e.g., active trigger points) • Counterirritant analgesia • Decreased perception of pain due to systemic sedation
	NEUROLOGICAL
Abnormal neuromuscular tone: spasticity, rigidity, clonus	• Normalized neuromuscular tone • Alteration of movement responses through proprioceptive and exteroceptive stimulation techniques • Balance of agonist and antagonist muscle function • Increased ease and efficiency of movement
	CARDIOVASCULAR
Decreased arterial supply	Increased arterial supply
Decreased venous return	Increased venous return
Increased blood pressure	Decreased blood pressure
Swelling: lymphedema	• Increased lymphatic return • Increased venous return • Decreased edema • Increased joint mobility
	PULMONARY
Impaired ability to clear sputum	• Increased respiration/gaseous exchange • Increased airway clearance/mobilization of secretions • Decreased dyspnea
Dyspnea	Decreased dyspnea due to increased airway clearance or increased perceived relaxation

(continued)

Table 2.1 *(continued)*

Impairment in body structures and functions	Outcomes
PULMONARY	
Decreased rib-cage mobility (other than bony abnormality)	• Increased rib-cage mobility • Increased muscle extensibility • Increased ventilation
PSYCHONEUROIMMUNOLOGICAL	
Stress	• Systemic sedation • Increased relaxation • Increased ability to monitor physical and psychological effects of stress
Depression	Improved mood
Altered patterns of sleep	Improved quantity and quality of sleep
GASTROINTESTINAL	
Gastrointestinal immobility secondary to sedentary status	Stimulated peristalsis
CENTRAL NERVOUS SYSTEM	
Reduced mental focus	Systemic arousal and enhanced mental focus
Failure to thrive in high-risk infants	Promoted weight gain and development through increased vagal activity, sensory organization
Lethargy	Sensory arousal and enhanced alertness

Adapted, by permission, from C. Andrade and P. Clifford, 2008, *Outcome-based massage: From evidence to practice,* 2nd ed. (Baltimore, MD: Lippincott Williams & Wilkins), 7-8.

Client-Centered Outcomes for Wellness Massage

Wellness encompasses a balance of body, mind, and spirit, and clients' self-perception of well-being that is distinct from their state of health (Andrade and Clifford 2008). Clients who present for wellness massage may not have medical conditions and associated impairments. Therefore, outcomes for wellness focus on the client's desired wellness goals, which can include optimized functioning of any body part or body system, prevention of injury, improved body awareness, enhanced mental focus, stress reduction or enhanced ability to deal with stress, and self-nurturing (Andrade and Clifford 2008; Grant et al. 2008).

When a client requests wellness massage, the therapist needs to confirm that this client does not have underlying impairments. For these clients, the successful achievement of wellness-related outcomes may first involve the treatment of these impairments. The Research Outcomes Database of the Canadian Interdisciplinary Network for Complementary and Alternative Medicine (IN-CAM) contains an extensive list of concepts related to wellness, as well as ways of measuring them (IN-CAM 2010). Table 2.2, derived from this database, lists possible domains, outcomes, and measures for wellness.

Whole Systems-Oriented Outcomes

The whole systems approach takes a broader view of the client within the context of the therapeutic environment and the therapist–client relationship, rather than

Table 2.2 Domains, Definitions, and Sample Outcomes for Wellness and Whole Systems

Domain	Definition	Sample outcomes
Physical	Related to the body	• Decreased pain • Decreased insomnia • Decreased fatigue • Improved functional status • Decreased disability
Social	Related to the life and relations of humans in their community	• Improved social functioning • Increased social support • Improved family relationships • Decreased loneliness
Psychological	Related to the mind, emotions, or other mental phenomena	• Increased general well-being • Decreased anxiety • Decreased depression • Increased relaxation • Improved coping skills
Spiritual	Related to the spirit or soul, as distinguished from the physical self	• Enhanced spiritual well-being • Improved mindfulness
Health-related quality of life	Related to ability to function in and derive satisfaction from a variety of roles in the presence of impaired health status	• Improved quality of life • Decreased effects of sickness • Improved functional status
Holistic	Related to outcomes on a global level	• Enhanced well-being • Improved wellness • Increased life satisfaction
Context	The set of circumstances encompassing the intervention or healing experience, such as the client–provider relationship	• Increased empathy • Increased positive attitudes to therapy • Increased trust in health care provider
Process	Related to the process of healing and personal transformation, such as learning	• Enhanced capacity for transformation • Enhanced personal growth
Individualized	Important to, and as identified by, the individual client or research participant	Various

From Andrade and Clifford 2008; INCAM 2010.

focusing on the client's medical condition or wellness goals alone (Ritenbaugh et al. 2003). Outcomes from this perspective consider a client's experiences of massage, psychosocial effects of the therapeutic environment, the client's expectations of the therapist, and the therapist's perspective. Within the realm of experiences of massage, for example, clients report improved body image, self-image, social identity, confidence, perceived relaxation, perceived well-being, and ability to cope with stress as a result of MT (Bredin 1999; Billhult, Stener-Victorin, and Bergborn 2007; Paterson et al. 2005; Price 2005). Furthermore, massage helps clients connect mind and body and feel good and cared for (Mulkins, Verhoef, and Cormier 2005). Clients also report desiring the following characteristics in a MT experience: personal time, a competent therapist, trust, holism, empowerment, effective touch, and relaxation (Smith, Sullivan, and Baxter 2009). Finally, from the therapists' perspective, the evidence has provided some insight into the positive and negative personal and professional experiences that influence a practitioner's professional choices (Herbert et al. 2007). Table 2.2 notes possible domains, outcomes, and measures for whole systems excerpted from the IN-CAM (2010) database.

INTEGRATING CLINICAL DECISION MAKING, OUTCOME-BASED MASSAGE, AND EVIDENCE-BASED PRACTICE

The clinical decision-making model in OBM is a repeatable, logical series of steps that therapists can use to (a) gather and analyze client information and (b) plan and progress treatment regimens (Andrade and Clifford 2008). It has four phases: the evaluative phase, the treatment planning phase, the treatment phase, and the discharge phase. Each phase has a different set of purposes and procedures. Therapists can use this clinical decision-making process to enhance the fit between clients' presenting issues and treatment techniques. In addition, they can use evidence throughout their clinical decision making to build their knowledge base and to support their choices of examination and treatment techniques. This will ultimately improve the quality of care, outcomes, and client satisfaction. The following case study illustrates this approach to integrating clinical decision making, OBM, and EBP (figure 2.1).

CASE STUDY

Evaluative Phase

The evaluative phase, illustrated by a case in this section, consists of the preparation necessary before treatment planning. During this important period, conscientious massage therapists acquire the general information they will need to maximize their effectiveness for a category of patients, as well as the more specific information pertinent to an individual patient belonging to that category.

Before Treatment

Since Michael plans to see a number of clients with fibromyalgia in his practice, he expands his clinical knowledge base by consulting the evidence on fibromyalgia (see chapter 16) to answer the following questions: Who gets fibromyalgia? How does fibromyalgia affect skeletal muscle? What are the symptoms of fibromyalgia?

Step 1: Review the Reason for Client Treatment

Patricia has made an appointment for massage therapy. Before Michael sees Patricia, he reviews the documentation that indicates she is seeking treatment of muscle pain and headaches associated with fibromyalgia.

Step 2: Propose Client Issue

Prior to meeting with his client, in order to guide his clinical thinking, initial assessment, and treatment and evaluation strategies, Michael first *proposes the client issue* that Patricia may be experiencing. He wonders if she is having a flare-up of fibromyalgia symptoms and consults the medical evidence on the diagnosis and prognosis of fibromyalgia. He then *asks answerable questions:* For women with fibromyalgia, is the assessment of tender points better suited to confirming the presence of fibromyalgia than self-reported muscle pain? What are some of the psychosocial issues for people with fibromyalgia?

(continued)

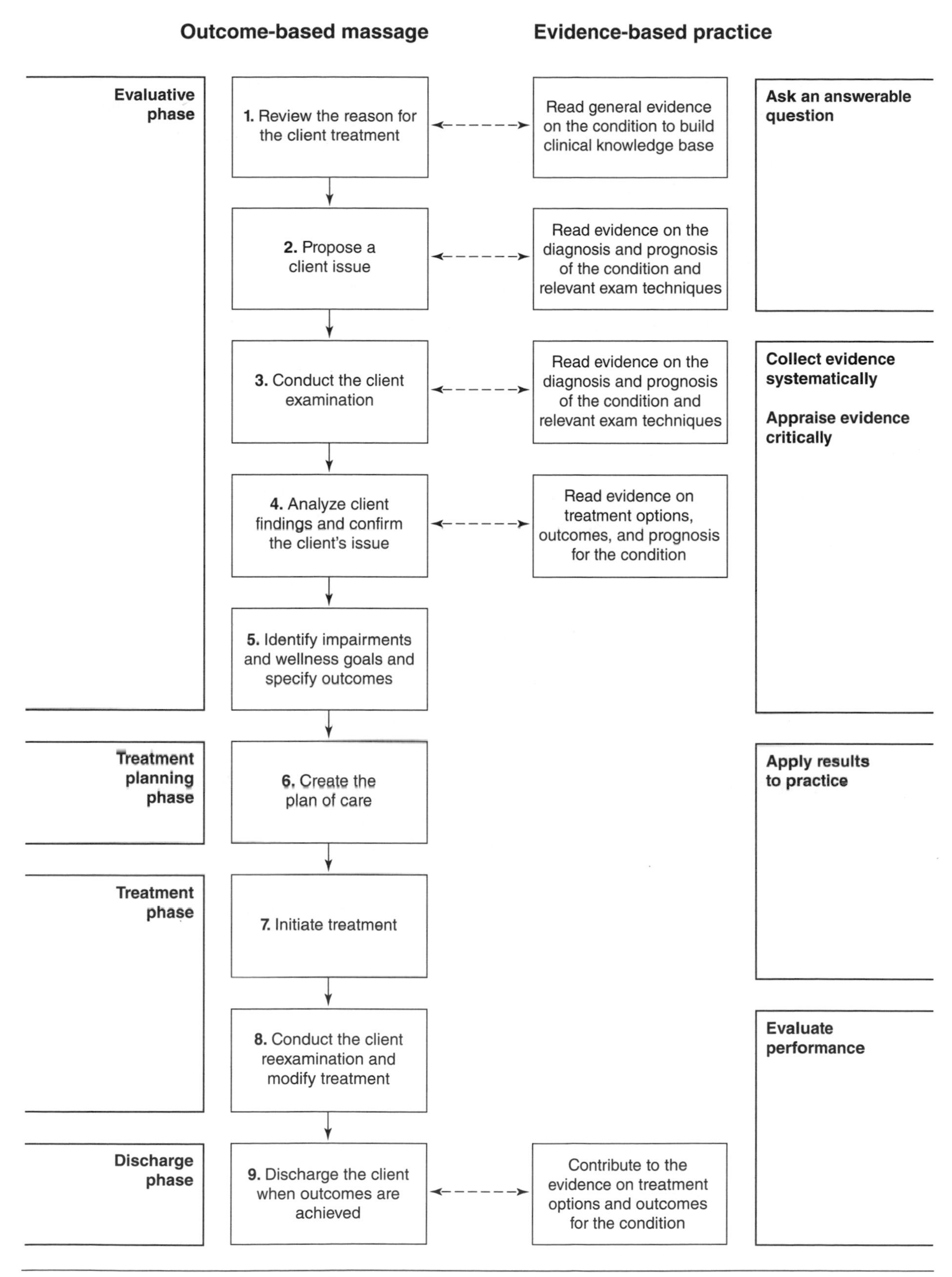

Figure 2.1 Integrating Evidence-Based Practice and Outcome-Based Massage Into Clinical Practice

Based on Andrade and Clifford 2008; Sackett et al. 2000.

Michael next delves into the evidence. He *collects evidence systematically* by searching public research databases available on the Internet (Google Scholar, PubMed, ERIC, and PEDro). Michael performs two searches: one with the search terms *fibromyalgia, diagnosis,* and *tender points,* and a second, using the terms *fibromyalgia* and *psychosocial.* He *appraises the evidence critically* by sorting his results into three groups, based on the quality of the evidence he thinks they will provide: peer-reviewed journals, practice guidelines from professional organizations in other health care professions, and non–peer reviewed Internet-based information.

Michael acquires two main insights from reading this evidence. The first is that assessment of tender points using manual palpation and the identification of at least 11 out of 18 possible tender points are necessary components for the assessment and diagnosis of fibromyalgia (Harden et al. 2007) . The second is that people with fibromyalgia frequently present with psychosocial distress and sleep disturbances (Field, Delage, and Hernandez-Reif 2003; Martinez-Lavin 2007). With this information, Michael prepares for his session with Patricia.

Steps 3 and 4: Conduct Client Examination and Analyze Client Findings

Patricia arrives for treatment complaining of muscle pain and cramps, disturbed sleep, fatigue, headaches, and anxiety. In addition, she explains that her flare-up of fibromyalgia symptoms may be the result of a hectic and stressful period at work. With Patricia's informed consent, Michael *conducts the client examination* with careful attention to tender-point assessment. He *analyzes examination findings*, which include 18 tender points, widespread muscular pain, muscle cramps, disturbed sleep, fatigue, headaches, anxiety, and altered body image. Based on these findings, Michael *confirms the client's issue* as a flare-up of fibromyalgia symptoms. Michael decides to treat Patricia and proceeds to the *treatment planning phase.*

Treatment Planning, Treatment, and Discharge Phases

Following the essential groundwork of the evaluative phase, a well-prepared massage therapist is ready to undertake the treatment planning, treatment, and, eventually, discharge phases. Each phase is important, presenting the massage therapist with opportunities to exercise professional judgment, optimize overall treatment, and increase patient well-being and satisfaction.

Step 5: Identify Impairments and Specify Outcomes

Michael reviews his examination findings and *identifies impairments,* including 18 tender points, pain in multiple muscle groups, muscle cramps in the lower extremities, interrupted sleep due to muscle pain and cramping, fatigue with and without activity, generalized anxiety, headaches, and altered body image. Then, to *specify outcomes,* he makes a list of appropriate treatment goals for these impairments, including Patricia's desired outcomes of decreased muscle pain and improved sleep, as well as decreased number of tender points, decreased cramping of muscles in the lower extremities, decreased complaints of fatigue, decreased anxiety, decreased frequency and intensity of headaches, and improved body image.

Step 6: Create the Plan of Care

Michael understands that his treatment will be most effective if he integrates the research evidence with his clinical expertise in pursuit of Patricia's desired outcomes. This leads to another brief round of collecting and appraising evidence.

From a new, refined literature search, Michael learns several additional directions in treatment. First, light pressure massage may be valuable in the early stages of the treatment and during flare-ups. However, neuromuscular and connective-tissue massage techniques with moderate to deeper pressure result in a greater reduction in muscular pain (Baranowsky et al. 2009; Brattberg 1999; Field, Delage, and Hernandez-Reif 2003; Holdcraft, Assefi, and Buchwald 2003; Wahner-Roedler et al. 2005). In addition, massage can also alleviate psychological distress and sleep disturbances in people with fibromyalgia (Brattberg 1999; Field et al. 2002; Ekici et al. 2009; Martinez-Lavin 2007). Furthermore, clients with fibromyalgia can use active range of motion, gentle stretching, and self-massage effectively for home care (Field, Delage, and Hernandez-Reif 2003; Rooks et al. 2007). Finally, he notes that clients seek personal time, a competent therapist, trust, holism, empowerment, effective touch, and relaxation in an MT experience (Smith, Sullivan, and Baxter 2009).

Michael uses this information to *apply results to practice* by identifying massage and complementary techniques that he can use to achieve each of the specified treatment outcomes. He integrates this material into the *plan of care* (also commonly referred to as the *treatment plan*) for Patricia, and then he documents the plan. The plan of care for Patricia will consist of brief treatments with light- to moderate-pressure massage techniques during initial sessions. It will progress to greater depth and duration of treatment as she improves her treatment tolerance. His areas of priority include the head, neck, chest, arms, and back. For home care, he suggests active range of motion of the neck and upper extremities, gentle stretching, and self-massage. Michael reviews this plan of care with Patricia, reaches an agreement that it is consistent with her desired outcomes for treatment, and obtains her informed consent. Although he does not share this with Patricia, he also plans to pay particular attention to building trust and empowering her in self-management to assist her in dealing with her condition.

Steps 7 and 8: Initiate Treatment, Conduct Reexamination, and Modify Treatment

Michael *initiates treatment* by implementing the plan of care. He *conducts client reexaminations* periodically throughout the treatment process, in order to *evaluate performance.* In doing so, he observes the results of his clinical actions and determines whether they were successful. He uses this information to gauge the effects of his treatment and Patricia's progress toward the desired treatment outcomes, and to guide him as he *modifies treatment.*

Step 9: Discharge

Michael continues a cycle of client reexamination, performance evaluation, and treatment modification until Patricia approaches achievement of her treatment outcomes. At this point, he initiates discharge planning and performs treatment and discharge planning in parallel, until his client examination indicates that Patricia has achieved her treatment outcomes. Michael *discharges* Patricia to a home care program of stretching, self-massage, and relaxation techniques. He also refers her to a local fibromyalgia society for ongoing personal support.

After he discharges Patricia, Michael notes her positive results. Michael takes a moment to *evaluate performance* by reviewing his clinical documentation on Patricia's examination and treatment. He concludes that moderate-pressure massage techniques, in combination with a home regimen of stretching, relaxation techniques, and self-massage, likely contributed to her decrease in pain and other fibromyalgia symptoms. He shares these results with professional colleagues, while maintaining client confidentiality, as a means of informally contributing to the evidence on massage treatment for fibromyalgia.

PRACTICAL ISSUES IN ADOPTING EVIDENCE-BASED AND OUTCOME-BASED APPROACHES IN MASSAGE

Several practical issues arise for evidence-based and outcome-based approaches. Therapists need to consider clinical practice and research when they adopt these methods.

Clinical Practice

Two essential practices are necessary to support the adoption of OBM and EBP in clinical practice: clinical documentation and time for contemplation. First of all, without detailed information on impairments, wellness goals, examination findings, treatment techniques, and outcomes, therapists will be unable to make valid judgments about what worked and what did not work in their treatments. The second critical practice is for therapists to have enough time in their daily work schedules to think about the clinical care they provide. Analyzing examination findings, treatment planning and progression, client documentation, and consulting the evidence all take time, and scheduling must reflect this.

Research

Therapists must overcome two major challenges if they wish to successfully adopt outcome-based and evidence-based approaches. These are the lack of practice guidelines for individual impairments or wellness goals and the limited number of measures for the outcomes related to massage. Massage treatment guidelines for individual impairments are the building blocks of research and clinical practice in OBM. They raise the standard of care and give researchers and therapists a more specific outcome than a general treatment goal related to a medical condition. Fortunately, the base of treatment guidelines for specific impairments is growing (Grant et al. 2008). Over time, this should be complemented by an increase in the creation of validated outcome measures relevant to MT.

DIRECTIONS FOR FUTURE RESEARCH

Many practicing therapists consider evidence-based and outcome-based approaches to be theories that apply to research, rather than to day-to-day clinical practice. In reality, using these two approaches enhances how we treat clients and the outcomes that we achieve with massage. To integrate an outcome-based approach into treatment, therapists need to do three things during treatment planning. First, therapists should identify the client's impairments and wellness goals. Second, they need to determine which outcomes they can achieve using MT. Finally, therapists need to select the treatment techniques that can produce the desired outcomes. Furthermore, to become more evidence-based in their treatment approach, they need to determine which evidence is most relevant to their work, and then use the massage techniques that have the best research evidence to support their potential outcomes. Researchers, in turn, should conduct outcome-based research on the effects of a given massage technique (or specific combinations of techniques) on selected impairments in order to build an appropriate body of evidence.

SUMMARY

The Information Age has raised the standards and expectations for all forms of healthcare and wellness promotion, including massage therapy. To be optimally effective, contemporary massage therapists need to be able to collect, evaluate, and synthesize different forms of evidence, and then use that information to guide all phases of treatment. The influence and importance of evidence-based and outcome-based approaches are already established. They will only continue to increase as massage therapy advances.

Critical Thinking Questions

1. Explain why the profession of massage therapy needs evidence-based and outcome-based approaches.
2. In what ways are the concepts of *levels of evidence, evidence house,* and *evidence funnel* similar? How do they differ? Explain how you would apply one of them to a specific case.
3. What is *wellness,* and how is it different from health?
4. What does the *whole-systems approach* consist of? How does it apply to massage therapy?
5. List, define, and explain the importance of each of the four phases of outcome-based massage.

REFERENCES

Achilles, R., and T. Dryden. 2004. *Massage therapy research curriculum kit.* Evanston, IL: Massage Therapy Foundation.

Andrade, C.K., and P. Clifford. 2008. *Outcome-based massage: From evidence to practice.* 2nd ed. Philadelphia: Lippincott Williams & Wilkins.

Baranowsky, J., P. Klose, F. Musial, W. Haeuser, G. Dobos, and J Langhorst. 2009. Qualitative systemic review of randomized controlled trials on complementary and alternative medicine treatments in fibromyalgia. *Rheumatol Int* 30: 1-21.

Billhult, A., E. Stener-Victorin, and I. Bergborn. 2007. The experience of massage during chemotherapy treatment in breast cancer patients. *Clin Nurs Res* 16: 85-99.

Brattberg, G. 1999. Connective tissue massage in the treatment of fibromyalgia. *Eur J Pain* 3: 235-244.

Bredin, M. 1999. Mastectomy, body image and therapeutic massage: A qualitative study of women's experience. *J Adv Nurs* 29: 1113-1120.

Ekici, G., Y. Bakar, T. Akbayrak, and I. Yuksel. 2009. Comparison of manual lymph drainage therapy and connective tissue massage in women with fibromyalgia: A randomized controlled trial. *J Manip Physiol Ther* 32: 127-133.

Field, T., J. Delage, and M. Hernandez-Reif. 2003. Movement and massage therapy reduce fibromyalgia pain. *J Bodyw Mov Ther* 7: 49.

Field, T., M. Diego, C. Cullen, M. Hernandez-Reif, W. Sunshine, and S. Douglas. 2002. Fibromyalgia pain and substance P decrease and sleep improves after massage therapy. *J Clin Rheumatol* 8: 72.

Finch, P. 2007. The evidence funnel: Highlighting the importance of research literacy in the delivery of evidence informed complementary health care. *J Bodyw Mov Ther* 11: 78-81.

Goodman, C.C., W.G. Boissonault, and K.S. Fuller. 2003. *Pathology: Implications for the physical therapist.* 2nd ed. Philadelphia: Saunders.

Grant, K., J. Balletto, D. Gowan-Moody, D. Healey, D. Kincaid, W. Lowe, and R. Travillian. 2008. Steps toward massage therapy guidelines: A first report to the profession. *Int J Ther Massage Bodywork* 1. www.ijtmb.org/index.php/ijtmb/article/view/5/23.

Harden, R., G. Revivo, S. Song, D. Nampiaparampil, G. Golden, M. Kirincic, and T. Houle. 2007. A critical analysis of the tender points in fibromyalgia. *Pain* 8: 147-56.

Herbert, C., L. Bainbridge, J. Bickford, S. Baptiste, S. Brajtman, T. Dryden, P. Hall, C. Risdon, and P. Solomon. 2007. Factors that influence engagement in collaborative practice: How eight health professionals became advocates. *Can Fam Physician* 53: 1318-1325.

Holdcraft, L.C., N. Assefi, and D. Buchwald. 2003. Complementary and alternative medicine in fibromyalgia and related syndromes. *Best Pract Res Clin Rheumatol* 17: 667-683.

Hymel, G.M. 2006. *Research methods for massage and holistic therapies.* St. Louis: Elsevier Mosby.

IN-CAM outcomes database. 2010. Canadian Interdisciplinary Network for Complementary and Alternative Medicine Research. www.outcomesdatabase.org.

Jonas, W. 2001. The evidence house. *Western J Med* 175: 79.

Martinez-Lavin, M. 2007. Biology and therapy of fibromyalgia. Stress, the stress response system, and fibromyalgia. *Arthritis Res Ther* 9: 216-216.

Menard, M. 2008. Research literacy is a critical skill for practitioners. *Massage Magazine.* 151: 44-45.

———. 2009. *Making sense of research.* 2nd ed. Toronto, ON: Curties-Overzet .

Menard, M., and C. Piltch. 2009. The case for research: The role research plays in creating and maintaining an evidence-informed profession. *Massage Ther J* 48: 99-102.

Moyer, C.A., T. Dryden, and S. Shipwright. 2009. Directions and dilemmas in massage therapy research. *Int J Ther Massage Bodywork* 2: 15-27.

Mulkins, A.L., M. Verhoef, and E. Cormier. 2005. The benefits of massage in Vancouver's inner city. *Massage Ther J* 44: 102-109.

Paterson, C., J. Allen, M. Browning, G. Barlow, and P. Ewings. 2005. A pilot study of therapeutic massage for people with Parkinson's disease: The added value of user involvement. *Complement Ther Clin Pract* 11: 161-171.

Price, C. 2005. Body-oriented therapy in recovery from child sexual abuse: An efficacy study. *Altern Ther Health Med* 11: 46-57.

Ritenbaugh, C., M. Verhoef, S. Fleishman, H. Boon, and A. Leis. 2003. Whole system research: A discipline for studying complementary and alternative medicine. *Altern Ther Health Med* 9: 32.

Rooks, D., S. Gautam, M. Romeling, M. Cross, D. Stratigakis, B. Evans, D. Goldenberg, M. Iversen, and J. Katz. 2007. Group exercise, education, and combination self-management in women with fibromyalgia: A randomized trial. *Arch Intern Med* 167: 2192.

Sackett, D., S. Straus, W.S. Richardson, W. Rosenberg, and R.B. Haynes. 2000. *Evidence-based medicine: How to practice and teach EBM.* Edinburgh: Churchill Livingstone.

Smith, J.M., S.J. Sullivan, and G.D. Baxter. 2009. The culture of massage therapy: Valued elements and the role of comfort, contact, connection and caring. *Complement Ther Med* 17: 181-189.

Wahner-Roedler, D., P. Elkin, A. Vincent, J. Thompson, T. Oh, L. Loehrer, J. Mandrekar, and B. Bauer. 2005. Use of complementary and alternative medical therapies by patients referred to a fibromyalgia treatment program at a tertiary care center. *Mayo Clin Proc* 80: 55-60.

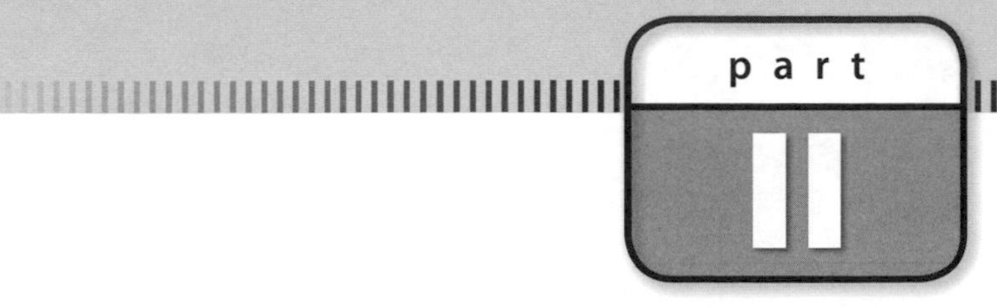

RESEARCH METHODS

How will our understanding of massage therapy progress? The chapters presented here provide an overview of the major approaches to research that apply to massage therapy. The strengths and limitations of both the quantitative and qualitative approaches to research are discussed in detail, while the final chapter illustrates how those approaches can be integrated within an individual study to more fully capture the complexity of massage therapy as it occurs in the real world.

chapter 3

Quantitative Research Methods

Christopher A. Moyer, PhD
Kimberly Goral, MS, NCTMB

"Whenever you can, count." So said Sir Francis Galton (1822-1911), a titanic figure in the history of science and statistics, in what is essentially an endorsement of quantitative research methods. Galton's advice recognizes that there will be a time when counting does not make sense. For these instances, we have qualitative (see chapter 4) and mixed methods (see chapter 5) approaches. But when counting, or *quantification* (to use the more technical term), does make sense, it offers clear advantages. Most modern researchers would agree with his assertion that we should count when we can.

quantification

▸ The technical term for counting, or for measuring something numerically, which is of great value in science.

WHY USE QUANTITATIVE METHODS?

Quantification—to assign meaningful and appropriate numerical values to what is observed—should be used whenever possible because it has inherent strengths and makes important scientific procedures possible. Key among its strengths are objectivity and precision; two of the scientific procedures it makes possible are replication and cumulation.

Objectivity

Imagine that we ask someone how much he slept last night. "I was really tired. I slept a really long time last night," he replies. This answer may be true, but how useful is it? Their answer is *subjective*; it is based on and framed by that person's inner experience, which is not something we can examine directly. As such, we do not know if the "really long time" that the person slept was 4 hours, 8 hours, 12 hours, or some other duration. A different question, based on a widely understood approach for quantifying sleep—How many hours did you sleep last night?—would potentially yield a more *objective* answer, based on observable phenomena in the world outside of himself. Assuming the person has a reasonably accurate clock and took notice of it, he might tell us, "Oh, I slept about 7 hours last night, which is a lot more than my usual 5 hours of sleep." Even this very basic objective measurement gives us the possibility of checking its accuracy or comparing it directly with something else, such as the amount a different person slept last night. We would not have to depend on the idiosyncratic and unobservable inner experience of the person.

subjective

▸ Based on a person's perspective and inner experience, and therefore unavailable for direct examination by others.

objective

▸ Based on observable phenomena, and therefore not dependent on an individual observer's perspective or inner experience.

Precision

What if we needed to know exactly how long somebody slept, perhaps because we are doing research to see if massage therapy (MT) can increase sleep duration? In other words, what if we need to know with precision? The only way to obtain precision is with careful measurement. In our previous example, asking a person how many hours he slept is a type of measurement, though not a precise one. However, if we needed to, we could measure sleep duration very precisely by other means, all of which would necessarily be quantitative. Research participants might be asked to wear an actigraph, a wristwatch-like device that makes a precise recording of a person's movements. For example, the time a person falls asleep or wakes up, within a range of a few minutes, can be inferred from the pattern of movements stored electronically in the actigraph's circuits. Or, the research participants might get connected to electroencephalographic equipment that monitors brain wave activity, which is capable of showing the exact second that a person transitions from wakefulness to sleep, or vice versa. Such precision is only possible when we carefully quantify the objects or phenomena we are interested in.

Replication

It is insufficient in science to obtain a particular result once. The same research procedures, including when they are performed by other researchers at a different time and place, need to yield consistent results for the scientific community to be confident that a true discovery has been made. This process of redoing a study and obtaining consistent results is called replication. Determining if one or more results replicate a previous result is made easier by the objectivity and precision associated with quantifiable outcomes.

Cumulation

A single study rarely, if ever, provides a definitive answer to a research question in the health sciences. One of the most important reasons for this is that most individual studies are too small—that is, they do not make use of enough participants—to reach definitive conclusions by themselves. Because each additional participant increases the time and money needed to complete a study, most MT studies have contained fewer than 50 participants, even though it may be necessary to have several hundred participants to convincingly examine certain research questions. For this reason, it is almost always the case that the findings from a set of studies on the same topic need to be accumulated for a clear answer to emerge.

As an example, consider this question: Does MT reduce depression? Hou and colleagues (2010) located 17 individual studies that examined this important question in a quantitative fashion. The average size of these studies is a little less than 45 participants each, and two of the studies make use of only 20 participants, which means they have very little power, in the statistical sense, to clearly answer the question. But considered together, this set of studies is akin to a superstudy with 756 participants! By weighting and then averaging the quantitative results of each individual study, the cumulative result is a very clear answer to the question. The answer is yes; on average, MT is quite effective in reducing depression. This same approach, in which the quantified results of individual MT studies are mathematically combined, has been used to powerfully assess the effects (or, in some cases, lack of effects) of MT on anxiety, mood, various forms of pain, blood pressure, and heart rate (Moyer, Rounds, and Hannum 2004), infant growth and development (Vickers et al. 2004), mechanical neck disorders (Haraldsson et al. 2006), low back pain (Furlan et al. 2009), and levels of the stress hormone cortisol (Moyer et al. 2011).

COMMON FORMS OF QUANTIFICATION ENCOUNTERED IN MT RESEARCH

Statistics, the effective use of numerical data, is a field unto itself. As such, a full treatment of statistics is beyond the scope of this chapter. In any case, it is not necessary. A working knowledge of quantitative research, sufficient for understanding most MT research, can be acquired by learning some of the fundamental concepts. These include descriptive statistics and inferential statistics.

Descriptive Statistics

Descriptive statistics are, just as the name implies, those statistics that describe a dataset. Most of what we might need to know about a dataset containing dozens, hundreds, or even thousands of numbers can be summarized with just two types of statistics: one that indicates the dataset's *central tendency* and one that indicates its *variability* around that central tendency.

While three different statistics can be used to indicate central tendency, by far the most frequently used and important to understand is the *mean*. The mean of a set of numbers is calculated by first summing the value of every entry in the set, and then dividing this sum by the number of entries in the set. This operation will already be familiar to anyone who has averaged something mathematically. If the three massage therapists employed at clinic A are 32, 35, and 38 years old, we can calculate the mean age of the massage therapists at clinic A as follows:

$$(32 + 35 + 38) = 105;\ 105 \div 3 = \text{Mean age of 35 years}$$

Other indicators of central tendency are the *median,* the value that occurs precisely midway in an ordered number set, and the *mode,* the most frequently occurring value in a number set. While both of these have their uses, in practice, they are encountered much less frequently than the mean, and so they are not discussed further here.

Notice that, if we only knew that the mean age of the therapists at clinic A is 35 years, we would still know nothing about the variability in their ages. Indeed, we can easily imagine another clinic with three therapists, clinic B, where the mean age is exactly the same, but where the spread in the therapists' ages is considerably greater.

Age	Clinic A	Clinic B
Youngest	32	23
2nd youngest	35	35
3rd youngest	38	47
Mean age	**35**	**35**

Researchers summarize the variability in a dataset by calculating the *variance* or the *standard deviation*. Conceptually, these are very similar to each other.

To quantify the variability in a dataset, we must first calculate the difference between each value and the mean for the set. Some of these values will be negative,

central tendency
▸ A general term for the various ways of determining the midpoint of a set of numbers. Specific measures of central tendency include the mean, median, and mode.

variability
▸ A general term for the extent to which a set of numbers spreads out from the set's midpoint.

mean
▸ The most frequently used measure of central tendency; it is calculated by first summing the value of every entry in the set, then dividing this sum by the number of entries in the set.

median
▸ A specific measure of central tendency; it is the value that occurs precisely midway in an ordered number set.

mode
▸ A specific measure of central tendency; it is the most frequently occurring value in a number set.

variance
▸ A specific measure of variability in a number set. The difference between each number in the set from the mean of the set is computed and then squared, after which the squared differences are summed, and the sum is divided by the number of cases in the set.

standard deviation
▸ A specific measure of variability; it is the square root of the variance.

and some will be positive. To illustrate, here is the result of this first step for the therapists' ages from clinic A:

Age	Clinic A ages	Difference from mean (35)
Youngest	32	−3
2nd youngest	35	0
3rd youngest	38	3

Next, each of these differences is squared, that is, multiplied by itself. Note that all of these resulting values will be positive, because a negative number multiplied by itself yields a positive product. We then add each of these to get a sum of squared differences:

Age	Clinic A ages	Difference from mean (35)	Squared difference from mean
Youngest	32	−3	9
2nd youngest	35	0	0
3rd youngest	38	3	9
Sum of squared differences			**18**

If we divide this sum of squared differences (18) by the number of number of cases that contributed to it (3), the resulting number is the variance for this dataset. For this dataset, the variance in age is 6. A smaller variance would indicate less variability around the mean, and a larger variance would indicate greater variability; as such, we can use this statistic to compare the variability of different datasets, just as we can use the mean to compare the central tendencies of various datasets.

The standard deviation is simply a transformation of the variance. In many cases, it makes better conceptual sense than the variance statistic that is based on squared values, because the standard deviation is standardized by the fact that we undo the effect of the previous squaring procedure. To calculate the standard deviation, we take the square root of the variance.

$$\sqrt{6} = 2.45$$

So, the mean age of the therapists at clinic A is 35 years, and the standard deviation of their ages is 2.45 years. The exact same procedures are applied to the dataset for clinic B:

Age	Clinic B ages	Difference from mean (35)	Squared difference from mean
Youngest	23	−12	144
2nd youngest	35	0	0
3rd youngest	47	12	144
Sum of squared differences			**288**

Variance:

$$288 \div 3 = 96$$

Standard deviation:

$$\sqrt{96} = 9.80$$

This table shows that their mean age is also 35 years, as we calculated previously, but that the standard deviation of their ages is 9.80 years. This considerably larger standard deviation indicates that there is more variability in the therapists' ages at clinic B.

We illustrated the calculation of these descriptive statistics with a step-by-step method, but this does not mean you should always do such calculations yourself. Indeed, it is sometimes impossible, in a practical sense, to do this with datasets that are large enough to be interesting. Fortunately, the widespread availability of computers means that we do not have to. The important thing is to have a sense of what these statistics refer to and how they are used. Do not be daunted if this does not come easily. In our experience, you will gradually acquire a familiarity and intuitive sense of these statistics and the procedures behind them as you increasingly become a research consumer.

Inferential Statistics

Inferential statistics are also aptly named, since their purpose is to help us to make an inference about the wider world from the very small part of it that we are able to examine directly in a research study. More specifically, we use inferential statistics to help us say something about the *population,* or all the members belonging to a particular category, based on a *sample,* which is a representative portion of that population.

population

▸ In statistics, all of the members that belong to a particular category.

sample

▸ In statistics, a representative subset of the population.

For example, we might be interested to know the effect of a 20-minute scalp massage on tension headache. To know this effect with total certainty, we would need to include every person who experiences tension headache in our study. This is obviously impossible. In reality, we might only be prepared to work directly with 30 participants; even if we have the time and money to do an enormous study with hundreds of participants, this is still only a small fraction of all the cases of tension headache that exist. Because we can never study every case that belongs to the entire population, we can never arrive at an answer with 100% certainty. However, we can use the findings from our sample to make a probabilistic estimate of what we would have found if we actually had been able to study every case in the population. This task—making inferences about a population based on a sample of that population—is the purpose of inferential statistical tests.

Many different types of inferential statistical tests actually exist. The specific one that a researcher uses depends on the exact research design that has been used. A detailed accounting of the many types of inferential statistical tests is beyond the scope of this chapter. Fortunately, present purposes are better served by a basic explanation of what all inferential statistical tests have in common, which is a result that takes the form of a probability, or p-value.

Understanding what a p-value represents is important. It is the probability that a result as strong or stronger than that which was observed could have occurred even if there is actually no true effect in the population. For example, the result of a hypothetical study might read, "after receiving a 20-minute session of scalp massage, participants' reported level of tension headache pain, assessed with a 10-point scale, was lower than it was prior to having received the treatment ($p < .05$)." This means that the researchers conducted an inferential statistical test that was based on the number of participants, the mean and standard deviation of their self-reports of tension-headache pain scale before scalp massage, and the mean and standard deviation of these self-reports following scalp massage. A result of that test indicating that a result was as strong or stronger than the one they actually observed in their sample would occur less than 5% of the time if scalp massage is actually ineffective, on average, in the whole population. In this hypothetical example, the observed result would give the researchers a high degree of confidence that their participants' tension headache pain was systematically lower after treatment compared to its level before treatment, and was not merely the result of random fluctuation in the data.

statistical significance

▸ The determination that a pattern of results indicates an underlying effect, and is not entirely due to chance.

While it is possible to get results with probabilities much smaller than $p < .05$, this value is the traditional cutoff used to determine *statistical significance,* which indicates that some effect has likely been discovered. Note that it is conceptually impossible to ever obtain a p-value of zero, which would represent total certainty of an effect's existence. This is because inferential statistical tests are always concerned with making an inference about a population having only studied the sample, a small but representative proportion of the total population.

It is also very important to understand what a p-value does not tell us. By itself, it does not tell us the magnitude of the effect. It may be true that tension headache pain is lower following scalp massage, but how much lower? Is the effect strong enough to make it worth seeking out and paying for the treatment, or is it so small that one might not even notice it under normal conditions? Is it better than other treatments, such as taking a dose of aspirin? Nor does the p-value tell us if the researchers were even asking the right question in the first place. It only tells us, in a mathematical and probabilistic sense, if some effect is likely to exist. In our hypothetical tension headache study, the statistically significant result only tells us that pain levels are lower at the end of the study. It does not tell us the specific cause of that reduction, which may have been the result of the scalp massage, or a placebo effect, or even the mere passage of time. A more sophisticated research design, including a control group, is needed to eliminate those last two possibilities.

In short, inferential statistical tests, and their resultant p-values, can be very useful scientific tools, but they also have the potential to be misunderstood or even misused. The latter has sometimes happened in MT research (Moyer 2007). When interpreting a p-value, always take the time to determine what specifically is being tested. Consider all the possible explanations for a finding, which is a function of the study design rather than a statistical test.

COMMON QUANTITATIVE RESEARCH DESIGNS TO EXAMINE MT

Several quantitative research designs are commonly encountered in MT research. The one a researcher uses depends on a variety of factors, including the specific hypotheses being tested; the available resources, including money, time, materials, setting, and participants; and, in some cases, ethical considerations. For these reasons, it may not be accurate to say that one design is better than another, because a thoughtful researcher chooses the research design in accordance with the limitations presented by the real world. On the other hand, it is true that some research designs are more definitive than others, in that they reduce the number of possible explanations for the observed outcome.

In the examples that follow, we present several hypothetical studies that attempt to answer the research question "Does MT reduce pain?" Pain, in these examples, has been measured on a 10-point self-report scale, where 0 represents no pain and 10 represents the worst pain possible. In fact, this is how pain is often measured in both clinical and research settings. Note, though, that our examples would work equally well for any outcome that can be quantified. The fundamental principles being illustrated would stay the same if the outcome was range of motion in degrees as measured with a goniometer, heart rate in beats per minute assessed with a medical monitor, or anxiety level scored on a standardized psychological survey.

The most basic quantitative research design is a case study, in which a single participant is studied. To answer the question "Does MT reduce pain?" we could have a person quantify their level of pain before and after MT treatment. Figure 3.1 displays a result we might expect.

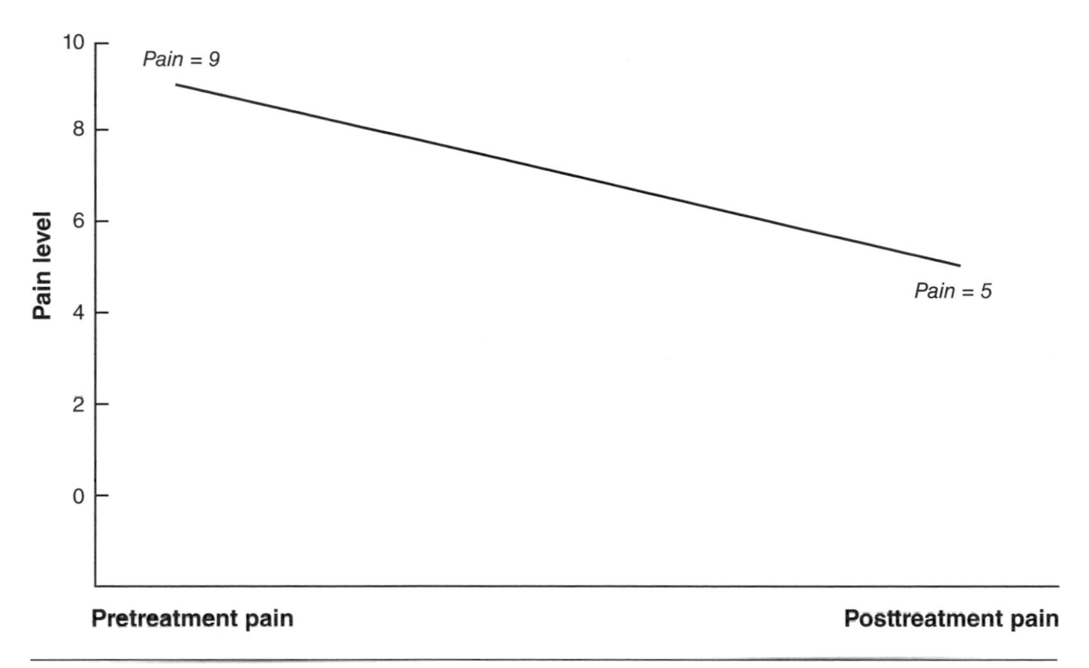

Figure 3.1 Self-reported pain in a single person who has received massage therapy. These hypothetical data are representative of a basic case study.

This is an encouraging result, at least for the client being studied, but it leaves a lot of questions unanswered. A key issue we might consider is whether this result is unique to this person, or if it represents an underlying pattern of pain reduction in response to MT that might be revealed if we studied a number of people. In addition, having multiple participants would give us the possibility of testing our results with statistical methods. These possibilities are illustrated in the next example.

In a within-group study, multiple participants all receive the same intervention. Their values before and after that intervention are compared with each other to determine if a change took place. All the details are the same as they were in the case study example, except we now have 10 subjects being studied, not just 1. (There is nothing special about the number 10. This number was chosen simply to create an easily visualized and realistic example. A within-group study can have any number of participants greater than 1.) Note that there is variation in their pain levels both prior to and following MT. This is to be expected, since no two people are exactly alike. Because of this variation, we can meaningfully calculate some descriptive statistics. The hypothetical data are displayed in figure 3.2.

Prior to treatment, the group's mean pain level is 7.7, with a standard deviation of 1.8. Following treatment, their mean pain level appears to be lower, at 4.0, while the variation in their pain level appears to be about the same, with a standard deviation of 1.9.

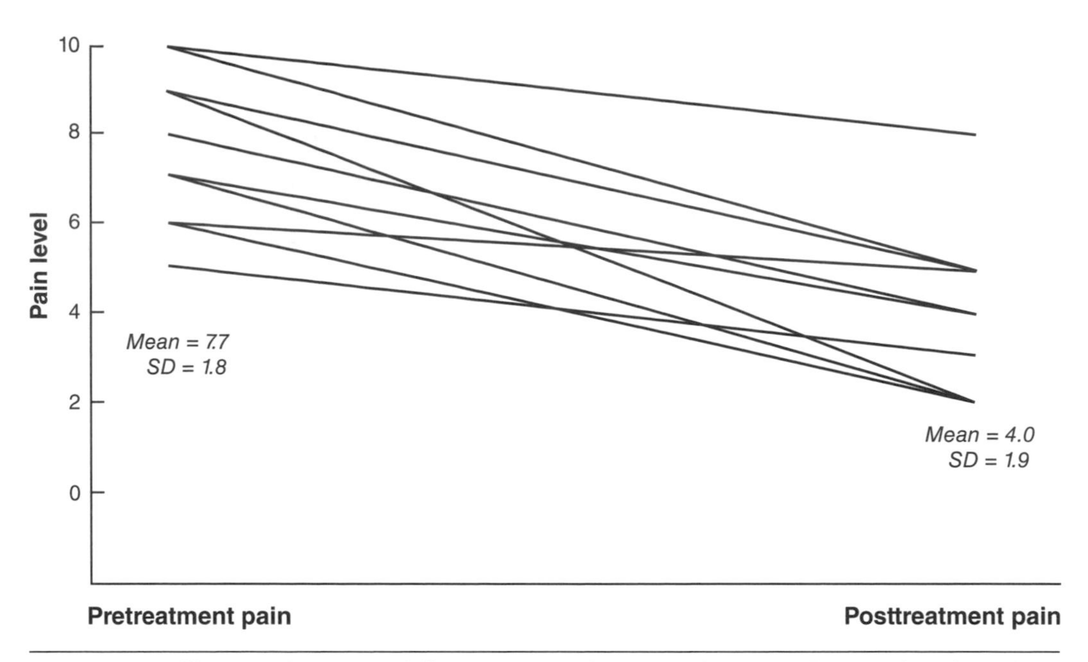

Figure 3.2 Self-reported pain in 10 different persons who received massage therapy. These hypothetical data represent a series of case studies, or a within-group research design. The massage group has significantly less pain after treatment (mean = 4.0) than at the beginning of treatment (mean = 7.7); paired $t(18) = 1.83$, $r = .53$, $p < .001$.

Given that there is variation in the data, an important question we would like to have answered is this: Does the 3.7-point reduction in pain level represent a true, systematic change during the treatment period, or could it be merely the result of random variation? An inferential statistical test, and its resultant p-value, can help us decide. Figure 3.3 displays a graphical summary of the 10 participants' data and the detailed results of an appropriate inferential statistical test (in this instance, a paired-samples t-test).

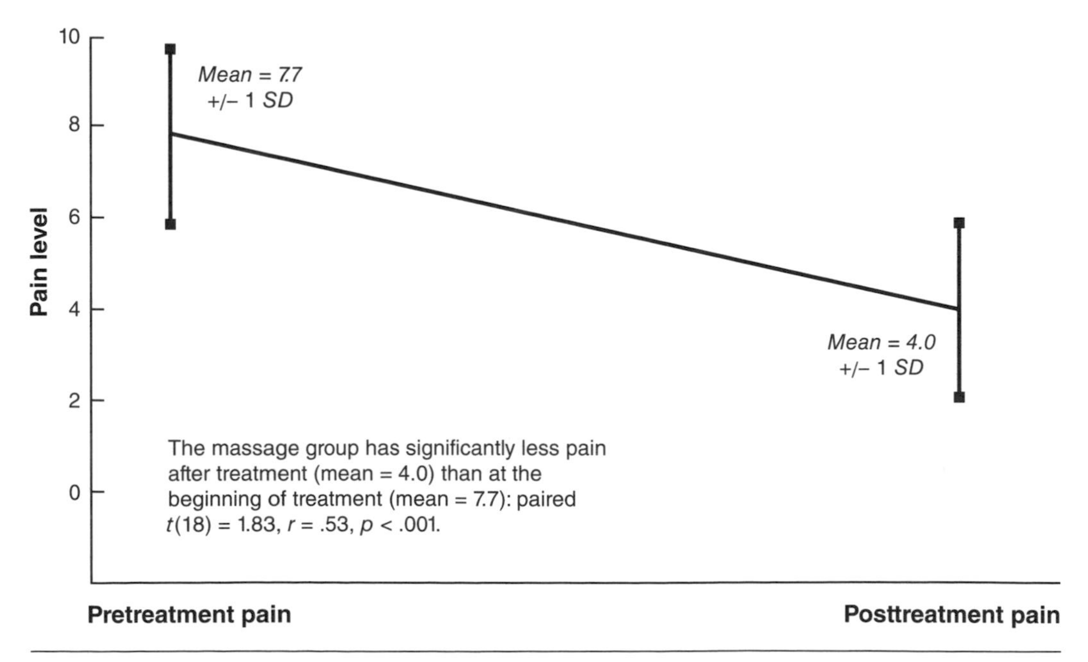

Figure 3.3 Central tendency (means), variation (SD, or standard deviations), and inferential statistical analysis of self-reported pain in 10 different persons who received massage therapy. These hypothetical data represent a series of case studies, or a within-group research design.

The resultant p-value is less than one-tenth of 1%. In other words, while it is not completely impossible that the observed reduction is the result of random variation, the likelihood that we would have observed such a strong result strictly due to random variation is less than 1 chance in 1,000. We can reasonably reject the possibility that such a change was due only to randomness, and can have great confidence that the observed reduction is systematic and that it represents a true effect.

But what is the effect? Note that we did not conclude that the reduction of pain had to have been the effect of MT. The reason for this is that there are several other possible explanations. The tiny p-value of the statistical test only tells us that something systematic probably happened. It cannot tell us what that was. Our ability to figure that out is a function of the research design itself. The reduction could have been due to the personal attention the participants received while receiving MT. Or, it could have been due to their expectation that the treatment would help them, which we know can produce powerful effects all by itself. It is also possible that the mere passage of time systematically caused the participants' pain to lessen. After all, nearly every pain we ever experience begins to go away all by itself. Any combination of these could have produced the change we observed even if MT provided no effect by itself.

To more precisely test the effect of MT itself, we need a different research design. We need to arrange for some people to receive MT just as they have in the within-group example, but we also need some people to experience as many of those confounding variables—attention, placebo, and the passage of time—as possible without getting MT. If the only difference between our two groups is whether or not they received MT, any difference in outcomes would have to be the effect of MT. This is the logic behind a between-groups study, which is also referred to as a *randomized controlled trial* or a *randomized clinical trial* (Both of these terms are abbreviated as RCT, which is how we will refer to this study design). Because an RCT has the greatest potential to reduce the influence of extraneous and confounding variables (Hymel 2006), it is widely regarded to be the gold standard for treatment research (Creswell 2009).

randomized controlled trial (RCT)

▸ A specific research design in which participants are randomly assigned to a treatment or control group. RCTs are very useful because they have the greatest potential to reduce the influence of extraneous and confounding variables so that the true effect of a treatment can be most accurately determined.

The randomization in RCT refers to the method for forming groups. Consider for a moment what might happen if we used a nonrandom, systematic approach to forming groups. For example, what if we let research participants decide for themselves whether they would prefer to be in the group that will receive MT or in the group that will receive some other treatment or no treatment at all? It is very possible that people with the greatest enthusiasm for MT would choose to be in the MT group, and those with apprehension about receiving MT would opt to be in the other group to which MT will be compared. The two groups would differ in an important way before any treatment is even administered. This means we could not be sure at the end of the study that any difference in outcomes had not been caused by a preexisting difference in our participant groups. To eliminate this possibility, it is always preferable, when possible, to use a random process for the creation of groups. Using the flip of a coin or a similarly random process gives us the greatest chance that our groups will not be systematically different from each other in a way that could influence their response to treatments.

A control group is the other main key component of an RCT. Its inclusion in the study controls for the possible influence of attention, placebo, time, or any other confounds that otherwise prevent us from seeing the precise effect of the treatment we are studying. At the conclusion of our study, we can compare the group that received treatment with the control group. Note that this is fundamentally different from the comparison we made in the example of the within-group study, where the same participants were compared to an earlier version of themselves.

Let us consider an example. This time we begin with 20 participants. (As before, there is nothing special about this number. We have chosen it only to most effectively illustrate the similarities and differences between this and the within-group study.) Coin flipping, a random process, is used to determine which subjects will receive MT and which ones will be members of the control group that will experience a time-matched wait-list control condition. This means they will be offered the MT after their control data has been collected. Figure 3.4 displays a pattern of hypothetical data that might result from such an RCT.

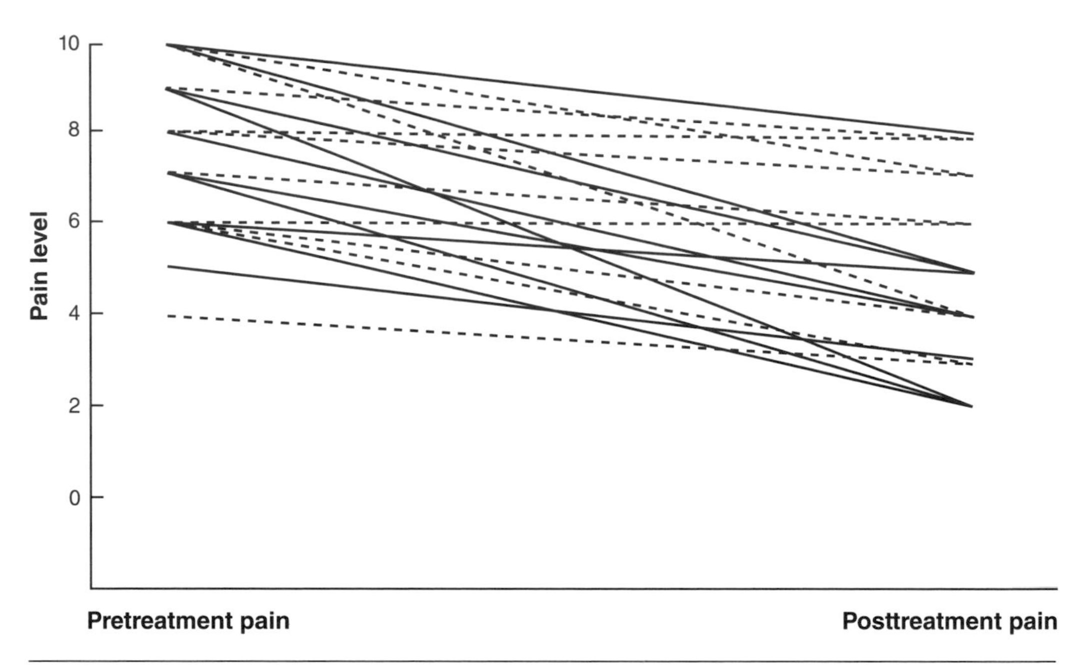

Figure 3.4 Self-reported pain in 10 persons who received massage therapy (solid lines), and 10 other persons who were in a time-matched wait-list control condition (dashed lines). These two different groups were formed randomly. These hypothetical data represent a randomized controlled trial.

Before even performing any analyses, we can see one effect very clearly: Nearly everyone, regardless of whether they received MT, has improved. Such a pattern is frequently observed in actual RCTs, serving to illustrate the importance of control groups in research. In many instances, and for a variety of reasons, people get better even without treatment. It is essential to account for this if we want our research findings to be as accurate and informative as possible.

While that overall trend is interesting, what we really want to know is if MT outperformed the control group. This is not easy to determine when viewing the raw data. As we did before with our within-group study example, we now clarify matters by displaying the data according to its descriptive statistics. Then, we analyze it by performing some inferential statistical tests. This is displayed in figure 3.5.

For the purposes of illustration, we have used the exact same values for the MT group as we used in our within-group study example. However, the addition of a control group shows us that the results from the within-group design might cause us to overestimate the true effect of MT, since we can see that participants in the control group also got better during the same time period without having received any treatment at all. So, how do the two groups compare?

Though it is not strictly necessary, we might want to begin by comparing their pain levels at the beginning of the study. We do not expect them to be different,

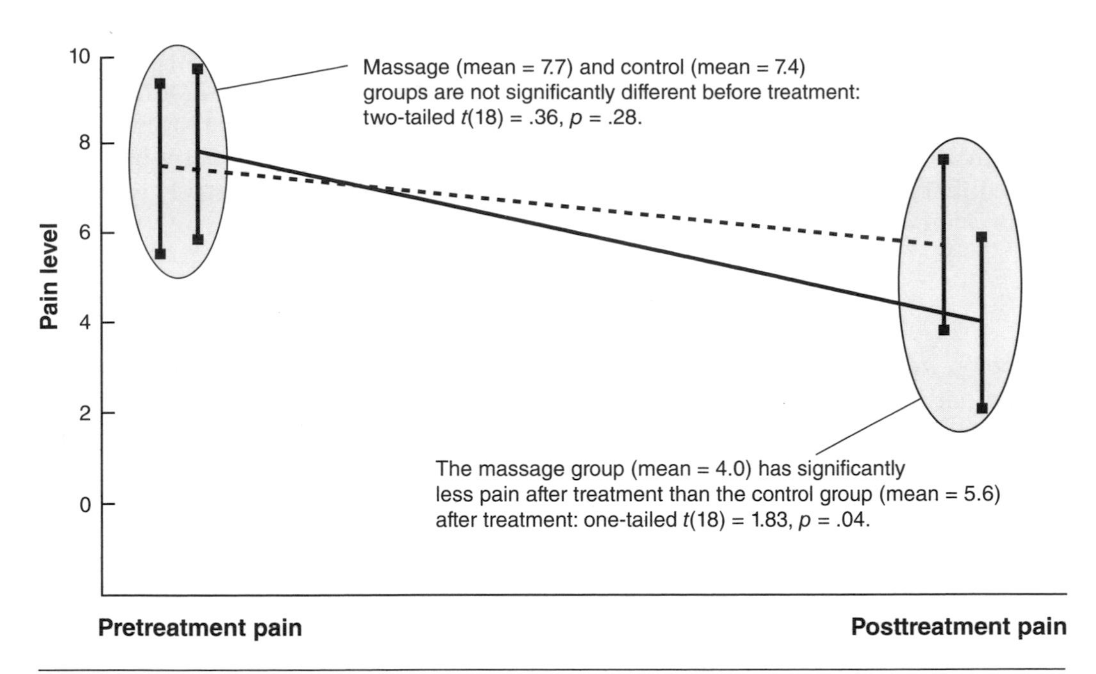

Figure 3.5 Descriptive display and inferential statistical analysis of self-reported pain in 10 persons who received massage therapy (solid lines), compared against 10 persons who were in a time-matched wait-list control condition (dashed lines). These two different groups were formed randomly. These hypothetical data represent a randomized controlled trial.

because at that point in time we have treated everyone exactly the same. Any difference would be due to pure chance. Nevertheless, an inferential statistical test to compare the pretreatment pain levels of the MT and control groups permits us to check this assumption. The result of this test (specifically, a two-tailed independent samples t-test, which is "two-tailed" because if a difference exists, we have no reason to predict that it will be in favor of a particular group) yields a p-value of 28%. This is greater than the 5% cutoff that is traditionally used to find a significant difference in clinical research. So, we are reassured that our randomly formed groups probably did not differ, in a statistical sense, in their mean pain levels.

On to the more interesting question: Do the groups differ at the end of the study? We conduct an inferential statistical test on the posttreatment data (specifically, a one-tailed independent samples t-test, which is "one-tailed" because we do expect the difference, if there is one, to be in the direction that favors the MT group) and obtain a p-value of 4%. Because this p-value is smaller than the traditional 5% cutoff to establish statistical significance, we conclude that MT actually does provide pain relief above and beyond that provided by mere waiting, as experienced by the control group. In other words, if MT actually provided no true benefit in excess to that of the control condition, there is only a 4% likelihood that we would have observed such a strong difference in favor of MT at the end of the study, with this number of participants, due only to random variation of the data.

Research designs more complicated than this are also possible. Nothing prevents us from having three or more groups or from taking measurements at multiple time points. The complexity of the statistical analyses increases as the complexity of the research designs increases, but the fundamental principles are the same as those we have illustrated up to this point. Inferential statistical testing, correctly applied, helps us determine if a pattern of results observed with a sample does, or does not, represent some actual effect in the larger population that the sample represents. At the same time, it is essential to specifically determine if there are alternate explanations for the result of any particular inferential statistical test. A statistically significant p-value by itself tells us very little. To correctly interpret it, we must also understand how it is limited by the design of the study to which it has been applied.

SUMMARY

On being introduced to quantitative research methods and their accompanying statistical methods, many people experience fear and a desire to avoid these subjects (Salkind 2007). This is unfortunate for professionals, such as massage therapists, whose work is concerned with health and wellness, since quantitative approaches dominate the research literature even as an appreciation for qualitative approaches increases. In addition, there simply is no substitute for the understanding that is possible when quantitative data are analyzed thoughtfully and displayed with clarity (Tufte 2001).

The good news is that fear and avoidance are lessened, and our comfort and familiarity are increased, simply by steady exposure. Massage therapists who wish to gain cutting-edge knowledge of their profession need to be active research consumers and need to be able to extract information from quantitative research reports. In doing so, keep in mind you do not need to be a statistician to benefit from reading quantitative research reports. Nor is it necessary to grasp all of the statistical minutiae of a study in order to understand the main findings. A basic understanding of the fundamentals of descriptive and inferential statistics, combined with careful thinking about the possible limitations of the study you are reading, will take you a long way in being an intelligent and informed consumer of MT research.

Quantitative research methods have a long history. They have been used extensively in all scientific fields. Quantitative research methods are of particular value due to their potential to reduce subjectivity, enhance precision, and permit replication and cumulation. Though it is easy to be intimidated by the amount and complexity of the mathematics necessary to master these methods, the basic familiarity and comfort level required for research literacy can be acquired simply through careful and continued exposure to reports of quantitative research. Acquisition of such familiarity and comfort should be a goal for professional massage therapists, since quantitative research methods have had, and will continue to have, a major effect on massage therapy research and the advancement of the profession.

Critical Thinking Questions

1. List and describe the four key strengths of quantitative research methods.
2. What is the *central tendency* of a dataset? List and describe the three specific ways to quantify the central tendency.
3. Describe what a *standard deviation* is, and how it is useful. Do this in a nontechnical way, so that a person without a mathematical background could meaningfully understand your answer.
4. Describe *statistical significance* and how is it used to interpret results. Do this in a nontechnical way, so that a person without a mathematical background could meaningfully understand your answer.

5. How does a *randomized controlled trial (RCT)* differ from a within-group study design? Explain how and why an RCT is better than a within-group study design.
6. Create three massage therapy research questions of interest to you that would be best answered using an RCT methodology.

REFERENCES

Creswell, J.W. 2009. *Research design: Qualitative, quantitative, and mixed method approaches*. Thousand Oaks, CA: Sage.

Furlan, A.D., M. Imamura, T. Dryden, and E. Irvin. 2009. Massage for low back pain: An updated systematic review within the framework of the Cochrane back review group. *Spine* 34(16): 1669-1684.

Haraldsson, B.G., A.R. Gross, C.D. Myers, J.M. Ezzo, A. Morien, C. Goldsmith, P.M. Peloso, G. Bronfort, and Cervical Overview Group. 2006. Massage for mechanical neck disorders. *Cochrane Db Syst Rev* 3: CD004871.

Hou, W.H., P.T. Chiang, T.Y. Hsu, S.Y. Chiu, and Y.C. Chieh. 2010. Treatment effects of massage therapy in depressed people: A meta-analysis. *J Clin Psychiatry* 71(7): 894-901.

Hymel, G.M. 2006. *Research methods for massage and holistic therapies*. St. Louis: Elsevier.

Moyer, C.A. 2007. Between-groups study designs demand between-groups analyses: A response to Hernandez-Reif, Shor-Posner, Baez, Soto, Mendoza, Castillo, Quintero, Perez, and Zhang. *Evid Based Complement Alternat Med* 6(1): 49-50.

Moyer, C.A., J. Rounds, and J.W. Hannum. 2004. A meta-analysis of massage therapy research. *Psychol Bull* 130(1): 3-18.

Moyer, C.A., L. Seefeldt, E.S. Mann, and L.M. Jackley. 2011. Does massage therapy reduce cortisol? A comprehensive quantitative review. *J Bodyw Mov Ther* 15(1): 3-14.

Salkind, N.J. 2007. *Statistics for people who (think they) hate statistics*. 3rd ed. Thousand Oaks, CA: Sage.

Tufte, E.R. 2001. *The visual display of quantitative information*. 2nd ed. Cheshire, England: Graphics Press.

Vickers, A., A. Ohlsson, J.B. Lacy, and A. Horsley. 2004. Massage for promoting growth and development of preterm and/or low birth-weight infants. *Cochrane Db Syst Rev. 2004* 2: CD000390.

chapter 4

Qualitative Research Methods

Carla-Krystin Andrade, PhD, PT
Paul Clifford, BSc, RMT

Massage is a complex intervention with physiological, psychological, social, and spiritual components (Andrade and Clifford 2008). Consequently, researchers need to be able to study both the specific effects of massage, such as neurological or cardiorespiratory effects, and the nonspecific effects, including the therapeutic relationship and environment. Qualitative methods are particularly well suited to the study of the psychosocial outcomes and nonspecific effects of massage. This chapter provides an overview of the theory underlying qualitative research and of selected qualitative research methods. It then expands on the methods and uses of qualitative research within massage therapy (MT).

WHY DO WE NEED QUALITATIVE RESEARCH?

Qualitative research uses rich narrative data and a flexible research design to provide in-depth descriptions and insight into phenomena in their natural context (Andrade and Clifford 2008; Bryman 2004; Cassidy 2002; Denzin and Lincoln 2005; Kania, Porcino, and Verhoef 2008; Lincoln and Guba 1985; Pope and Mays 1995; Verhoef, Casebeer, and Hilsden 2002). It explores, documents, and focuses on people's perceptions, experiences, and views, as well the meanings that they give to them. Its goal is to provide a deep understanding of clients' experiences, rather than a quantified answer to a question, a confirmation of a hypothesis, or generalizable laws.

qualitative research
▸ Method of inquiry that emphasizes the collection of data that is not quantifiable, narrative, experiential, and observational methods.

Qualitative research methods have been invaluable in the social sciences, where the goal is often to explore and document psychological and social processes involved in human interactions. By contrast, quantitative research methods have been more dominant in health care, which has its roots in the basic sciences (Andrade and Clifford 2008; Cassidy 2002; Grypdonck 2006; Kania, Porcino, and Verhoef 2008; Pope and Mays 1995; Verhoef, Casebeer, and Hilsden 2002). Recently, health care researchers have begun to accept the value of qualitative methods for expanding our understanding of the human interactions and experiences within the field. Furthermore, they are recognizing that qualitative research can enable us to study complex topics in areas where there is little prior investigation and where quantification alone cannot increase our understanding of the issues.

UNDERSTANDING QUALITATIVE RESEARCH

Social scientists developed qualitative research methods for their investigations of human interactions. They did so because they found that existing quantitative methods, developed for the physical sciences, were not always well suited to studying highly variable and idiosyncratic human behaviors. Debate is ongoing about the different assumptions that underlie qualitative and quantitative approaches and the ways in which we can use these methodologies within health care research. This chapter introduces some of the basic issues and chapter 5, which focuses on mixed methods research, provides more detail.

Paradigms

paradigm

▸ A world view, or a set of beliefs and rules, that guides the decisions that researchers make; a theoretical or philosophical framework.

A *paradigm* is a world view, or a set of beliefs and rules, that guides the decisions that researchers make (Bryman 2004; Kuhn 1970). For some researchers, qualitative research is based on a different, and mutually exclusive, paradigm than quantitative research (Armitage and Keeble 2007; Bryman 2004; Denzin and Lincoln 2005; Lincoln and Guba 1985). Consequently, they see them as having two incompatible paradigms that researchers cannot combine. Other researchers argue that this polarized view of two different paradigms unnecessarily limits the ways in which we can combine qualitative and quantitative research (Pope and Mays 1995; Tashakkori and Teddlie 2002; Tashakkori and Teddlie 1998). Another position taken by some researchers is that we need a third research paradigm, such as pragmatism, to support a framework that integrates the best of qualitative and quantitative research (Armitage and Keeble 2007; Creswell 2003; Onwuegbuzie, Johnson, and Collin 2009). Regardless of one's philosophical position, there is value in understanding the basics of the qualitative and quantitative paradigms.

The Quantitative Paradigm

quantitative paradigm

▸ The position that an objective reality exists that is independent of peoples' perceptions.

The *quantitative paradigm* suggests that there is a single reality that exists independently of people and a single truth or accurate representation of this reality (Denzin and Lincoln 2005; Lincoln and Guba 1985; Pope and Mays 1995). The extension of this belief is that researchers can stand back from reality in order to observe and measure it using objective instruments. As a result, the goal of quantitative researchers is to test hypotheses about how things work and to generate laws that they can apply to other situations.

The Qualitative Paradigm

qualitative paradigm

▸ The position that a subject's personal perceptions define reality, such that no objective reality exists that is independent of human perceptions.

By contrast, the *qualitative paradigm,* which is intended for studying human interactions and social constructs, proposes that people define reality; reality does not exist separately from people (Denzin and Lincoln 2005; Kania, Porcino, and Verhoef 2008; Lincoln and Guba 1985; Pope and Mays 1995). Qualitative researchers focus, therefore, on capturing each subject's point of view, with as much rich description as possible, and on analyzing that information within that person's social context. They use subjective measures and tolerate, or actively seek, different perspectives on the phenomena they are studying. They do this with the goals of gaining a deep understanding of the person or phenomenon that they are observing and generating hypotheses for future study.

QUALITATIVE RESEARCH METHODOLOGIES

Qualitative research methodologies differ from quantitative research methodologies in several ways (Denzin and Lincoln 2005; Glaser and Strauss 1967; Goetz and LeCompte 1984; Groenewald 2004; Lincoln and Guba 1985; Menard 2009; O'Reilly 2005; Portney and Watkins 2008). First of all, qualitative research methodologies are inductive in the sense that they move from observation to hypothesis, rather than using the quantitative approach of testing a hypothesis with observations. Next, they use purposive sampling, rather than quantitative sampling methods, as a means of selecting participants or other data sources that will reveal critical issues related to the phenomenon of interest. In addition, they have an emergent design in which the researcher modifies the sampling and data collection methods in response to the findings that arise. This differs from the quantitative approach of carrying out a predefined set of research procedures. Furthermore, their data collection most often takes place in the natural environment where the behaviors or phenomena that are the subject of the research actually take place, rather than in a laboratory or a highly controlled clinical environment, as is often the case in quantitative research. Finally, they use an iterative approach to data analysis, in which they perform repeating cycles of data analysis to refine the key findings. They also base their interpretation of findings on the specific context and people they are studying. In contrast, the quantitative goal is to generalize findings to other people and settings. Many types of qualitative research methodologies, or research designs, exist. The most common are grounded theory, ethnography, and phenomenology.

Grounded Theory

Grounded theory, developed by Glaser and Strauss (1967), involves the generation of theory from participants' responses (Corbin and Strauss 2007). This differs from the quantitative approach of using participants' responses to verify preexisting theories. Researchers performing grounded theory research collect data from the participants through interviews, observations, and documents. They then transcribe participants' responses and use comparative analysis techniques to sort and categorize the data, identify patterns, and develop a theory. In this way, researchers create a new theory that is grounded in the descriptions of participants' experiences and perceptions. Researchers' ability to do this successfully depends on their theoretical sensitivity, or attentiveness to the nuances and deeper meanings of the data they are analyzing. Herbert and colleagues (2007) used this approach to identify themes that illustrate the ways in which the childhood and adult experiences of eight healthcare professionals shaped their choice to participate in collaborative practice within their careers (box 4.1).

Ethnography

An *ethnography* is a description of a culture (Byrne 2001b; Denzin and Lincoln 2005; Goetz and LeCompte 1984; Hall 2010; O'Reilly 2005). This approach describes and interprets the activities of a group of people who have something in common. Ethnographic research is based on direct observations of people in a naturalistic setting. The goal of ethnography is to describe the culture from the participants' point of view without imposing the researcher's own conceptual framework on the findings. Paterson and colleagues (2008) used this approach to describe the challenges, successes, and value of implementing MT educational and treatment programs in a remote aboriginal community in Hopevale, Australia (box 4.2).

ethnography

▸ A qualitative research method aimed at understanding customs or a culture.

BOX 4.1

Example of Grounded Theory Research in Massage

Background	The paper examines why health professionals from different backgrounds are motivated to engage in collaborative practice.
Research question	Why do health professionals choose to practice in a collaborative way?
Sample	Self-selected group of 8 women from 5 different health professions.
Methods	Participant/researchers interviewed each other in pairs for 30 to 45 min. They transcribed the interviews verbatim and analyzed the data for key themes and subthemes.
Findings	The key attitudes, skills, and personal qualities that they identified as being necessary for collaborative practice included maintaining an open mind, listening, humility, and confidence. Family background, childhood experiences, role models, and previous experience in both collaborative and noncollaborative work environments influenced the choice to practice collaboratively. Finally, the act of sharing personal stories was helpful in establishing trust and collaboration between the participants.

Based on Herbert et al. 2007.

BOX 4.2

Example of Ethnographic Research in Massage

Background	The paper describes an ambitious project to bring both massage training and massage therapy clinics to 17 aboriginal communities in a remote region of Australia.
Research question	How would training aboriginal massage therapists and their practice in the community affect cultural and personal health and well-being?
Sample	Members of 17 aboriginal communities in a remote region of Australia.
Methods	During several 8-week blocks during 1 year, the researchers trained local health care workers to a standard level of massage proficiency. They also provided massage in small clinics, at day cares, and at various community events. Researchers gathered data through self-report questionnaires of clients, direct observation of individual and communal massage sessions, and semistructured interviews of participants.
Findings	The report notes that the project improved the confidence of the people who participated in the massage training. In addition, those participants who received massage reported improvements in chronic physical symptoms and emotional well-being.

Based on Paterson et al. 2008.

Phenomenological Studies

Phenomenological studies describe a specific aspect of a group's lived experiences. They are concerned with how members of the group interpret and make sense of their life experiences, as opposed to merely describing those experiences (Byrne 2001a; Groenewald 2004; Smith, Flowers, and Larkin 2009). In other words, the aim is to describe what people's life experiences mean to them. Researchers first gather the raw descriptions of participants' experiences through in-depth interviews or other data, such as personal journals, poems, or photographs that communicate the participants' lived experiences. Then they analyze and interpret the data with the goal of identifying patterns that show the structure and meaning participants give to their experiences. Billhult and colleagues (2007) took this approach to describe the phenomenological experience of 10 women who received massage while undergoing chemotherapy for breast cancer (box 4.3).

phenomenological studies

▸ A qualitative research method to describe a specific aspect of the lived experiences of a person or a group.

BOX 4.3

Example of Phenomenological Research in Massage

Background	The paper describes the meaning that breast cancer patients undergoing chemotherapy treatment give to the experience of having a massage.
Research question	What is the experience of massage for breast cancer patients undergoing chemotherapy?
Sample	10 Swedish women with diagnosed breast cancer at various stages who were scheduled to undergo chemotherapy.
Methods	Effleurage with oil was given by hospital staff with experience in massage. Treatment lasted 20-30 min. and was applied to the client's choice of feet and distal legs or hands and distal arms. Researchers interviewed participants once after the last massage.
Findings	Analysis of patients' comments resulted in 5 themes: distraction from a frightening experience, a change from negative to positive experiences, relaxation, feeling cared for, and feeling good.

Based on Billhutl, Stener-Victorin, and Berghorn 2007.

QUALITATIVE DATA COLLECTION METHODS

Researchers use qualitative data collection methods to obtain detailed, rich, narrative data about participants, their contexts, their perceptions, and their experiences (Byrne 2001a; Corbin and Strauss 2007; Denzin and Lincoln 2005; Groenewald 2004; Kania, Porcino, and Verhoef 2008; Lincoln and Guba 1985; O'Reilly 2005; Patton 2002). In qualitative research, the researcher serves as the primary instrument for data collection, rather than relying on external instruments and standardized measures. Observation, interviews, focus groups, and document analysis are four commonly used methods of gathering data for qualitative research. Furthermore, researchers can use triangulation, or a systematic combination, of several data collection methods and data sources to increase the depth of their understanding of the phenomena under investigation.

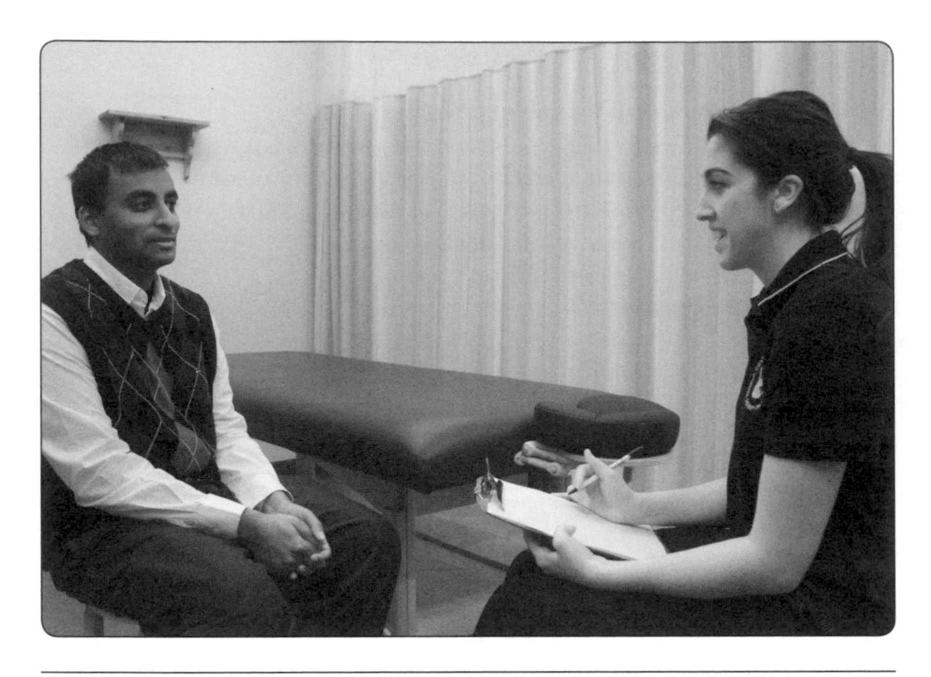

Interviews allow participants to report their perceptions and experiences in their own words and often yield rich, detailed insights.

Photo courtesy of J. Styles.

Interviews

Interviews allow participants to report their perceptions and experiences in their own words (Corbin and Strauss 2007; Denzin and Lincoln 2005; Groenewald 2004; Frechtling Westat 2002; Portney and Watkins 2008). Interview formats can be unstructured, semistructured, or structured, depending on the extent to which the researcher plans and organizes the questions beforehand. Interviews are advantageous in that they yield rich, detailed data and insights. They also permit researchers to explore and clarify in-depth issues with the participants. Disadvantages include the need for well-trained interviewers and the difficulty of transcribing and analyzing interview data.

Observation

Observational techniques are those methods by which the researcher gathers data by watching the participants and their actions in their natural setting (Corbin and Strauss 2007; Denzin and Lincoln 2005; Groenewald 2004; National Science Foundation 2002; Portney and Watkins 2008). Advantages include the opportunity to collect direct information about the behavior of individual participants and groups in their natural setting and to permit the researcher to enter into and understand the participants' situation. The disadvantages of observation are that the process can be expensive and time consuming. It requires highly trained observers, and it may itself affect the behavior of participants.

Focus Groups

focus group

▸ A qualitative research method in which a small group of study participants is assembled to engage in a structured discussion of a topic.

Focus groups are a gathering of a small number of participants for a structured discussion of a topic, which is combined with observation of the participants (Corbin and Strauss 2007; Denzin and Lincoln 2005; Groenewald 2004; National Science Foundation 2002; Portney and Watkins 2008). An advantage of a focus group is that the responses of one participant may trigger responses of other participants, thereby generating a process that leads to new insights. Disadvantages include the effect of peer pressure on participants' responses, lack of time for each person's response, and the need for skilled facilitators.

Document Analysis

Document analysis of existing public or personal documents can be a rich source of background data on a group of participants that cannot be obtained through interviews or observations (Corbin and Strauss 2007; Denzin and Lincoln 2005; Groenewald 2004; National Science Foundation 2002; Portney and Watkins 2008). The advantages are that document analysis is useful for determining participants' values and interests, the political climate, pertinent public attitudes, and trends.

The disadvantages are that it can be a time-consuming process, and the documents may be inaccurate or incomplete.

EVALUATING THE TRUSTWORTHINESS OF QUALITATIVE RESEARCH

What are the rules for judging sound qualitative research? Quantitative researchers developed the standards of internal and external validity, reliability, and objectivity for this purpose (Portney and Watkins 2008). Correspondingly, qualitative research can be judged using modifications of these standards that are suited to the nature of qualitative research methods and data; these are credibility, transferability, dependability, and confirmability (Denzin and Lincoln 2005; Lincoln and Guba 1985; Pope and Mays 1995).

Credibility refers to whether we can believe the findings and conclusions of the research. Researchers can perform a variety of activities to increase the credibility of research. In the field, they can increase the amount and types of information they gather from participants through prolonged engagement with participants, repeated observations, and the combination of data from different sources and methods (triangulation). Peer debriefing, an ongoing discussion of the research design and findings with a peer who is external to the project, can assist in keeping the researcher on track during the research process. Researchers can use the analysis of data from negative cases, which seem to contradict the findings from other participants, to test the boundaries and soundness of their interpretations. Finally, using member checks (the process of testing data), analytic categories, interpretations, and conclusions with members of those groups from whom the data were originally obtained gives researchers an opportunity to see if their interpretations are consistent with the views of the participants.

Transferability, the extent to which research findings can be applied to other situations, can be maximized through the use of thick description. *Thick description* involves a detailed description of the participants and their context, allowing other researchers and readers of the study to decide if they can use the findings within their own settings.

Dependability is assured by using multiple, overlapping methods of data collection (triangulation), and by having an external person conduct a dependability audit to review the data records, the research methods, and findings. Researchers can use a reflexive journal (a log of their ideas and responses to the research process, the dependability audit, and triangulation of data collection methods) to improve *confirmability,* or the extent to which they can confirm their findings.

credibility

▸ In qualitative research, the degree to which we can believe the findings and conclusions of research.

transferability

▸ In qualitative research, the degree to which research findings can be extended and applied to other situations.

dependability

▸ In qualitative research, the degree to which data are consistent across different methods.

confirmability

▸ In qualitative research, the degree to which research findings can be agreed on and supported by others.

READING QUALITATIVE RESEARCH ARTICLES

Clinicians and other consumers of research can assess the relative strengths and weaknesses of a qualitative research study for themselves by asking good questions while reading research articles (Andrade and Clifford 2008; Greenhalgh and Taylor 2001; Pope and Mays 1995; Menard 2009). Table 4.1 includes some questions that clinicians can use to guide their reading.

The Introduction

Clinicians can glean the purpose of the study from the introduction. In reading the introduction, they can determine if there is a clear clinical problem or gap in the previous research that provides a sound rationale for the study. In addition, they

Table 4.1 Questions to Consider When Reading Qualitative Research Articles

Section	Questions
Introduction	• Is the clinical issue/problem or the gap in the research clearly stated? • Do the authors provide a complete and up-to-date literature review? • Did the authors examine other studies that focus on similar designs, populations, and outcomes? • Does the literature review provide support for the clinical problem or research gap? • Is the problem clinically relevant? • Do the authors provide a stated model or paradigm that forms the theoretical basis for the study? • Are the purposes or research questions clearly stated and supported by the literature?
Methods	• Are the participants and the context in which they live well described? • Do the researchers describe their research methods in enough detail for you to evaluate them? • Are the researchers qualified to use the methods described in their study? For example, are they experienced interviewers? • Do the authors clearly describe their sample, the justification for the sample, and the sampling approach for you to determine if any biases or errors in recruiting are present? • Are the treatment procedures and training of the people delivering the intervention described clearly enough so that you could reproduce them? • Do the research methods allow the researcher to address the purpose of the study? • Do the researchers use rigorous and appropriate methods for collecting high-quality data? • Do the researchers describe techniques they use to increase the trustworthiness or quality of their results and interpretations? • Have the researchers accounted for all of the participants or did some of them leave the study? • Does the data analysis match the design and purposes of the study? • Does the researcher describe the data analysis techniques clearly and include adequate justification for the choice of techniques? • How were the themes, categories, concepts, and conclusions generated from the data? • Did the researchers seek negative cases that would test their assumptions?
Results	• Do the authors clearly report key findings from data analysis or are data missing? • Are the findings consistent with the stated purpose and procedures? • Could the researchers have reasonably obtained the reported results using the procedures they outlined? • Are the results credible, given the question and the methods? • Do the researchers include enough samples of the original data to be able to show the relationship between their interpretations and the participants' reports?
Discussion/ conclusions	• Are the conclusions what you would expect from the authors' stated results and purposes? • Do the authors relate their findings to existing literature and clinical practice when explaining their conclusions? • Do the authors provide a logical explanation for their results or lack of results? • Do the authors outline limitations of their design and suggest improvements? • Do the authors provide directions for future research suggested by their study? • Are the findings applicable to your setting and client population? • Would you change the way you practice based on this study?
General questions	• Is it a peer-reviewed journal with blinded reviewers? • Are the background and experience of the researchers appropriate for the study? • Is there any bias resulting from the agencies that funded the study?

Adapted, by permission, from C. Andrade and P. Clifford, 2008, *Outcome-based massage: From evidence to practice,* 2nd ed. (Philadelphia: Lippincott Williams & Wilkins), 42.

can examine the clinical population and clinical issues that the study addresses and decide if these are relevant to their own clinical practice.

Research Methods

The methodology section often holds the key to the credibility of the study. Clinicians should consider several important issues. First of all, clearly defined procedures for interventions and the training of the clinicians providing interventions will assist clinicians in determining the following:

- Whether the interventions are relevant for their own clinical populations.
- If the researchers delivered the interventions correctly.
- If clinicians could reproduce the interventions in their own clinical practice.

Second, clinicians can consider the characteristics of the study sample and judge whether they represent the relevant clinical population, or if the researchers selected them in a manner that may distort, rather than clarify, the findings. Third, clinicians can peruse the research procedures to identify if they are well described and logical, and whether they enable the researchers to address the question or purpose stated in the introduction. Finally, clinicians need not shy away from the data analysis section. Even without advanced research knowledge, clinicians should be able to make sense of the basic intent of the analysis and evaluate whether the researchers analyzed the relevant data.

Research Results

Whether results are in a narrative, tables, charts, or other diagrams, they must be well organized and easily understood. The main issue for clinicians is whether the researchers could have reasonably obtained their results using the procedures they described. From there, clinicians can locate the positive and negative findings that the researchers report. Clinicians are wise to return to the results section as they read the discussion and conclusion to see if the researchers' findings do, in fact, support their conclusions.

Discussion and Conclusions

Armed with a basic analysis of the study, clinicians can review the researchers' conclusions with critical eye. Do the authors give logical explanations for their findings or lack of findings? Do they use the existing literature to support their arguments? Are there gaps in the logic of their conclusions or limitations to the study design? These are some of the questions clinicians can consider at this point. Finally, they can focus on identifying the relevance of the study's findings for their own clinical practice.

USING QUALITATIVE RESEARCH METHODS IN MASSAGE THERAPY

What aspects of MT can be studied using qualitative research? If massage is a holistic treatment that addresses the mind, body, and spirit, then we need research methods that enable us to document mental, physical, spiritual, and social processes. The strengths of qualitative research are its ability to capture participants' internal processes (assumptions, beliefs, untaught practices, perceptions, and meanings) and the nonspecific effects of massage that reflect the interaction between the context in which massage occurs and the process of delivering massage interventions (Cassidy 2002; Grypdonck 2006; Kania, Porcino, and Verhoef 2008; Verhoef, Casebeer, and Hilsden 2002). Researchers can capitalize on these strengths and use qualitative methods to answer appropriate questions that will continue to increase our understanding of massage and its outcomes.

Questions for Qualitative Research

Cassidy (2002) proposes the four fields model, which identifies the domains of research on massage to answer two key questions: Does massage work? Is it useful to people? Within this model, the domains of sociocultural effectiveness, within-practice effectiveness, and comparative effectiveness are more appropriate for qualitative research than is the domain of physiological effectiveness. By focusing on the first three domains, researchers can answer a number of questions using qualitative research methods, such as those outlined in table 4.2. These questions can lead to insights into the context, structure, process, and outcomes of MT that cannot be achieved through quantification (Cassidy 2002; Grypdonck 2006; Kania, Porcino, and Verhoef 2008; Verhoef, Casebeer, and Hilsden 2002). They can also reveal the inner workings of people and the language they use to describe their experiences. Finally, they can explain the relationship between people's inner experiences and outcomes. They can also provide baseline data to inform the development of quantitative questions and measures for massage.

Qualitative Research Findings on Massage

Qualitative research in MT is an emerging area; consequently, the body of literature is still small and the quality of the studies varies. Nevertheless, there is increasing evidence that massage techniques may produce important psychological outcomes, such as the reduction of stress, depression, and anxiety in many different populations (Moyer, Rounds, and Hannum 2004). In addition, within the realm of the clients' experiences of massage, many report that massage contributes to improved body image, self-image, social identity, confidence, perceived relaxation, perceived well-being, and ability to cope with stress (Bredin 1999; Billhult, Stener-Victorin, and Bergborn 2007; Paterson et al. 2005; Price 2005). Furthermore, clients report that massage helps increase their perception that their mind and body are connected, and that it leaves them feeling both good and cared for (Mulkins, Verhoef, and Cormier 2005). Clients also report that they value specific characteristics of MT, such as personal time, a competent therapist, trust, a holistic approach, empowerment, effective touch, and relaxation (Smith, Sullivan, and Baxter 2009). In addition, qualitative research gives us some insight into the massage therapists' perspective, such as the positive and negative personal and professional experiences that influence a practitioner's professional choices (Herbert et al. 2007). These studies and their findings underscore the importance of qualitative research in MT.

IMPLICATIONS FOR MASSAGE THERAPY

The complexity of massage requires alternatives to traditional quantitative research methods. Yet the difference between qualitative and quantitative research methods goes beyond the use of words versus use of numbers. Done well, qualitative research gives us a deeper understanding of the perceptions and experiences of

Table 4.2 Examples of Research Questions

Domain from four field model (Cassidy 2002)	Area (Kania, Porcino, and Verhoef 2008)	Observation (Kania, Porcino, and Verhoef 2008)	Example of a qualitative question
Sociocultural effectiveness: Questions that deal with how people perceive and evaluate the field of massage therapy and explain it to themselves or others, such as demographics, costs of care, epidemiology, education and outreach, law and politics, and history of the field.	Structure of care	People with chronic medical conditions are seeking massage therapy.	What are clients' reasons for seeking massage therapy treatment when they have a chronic medical condition?
		Massage therapists practice in a growing variety of settings.	What are physicians' and nurses' perceptions of the value and role of massage therapists in a skilled nursing facility?
			What contributes to patient satisfaction with massage therapy in different practice settings?
	Process of care	Many massage therapists are trained to perform orthopedic assessments.	What are massage therapists' perceptions of their training and competency in performing orthopedic assessments?
		Delivering massage therapy requires an understanding of personal boundaries.	How do massage therapists develop an understanding of personal boundaries during massage therapy training and practice?
Within-practice effectiveness: All questions that deal with issues about the practice of massage, including comparisons of intervention techniques, duration and frequency of sessions, and the effect of the practitioner on result of care.	Outcomes of care	Massage therapy reduces musculoskeletal pain.	How do clients with fibromyalgia describe the effect of massage therapy on their musculoskeletal pain?
		Massage therapy reduces the negative side effects of cancer treatment.	How do women who have undergone mastectomy describe their experiences of receiving massage therapy?
		Many clients use massage therapy for issues related to wellness.	What does *wellness* mean to healthy massage therapy clients and how do they describe the effects of massage therapy?

the people who give or receive MT treatments. It can provide insights into the contexts, processes, and outcomes of MT that may be impossible to adequately summarize through quantification. It can also help researchers refine quantitative research questions and elaborate on the findings of quantitative research. Finally, massage therapists can consider qualitative methods to be rigorous, systematic methods with standards for trustworthiness. In short, researchers can use qualitative research methods with confidence to extend the body of evidence for MT.

SUMMARY

Qualitative research is the collection and analysis of word-based experiential and observational data. Researchers use methods of qualitative data collection to obtain detailed, rich, narrative data about participants, their contexts, their perceptions, and their experiences. Observation, interviews, focus groups, and document analysis are four of the most commonly used methods for gathering data in qualitative research. A combination of these methods can be used to increase the depth of understanding of the phenomena under investigation.

Standards for evaluating the trustworthiness of qualitative research methods include credibility, transferability, dependability, and confirmability. Qualitative research methods are best used to answer questions about psychosocial outcomes and nonspecific effects such as the following: What are clients' reasons for seeking massage therapy when they have a chronic medical condition? How do clients with fibromyalgia experience the effect of massage therapy on their musculoskeletal pain? Clinicians can assess the rigor and applicability of qualitative research studies to their practice by reading carefully and critically, and by asking themselves whether the interventions are relevant for their own clinical populations, if the researchers delivered the interventions correctly, and if the interventions are relevant to their own clinical practice. Given the complexity of massage therapy as an intervention, qualitative research studies have much to contribute to our overall understanding of massage therapy.

Critical Thinking Questions

1. How does qualitative research methodology contribute to our overall understanding of massage therapy?
2. What are the differences among grounded theory, ethnography, and phenomenology?
3. Describe four commonly used methods of qualitative data collection.
4. List and describe the four concepts that are used for judging qualitative research.
5. Generate a massage therapy research question that would best be addressed using qualitative research methods.

REFERENCES

Andrade, C.K., and P. Clifford. 2008. *Outcome-based massage: From evidence to practice.* 2nd ed. Philadelphia: Lippincott Williams & Wilkins.

Armitage, A., and D. Keeble. 2007. *Mutual research designs: Redefining mixed methods design.* Paper presented at the British Educational Research Association Annual Conference, Institute of Education. London: University of London.

Billhult, A., E. Stener-Victorin, and I. Bergborn. 2007. The experience of massage during chemotherapy treatment in breast cancer patients. *Clin Nurs Res* 16: 85-99.

Bredin, M. 1999. Mastectomy, body image and therapeutic massage: A qualitative study of women's experience. *J Adv Nurs* 29: 1113-1120.

Bryman, A. 2004. *Quantity and quality in social research.* 2nd ed. London: Routledge.

Byrne, M. 2001a. Understanding life experiences through a phenomenological approach to research. *AORN J* 73: 830-832.

———. 2001b. Ethnography as a qualitative research method. *AORN J* 74: 82.

Cassidy, C.M. 2002. *Methodological issues in investigations of massage/bodywork therapy.* Evanston, IL: American Massage Therapy Association Foundation.

Corbin, J., and A. Strauss. 2007. *Basics of qualitative research: Techniques and procedures for developing grounded theory.* 3rd ed. Thousand Oaks, CA: Sage.

Creswell, J.W. 2003. *Research design: Qualitative, quantitative and mixed method approaches.* 2nd ed. London: Sage.

Denzin, N.K., and Y.S. Lincoln., eds. 2005. *The SAGE handbook of qualitative research.* Thousand Oaks, CA: Sage.

Frechtling Westat, J. 2002. The 2002 *user friendly handbook for project evaluation.* Arlington, VA: National Science Foundation. www.nsf.gov/pubs/2002/nsf02057/nsf02057.pdf.

Goetz, J.P., and M.D. LeComte. 1984. *Ethnography and qualitative design in educational research.* New York: Academic Press.

Glaser, B.G., and A.L. Strauss. 1967. *The discovery of grounded theory: Strategies for qualitative research.* New York: de Gruyter.

Greenhalgh, T., and R. Taylor. 1997. How to read a paper: Papers that go beyond numbers (qualitative research). *Br Med J* 315: 740-743.

Groenewald, T. 2004. Phenomenological research design illustrated. *International Journal of Qualitative Methods* 3: 42-55

Grypdonck, M.H.F. 2006. Qualitative health research in the era of evidence-based practice. *Qual Health Res* 16: 1371-1385.

Hall, B. 2010. *How to do ethnographic research: A simplified guide.* www.sas.upenn.edu/anthro/anthro/cpiamethods.

Herbert, C., L. Bainbridge, J. Bickford, S. Baptiste, S. Brajtman, T. Dryden, P. Hall, C. Risdon, and P. Solomon. 2007. Factors that influence engagement in collaborative practice: How eight health professionals became advocates. *Can Fam Physician* 53: 1318-1325.

Kania, A., A. Porcino, and M.J. Verhoef. 2008. Value of qualitative research in the study of massage therapy. *Int J Ther Massage Bodywork* 1. www.ijtmb.org/index.php/ijtmb/article/viewArticle/26/34.

Kuhn, T. 1970. *The structure of scientific revolutions.* Chicago: University of Chicago Press.

Lincoln, Y.S., and E.G. Guba. 1985. *Naturalistic inquiry.* Newbury Park, CA: Sage.

Menard, M. 2009. *Making sense of research.* 2nd ed. Toronto, ON: Curties-Overzet.

Moyer, C.A., J. Rounds, and J.W. Hannum. 2004. A meta-analysis of massage therapy research. *Psych Bull* 130: 3-18.

Mulkins, A.L., M. Verhoef, and E. Cormier. 2005. The benefits of massage in Vancouver's inner city. *Massage Ther J* 44: 102-9.

Onwuegbuzie, A.J., R.B. Johnson, and K. Collin. 2009. Call for mixed analysis: A philosophical framework for combining qualitative and quantitative approaches. *International Journal of Multiple Research Approaches* 3: 114-139.

O'Reilly, K. 2005. *Ethnographic methods.* New York: Routledge.

Paterson, C., D. Vindigni, B. Polus, T. Browell, and C. Edgecombe. 2008. Evaluating a massage therapy training and treatment programme in a remote Aboriginal community. *Complement Ther Clin Pract* 14: 158-167.

Paterson, C., J. Allen, M. Browning, G. Barlow, and P. Ewings. 2005. A pilot study of therapeutic massage for people with Parkinson's disease: The added value of user involvement. *Complement Ther Clin Pract* 11: 161-171.

Patton, M.Q. 2002. *Qualitative research and evaluation methods.* 3rd ed. Thousand Oaks, CA: Sage.

Pope, C., and N. Mays. 1995. Reaching the parts other methods cannot reach: An introduction to qualitative methods in health and health services research. *Br Med J* 311: 109-112.

Portney, L., and M. Watkins. 2008. *Foundations of clinical research: Applications to practice.* 3rd ed.Upper Saddle River, NJ: Prentice Hall.

Price, C. 2005. Body-oriented therapy in recovery from child sexual abuse: An efficacy study. *Altern Ther Health Med* 11: 46-57.

Smith, J., P. Flowers, and M. Larkin. 2009. *Interpretive phenomenological analysis: Theory, method and research.* Thousand Oaks, CA: Sage.

Smith, J.M., S.J. Sullivan, and G.D. Baxter. 2009. The culture of massage therapy: Valued elements and the role of comfort, contact, connection and caring. *Complement Ther Med* 17: 181-189.

Tashakkori, A., and C. Teddlie. 1998. *Mixed methodology: Combining qualitative and quantitative approaches.* Thousand Oaks, CA: Sage.

———. 2002. *Handbook of mixed methods in social and behavioral research.* London: Sage.

Verhoef, M.J., A. Casebeer, R. Hilsden. 2002. Assessing efficacy of complementary medicine: Adding qualitative research methods to the "gold standard." *J Altern Complem Med* 8: 275-281.

Mixed Methods Research

Marja Verhoef, PhD

Mixed methods research combines both quantitative and qualitative research. This chapter reviews the use of mixed methods research to assess the benefits of massage therapy and looks at the various ways in which qualitative and quantitative research can be combined. Several examples illustrate the various aspects of mixed methods research.

Massage therapy can be seen as a complex intervention consisting of physiological, psychological, social, and spiritual components (Andrade and Clifford 2008). In addition, many contextual factors affect the outcomes of massage therapy and may enhance or worsen its outcomes. Examples include the therapeutic intent of the practitioner, the patient's characteristics, such as beliefs, expectations, and preferences, as well as the relationship between the patient and the provider. When studying the influence of massage therapy, it is important to capture this complexity and to consider a mixed methods design in which both quantitative and qualitative research methods are combined. Of course, which specific methodological approach is used ultimately depends on the research question (Muncey 2009). For example, if the question is about the number of people using massage therapy, or the strength of the association between scores on a pain scale before and after receiving massage therapy, a quantitative research design will be appropriate. If the question is how and why people make the decision to access massage therapy, a qualitative research design will be the best choice. However, sometimes research questions are more complex. For example, does massage therapy after major trauma improve people's quality of life? If so, what was it about the treatment that made the difference? In this case, both quantitative and qualitative inquiry would be required, since either alone would fall short in addressing these questions.

Mixed methods research is defined as "research that collects both qualitative and quantitative data in one study and integrates these data at some stage of the research process" (Halcomb, Andrew, and Brannen 2009, 9-10). Other terms are used as well, such as combined methods (Buchanan 1992), integrated methods (Coyle and Williams 2000), methodological pluralism (Barker and Pistrang 2005) and multimethod research (Stange 2004). The differences in terms are often related to the degree of methodological integration used in such research.

As the assumptions underlying quantitative and qualitative research are different (see chapters 3 and 4), some researchers have argued that these approaches are incompatible and cannot be combined (see Tashakkori and Teddlie 1998, chapter 1, for a discussion). However, renewed attention to qualitative research conducted between 1980 and 2000 has led to a more pragmatic approach that combines quantitative and qualitative research. Researchers, especially in the social sciences, have developed empirical approaches, such as mixed methods research, to understand problems that cannot easily be addressed by any other approach. These hybrid methods have provided the answers that were needed (Morgan 2008). This perspective has been defined as *paradigm relativism,* or "the use of whatever philosophical or methodological approach works for the particular research problem under study" (Tashakkori and Teddlie 1998, 5).

REASONS FOR USING A MIXED METHODS RESEARCH DESIGN

Many authors have addressed potential reasons for using mixed methods designs (Greene, Caracelli, and Graham 1989; Sandelowski 2000; Morgan 1998). The most common reasons are discussed in the following boxed element.

Reasons for Conducting Mixed Methods Research

Confirmation. Examine whether qualitative and quantitative data on the same phenomenon converge, and thus confirm the findings.

Complementarity. Examine whether data from one method elaborate, enhance, illustrate, or clarify the results of the other method.

Development. Use results from one method to help develop or inform the other method. Development broadly includes sampling and implementation, as well as measurement decisions.

Initiation. Seek contradiction, inconsistencies, and new perspectives, rather than consistency, to increase the breadth and depth of inquiry. This is usually applied in areas in which little is known.

Expansion. Extend the range of inquiry by using different methods to broaden the scope of the study.

It is important to note that various reasons may apply to the same study and may overlap. Complementarity is the most common reason for mixing qualitative and quantitative methods (Bryman 2006). Greene, Caracelli, and Graham (1989) have pointed out that the array of reasons for combining qualitative and quantitative methods ranges from very restricted (convergence) to wide and flexible (initiation and expansion). In massage therapy research, development, initiation, and expansion are becoming increasingly important due to the complexity of many healing systems. While these five reasons are most commonly referred to in the literature, some authors have used different ways of identifying reasons for mixing methods (Nastasi et al. 2007; Newman et al. 2003; Bryman 2006).

MIXED METHODS DESIGNS

Mixed methods designs "involve the collection or analysis of both quantitative and qualitative data in a single study in which the data are collected concurrently (simultaneously) or sequentially (consecutively), are given a priority, and involve the integration of the data at one or more stages in the process of research" (Creswell et al. 2003, 212). Therefore, all typologies of mixed methods research refer to (1) sequence, which indicates whether quantitative and qualitative data collection is concurrent or whether one comes before the other, and (2) priority, indicating whether quantitative or qualitative research is the dominant method versus the other, which is complementary (Creswell et al. 2003, Sandelowski 2000, Morgan 1998). A third component of interest is integration (Kroll and Neri 2009), which is perhaps the most important but least discussed component. It has been defined in many different ways, from "combining qualitative and quantitative research" (Creswell et al. 2003, 220) to "the knitting together of different approaches to research" (Andrew and Halcomb 2009).

In true mixed methods designs, qualitative and quantitative methods are purposefully integrated. Integration begins during the conceptual stages of the study. It must be reflected in the research question, so that it is clear how the different types of data will inform one another and how they provide answers to the research question. Integration can occur at various stages of the research process, mostly during data collection, data analysis, or data interpretation. Table 5.1 includes the most common mixed methods designs that have been reported in the literature, taking into account sequence and priority, and using common notation (Greene, Caracelli, and Graham 1989, Sandelowski 2000, Creswell et al. 2003). Not all potential designs are included in table 5.1. For example, Sandelowski (2000) notes that mixed methods research may consist of more than two phases. It may also be used in an iterative fashion. This could be the case for instrument development (see the section on instrument development on page 65).

Table 5.1 Common Designs for Mixed Methods Research

	Priority (qualitative or quantitative research)		
Sequence	**Quantitative**	**Qualitative**	**Equal (no priority)**
Concurrent	QUAN + qual	QUAL + quan	QUAN + QUAL
Sequential	QUAN → qual	QUAL → quan	QUAN → QUAL or QUAL → QUAN

QUAN and *QUAL* stand for the method that is dominant and that has priority. *Quan* and *qual* refer to the complementary, or secondary, method. Sequence is identified using an arrow (→) and concurrence with a + sign.
Based on Morgan 1998; Tashakkori and Teddlie 1998; Sandelowski 2000.

To date, the use of mixed methods research designs related to massage therapy is minimal. However, some studies are beginning to use this approach. Two examples are presented in boxes 5.1 and 5.2. The first study is an example of a situation in which complementarity is the reason for using a mixed methods design. In the second study, confirmation, expansion, and development appear to be the reasons for using mixing methods research.

CONDUCTING MIXED METHODS RESEARCH

This section addresses design components from the perspective of mixed methods research. It reviews methods of sampling, data collection and analysis, and instrument development, along with the advantages of adding qualitative inquiry to a randomized controlled trial (RCT). It also examines whole systems research, an approach that recognizes the inherent complexity of interacting components in an intervention such as massage therapy.

BOX 5.1

Massage Therapy Versus Simple Touch to Improve Pain and Mood in Patients With Advanced Cancer: QUAN + qual

Objective	To (1) evaluate the efficacy of massage for decreasing pain and symptom distress and for improving quality of life among persons with advanced cancer, and (2) to assess patient experiences with massage therapy and the treatment environment.
Methods	1. A 2-week single-blind randomized controlled trial (RCT) of massage therapy versus simple touch. 2. A detailed 6-page treatment form (requiring both qualitative and quantitative information) completed by the massage therapists before each treatment to document physical, psychological, and psychosocial issues, as well as patient–therapist communication.
Results	Both groups experienced significant improvement in pain and mood immediately after treatment, but massage therapy was superior to simple touch. Patients commented on areas that the therapist should avoid, voiced specific requests for treatment related to their symptoms, and shared the nature of their suffering and spiritual experiences. Results were not sustained beyond 3 weeks.
Conclusion	The qualitative reports provide important insights beyond the RCT results on how to enhance care for palliative cancer patients and to prepare for expressions of grief, fear, and anxiety related to dying, family conflicts, and uncertainty.

Based on Kutner et al. 2008; Smith et al. 2009.

BOX 5.2

Evaluating a Massage Therapy Training and Treatment Program in a Remote Aboriginal Community: The Hopevale Massage Therapy Project: QUAL + quan

Objective	To evaluate a massage training and treatment program (MTTP) in a remote aboriginal community (Hopevale) and to develop the frameworks, procedures, and processes necessary for future research.
Methods	Self-report health questionnaire, interviews with key informants (patients and community members), and participant observation.
Results	The quantitative data described the respondents' scores related to sociodemographic information, health, and well-being at baseline. Due to cyclones and floods, follow-up data collection was not conducted. The qualitative data indicated that the program had many individual benefits (e.g., symptom relief, increased well-being, treatment perceived as "something enjoyable"), as well as community-level benefits (e.g., increased participation, strengthening local health, and educational projects). Participant observation by the principal investigator confirmed these benefits.
Conclusion	The MTTP "interconnected with the people of Hopevale at three levels: individuals, the community, and the wider geographic, cultural, and political context." These findings provide a framework for future development and evaluation of the program, as well as suggest that participant observation may be one of the most appropriate designs for doing so.

Based on Paterson 2008, The Hopevale massage therapy project.

Sampling

Since no sampling techniques are unique to mixed methods research, combinations of qualitative and quantitative sampling strategies are used. While qualitative research typically involves purposeful sampling to enhance understanding of information-rich cases, quantitative research ideally involves probability sampling so that statistical inferences can be made. Sampling strategies in mixed methods use "both probability sampling (to increase external validity) and purposive sampling strategies (to increase transferability)" (Teddlie and Yu 2007, 201). External validity is the approximate validity with which we can infer that a presumed causal relationship (for example, between massage therapy and well-being) can be generalized (1) to and across different measures of the cause and effect and (2) across different types of persons, settings, and times. Transferability is a term used as a qualitative analogue (based on qualitative data) to external validity (Tashakkori and Teddlie 2003, 708, 716).

Teddlie and Yu (2007) provide a provisional typology of five different sampling strategies. The three most common strategies are described as follows. *Basic mixed methods sampling strategies* are types of random, or stratified, purposive sampling techniques (Sandelowski 2000). For example, participants in a large RCT of massage therapy may be divided into strata based on their outcomes (e.g., did the condition improve, stay the same, or deteriorate?). A purposive sample of respondents may then be drawn from each stratum to explore the experience of massage therapy. *Sequential sampling* is based on sequential designs. It uses quantitative sampling followed by qualitative sampling, such as for reasons of complementarity (see the section on adding qualitative inquiry to randomized controlled trials on page 65) or vice versa (such as in instrument development). *Concurrent sampling* uses probability and purposive sampling simultaneously (see box 5.1).

basic mixed methods sampling strategies

▸ Approaches for deriving a sample from a population that allow for the creation of additional, stratified samples based on outcomes.

sequential sampling

▸ A two-step sampling procedure consisting of a quantitative sampling, followed by a qualitative sampling.

concurrent sampling

▸ An approach to sampling that uses probability and purposive sampling simultaneously.

Data Collection

Mixed methods research combines data collection techniques associated with qualitative and quantitative research. Common qualitative techniques include interviews, focus groups, open-ended survey questions, and unstructured observations. Common quantitative data collection techniques include fully structured interviews or questionnaires and structured observation (Brannen and Halcomb 2009). Both unstructured and structured data can be used in a mixed methods

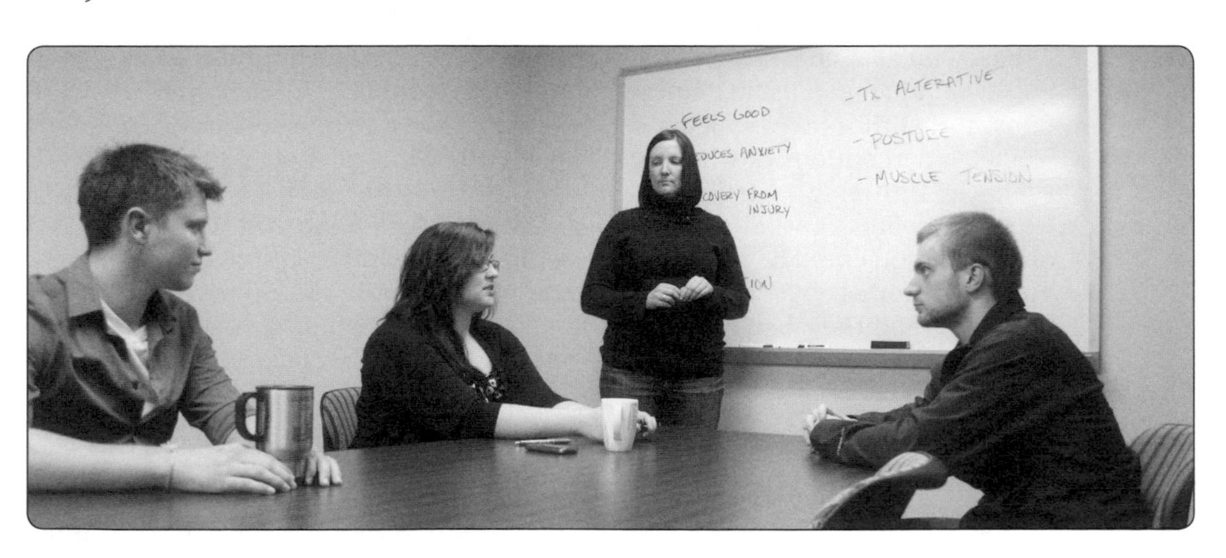

Focus groups are a common qualitative technique that can provide useful study data.

study to complement and inform each other. In addition, data collection instruments can also be mixed; examples include a survey with open-ended questions or an interview guide structured around prespecified topics. Similarly, observation can be partly prespecified and partly open ended.

Outcome instruments can also be mixed. For example, the MYMOP (Measure Yourself Medical Outcome Profile) and MYCAW (Measure Your Concerns and Wellbeing) both include open-ended and structured questions (Paterson 1996; Paterson et al. 2007). An excellent resource for both types of outcomes is the IN-CAM Outcomes Database (www.outcomesdatabase.org), which includes outcome measures of particular importance to complementary and alternative medicine (CAM) research. These are aimed at facilitating and supporting the assessment of CAM interventions through high-quality research that can improve clinical practice and inform policy.

Data Analysis

A study may collect both qualitative and quantitative data, analyze these using appropriate qualitative or quantitative techniques, and then compare or contrast these data to assist with interpretation (e.g., complementing, developing, expanding). Comparing such data can also help with understanding or resolving inconsistencies (for an example, see the section on adding qualitative inquiry to randomized controlled trials). However, there are also strategies that transform one type of data into the other. Two well-known strategies are *quantitizing* and *qualitizing* (Sandelowski 2000; Bazeley 2009).

quantitizing

▸ The conversion of qualitative data into numerical codes that can be analyzed statistically.

qualitizing

▸ The conversion of quantitative data into a narrative or descriptive format.

Quantitizing refers to converting qualitative data into numerical codes that can be analyzed statistically. In order to do so, verbal or visual data are reduced to items or variables that are intended to mean only one thing. Therefore, they can be represented numerically. For example, interview data on benefits of massage therapy can be grouped, coded, and then used as a variable in quantitative analysis. Quantitizing is also helpful when qualitative interviews are used to develop items for a new measuring instrument that can then be analyzed quantitatively.

Qualitizing refers to the process by which quantitative data are transformed into a narrative format or descriptive classification to profile participants. For example, beginning with scores from a measuring instrument such as a visual analogue scale, people can be profiled as mildly or severely affected by pain. These two groups can then be further described to develop verbal portraits or typologies (Sandelowski 2000).

Based on data collected in a qualitative study of women's approaches to gathering, evaluating, and using information on CAM treatments for menopausal symptoms, the authors developed a series of items for a follow-up survey to assess women's perceptions of what constitutes trusted information, using a five-point scale (quantitizing). Further quantitative descriptive analysis suggested that women's beliefs of what signifies good-quality information and trusted sources of information could be categorized as either pragmatic or intuitive (qualitizing). These categories could then be used to profile pragmatic and intuitive women and to understand their behaviors (Armitage et al. 2007). Other strategies for mixed methods analysis are discussed by Bazeley (2009) and Caracelli and Green (1993).

APPLICATIONS OF MIXED METHODS RESEARCH

Two common applications of mixed methods research include developing instruments and adding a qualitative component to randomized controlled trials. A third application is the role of mixed methods in whole systems research.

Instrument Development

The development of new instruments to measure a wide range of outcomes often uses mixed methods research. For example, the Consultation and Relational Empathy Measure (CARE; Mercer et al. 2004) assesses the consultation process based on a broad definition of empathy that is meaningful to patients, irrespective of their socioeconomic backgrounds. It was developed for the assessment of family physicians but appears to be applicable to other professions as well. Instrument items were developed based on theoretical work on the importance of empathy. This draft instrument was piloted in a diverse group of patients, followed by interviews with another group of patients to further inform face and content validity of the instrument. The instrument was then reviewed and discussed in a two-day meeting by practitioners, with guidance from a nurse with expertise in empathy research. Subsequently, the instrument was statistically tested for validity and reliability. This process of pilot testing, interviews, and psychometric assessment continued until the instrument was deemed sufficiently valid and reliable. It is only through such an iterative process that outcome instruments can be developed in a valid and reliable manner.

Adding Qualitative Inquiry to Randomized Controlled Trials

By far, the most common massage therapy research question is whether an intervention works (Cassidy 2002). Randomized controlled trials (RCTs) are commonly considered the best option for assessing this question. They are controlled experimental designs in which participants are randomly allocated to either the intervention or control group. While RCTs can be useful when the health condition of interest is clearly described, the treatment is well defined, and the circumstances of the patients are relatively similar, some maintain that RCTs are poorly suited for studying complex interventions, such as massage therapy, for the following reasons:

1. They do not take into account the underlying assumptions of massage therapy, such as the process of healing or therapeutic intent.
2. Massage therapy is a multicomponent individualized treatment that cannot be standardized.
3. Not all eligible study participants will want to be randomized.
4. Blinding and placebo control are nearly impossible.
5. RCTs exclude the nonspecific effects that are crucial in massage therapy.

As such, it could be advantageous to use a modified form of an RCT, such as a pragmatic trial, which allows individualization of the intervention (Menard 2009, 97-98).

If RCTs or pragmatic trials are used to evaluate massage therapy, the addition of qualitative data collection will be important to understand what is going on in the trial. Due to its limitations, it can be difficult to explain the results of an RCT. For example, an RCT of a yogic breathing and meditation intervention for participants living with HIV/AIDS (Brazier, Mulkins, and Verhoef 2006) resulted in some positive changes in well-being that lasted only for 1 or 2 weeks after the intervention. However, it also resulted in an increase in the experience and effect of stress over time. In the qualitative interviews, conducted after the RCT, participants explained that they were learning to feel everything, pleasant and unpleasant, with greater intensity. This process of greater self-awareness was not always comfortable or easy, and this caused both positive and negative experiences.

WHOLE SYSTEMS RESEARCH

Increasing recognition of the complex nature of interventions has led to the understanding that interventions such as massage therapy are complex systems. A complex system consists of multiple interacting components (patients, providers, treatments, and context). It is dynamic and nonlinear, and it evolves over time. This implies that the treatment system that evolves is not equal to the sum of its parts. Therefore, it cannot be understood by only comprehending the individual parts. Whole systems like massage therapy are defined as "approaches to health care in which practitioners apply bodies of knowledge and associated practices that maximize the patients' capacity to achieve mental and physical balance and restore their health, using individualized approaches to diagnosis and treatment" (Ritenbaugh et al. 2003). The patient–provider relationship plays an important role in this process.

Whole systems research (WSR) is defined as a framework specifically for the investigation of the effectiveness of whole systems of health care (Ritenbaugh et al. 2003). Within this framework, all aspects of any internally consistent approach to treatment, or to a whole system, need to be assessed. Since no one study can evaluate every aspect of a whole system, it is helpful to see WSR as a program of research that consists of various phases and multiple designs and methods. For example, one could begin to describe the important components of an intervention (the treatment options and patient characteristics, such as expectations, the patient–provider relationship, and so on). This could be followed by exploring the relationships between these factors, developing hypotheses about how, why, and under which circumstances the system works, and, finally, testing these hypotheses. In terms of methodology, mixed methods research would be an important part of such a program.

The Hopevale Massage Therapy Treatment Program (MTTP; see box 5.2) discussed by Paterson and colleagues (2008a) is an excellent example of a whole system that connects with the people of Hopevale at individual, community, cultural, and political levels. Identifying and exploring this complexity is the beginning of a longer term research program to evaluate the program and to assess its sustainability.

SUMMARY

Standard clinical practice research often falls short of effectively informing practice in a useful and meaningful way. Increasingly, research demonstrates that in real life, the patient, practitioner, treatment, and context interact to determine how well treatment systems, such as massage therapy, work. To assess which treatment regimens work, quantitative research is needed. To understand how and when the healing potential can be enhanced, qualitative research is needed. Mixed methods research takes both approaches into account. While it can be complex and expensive, it provides a more complete picture. Hence, treatment decisions based on mixed methods research ultimately have the potential to be more effective than those based on one approach only.

Massage therapy is a complex intervention that cannot be fully captured or adequately understood by a single research method or approach. For this reason, mixed methods research, which combines and integrates quantitative and qualitative approaches, is valuable. Its specific approaches to sampling, data collection, and data analysis, its potential to combine qualitative and quantitative data within the same study, and the broadened perspective made possible by whole systems research have the potential to expand our understanding of massage therapy and its inherent complexities.

Critical Thinking Questions

1. How can massage therapy research benefit from a mixed methods approach? Provide and describe at least three specific ways.
2. Consider an aspect of massage therapy of particular interest to you. Describe how this aspect of massage therapy could be investigated with a combination of qualitative and quantitative approaches within the same study.
3. Provide an example of massage therapy research data that could be meaningfully *quantized,* and explain how and why this would be done. Provide a different example of massage therapy research data that could be meaningfully *qualitized,* and explain how and why this would be done.
4. How can a mixed methods approach be used to inform instrument development? Describe how you might use such an approach to develop a measurement instrument that could address a need in massage therapy research or practice.
5. Describe *whole systems research,* and explain why it is a valuable framework for investigating massage therapy.

REFERENCES

Andrade, C.K., and P. Clifford. 2008. *Outcomes-based massage: From evidence to practice.* 2nd ed. Baltimore: Lippincott Williams & Wilkins.

Andrew, S., and E.J. Halcomb, eds. 2009. *Mixed methods research for nursing and the health sciences.* Oxford: Wiley-Blackwell.

Armitage, G.D., E. Suter, M. J. Verhoef, C. Bockmuehl, and M. Bobey. 2007. Women's needs for CAM information to manage menopausal symptoms. *Climacteric* 10(3): 215-224.

Barker, C., and N. Pistrang. 2005. Quality criteria under methodological pluralism: Implications for conducting and evaluating research. *Am J Commun Psychol* 35(3-4): 201-212.

Bazeley, P. 2009. Analysing mixed methods data. In *Mixed methods research for nursing and the health sciences,* eds. S. Andrew and E.J. Halcomb, 84-118. Oxford: Wiley-Blackwell.

Brannen, J., and E.J. Halcomb. 2009. Data collection in mixed methods research. In *Mixed methods research for nursing and the health sciences,* eds. S. Andrew and E.J. Halcomb, 67-83. Oxford: Wiley-Blackwell.

Brazier, A., A. Mulkins, and M. Verhoef. 2006. Evaluating a yogic breathing and meditation intervention for individuals living with HIV/AIDS. *Am J Health Promot* 20(3): 192-195.

Bryman, A. 2006. Integrating quantitative and qualitative research: How is it done? *Qual Res* 6(1): 97-113.

Buchanan, D.R. 1992. An uneasy alliance: Combining qualitative and quantitative research methods. *Health Educ Quart* 19(1): 117-135.

Caracelli, V.J., and J.C. Greene. 1993. Data analysis strategies for mixed-method evaluation designs. *Educ Eval Policy An* 15(2): 195-207.

Cassidy, C.M. 2002. *Methodological issues in investigations of massage/bodywork therapy.* Evanston, IL: American Massage Therapy Association Foundation.

Coyle, J., and B. Williams. 2000. An exploration of the epistomological intricacies of using qualitative data to develop a quantitative measure of user views of health care. *J Adv Nurs* 31(5): 1235-1243.

Creswell, J.W., V.L. Plano Clark, M.L. Gutmann, and W.E. Hanson. 2003. Advanced mixed methods research designs. In *Handbook of mixed methods in social and behavioral research,* eds. A. Tashakkori and C. Teddlie, 209-240. Thousand Oaks, CA: Sage.

Denzin, N.K., and Y.S. Lincoln. 1994. Introduction: Entering the field of qualitative research. In *Handbook of qualitative research,* eds. N.K. Denzin and Y.S. Lincoln, 1-17. Thousand Oaks, CA: Sage.

Greene, J.C., V.J. Caracelli, and W.F. Graham. 1989. Toward a conceptual framework for mixed-method evaluation designs. *Educ Eval Policy An* 11(3): 255-274.

Halcomb, E.J., S. Andrew, and J. Brannen. 2009. Introduction to mixed methods research for nursing and the health sciences. In *Mixed methods research for nursing and the health sciences,* eds. S. Andrew and E.J. Halcomb, 3-12. Oxford: Wiley-Blackwell.

Kroll, T., and M. Neri. 2009. Designs for mixed methods research. In *Mixed methods research for nursing and the health sciences,* eds. S. Andrew and E.J. Halcomb, 31-49. Oxford: Wiley-Blackwell.

Kutner, J.S., M.C. Smith, L. Corbin, L. Hemphill, K. Benton, B.K. Mellis, B. Beaty, S. Felton, T.E. Yamashita, L. Bryant, et al. 2008. Massage therapy versus simple touch to improve pain and mood in patients with advanced cancer: A randomized trial. *Ann Intern Med* 149(6): 369-379.

Menard, M.B. 2009. *Making sense of research.* 2nd ed. Toronto: Curties-Overzet.

Mercer, S.W., M. Maxwell, D. Heaney, and G.C. Watt. 2004. The consultation and relational empathy (CARE) measure: Development and preliminary validation and reliability of an empathy-based consultation process measure. *Fam Pract* 21(6): 699-705.

Morgan, L. 1998. Practical strategies for combining qualitative and quantitative methods: Applications to health research. *Qual Health Res* 8(3): 362-376.

———. 2008. Paradigms lost and pragmatism regained: Methodological implications of combining qualitative and quantitative methods. In *The mixed methods reader,* eds. V.L. Plano Clark and J.W. Creswell, 29-65. Los Angeles: Sage. Originally published in *J Mix Method Res* 1(1): 48-76, 2007.

Muncey, T. 2009. Does mixed methods constitute a change in paradigm? In *Mixed methods research for nursing and the health sciences,* eds. S. Andrew and E.J. Halcomb, 13-30. Oxford: Wiley-Blackwell.

Nastasi, B.K., J. Hitchcock, S. Sarkar, G. Burkholder, K. Varjas, and A. Jayasena. 2007. Mixed methods in intervention research: Theory to adaptation. *J Mix Method Res* 1(2): 164-182.

Newman, I., C.L. Ridenour, C. Newman and G.M.P. DeMarco. 2003. A typology of research purposes and its relationship to mixed methods. In *Handbook of mixed methods in social and behavioral research,* eds. A. Tashakkori and C. Teddlie, 167-188. Thousand Oaks, CA: Sage.

Paterson C. 1996. Measuring outcomes in primary care: A patient generated measure, MYMOP, compared with the SF-36 health survey. *BMJ* 312:1016-1020.

Paterson C., Thomas, A. Manasse, H. HYPERLINK "http://www.ncbi.nlm.nih.gov/pubmed?term=%22Cooke%20H%22%5BAuthor%5D&itool=EntrezSystem2.PEntrez.Pubmed.Pubmed_ResultsPanel.Pubmed_RVAbstract"Cooke. and G. Peace. 2007. Measure Yourself Concerns and Well-being (MYCaW): An individualised questionnaire for evaluating outcome in cancer support care that includes complementary therapies. *Complement Ther Med* 15(1): 38-45.

Paterson, C., D. Vindigni, B. Polus, T. Browell, and G. Edgecombe. 2008a. Evaluating a massage therapy training and treatment programme in a remote Aboriginal community. *Complement Ther Clin Pract* 14(3): 158-167.

———. 2008b. The Hopevale Massage Therapy Project: A community health development and training initiative for indigenous communities in Cape York. *Journal of the Australian Association of Massage Therapists* 6(2): 6-10.

Ritenbaugh, C., M. Verhoef, S. Fleishman, H. Boon, and A. Leis. 2003. Whole systems research: A discipline for studying complementary and alternative medicine. *Altern Ther Health M* 9(4): 32-36.

Sandelowski, M. 2000. Combining qualitative and quantitative sampling, data collection, and analysis techniques in mixed-method studies. *Res Nurs Health* 23(3): 246-255.

Smith, M.C., T.E. Yamashita, L.L Bryant, L. Hemphill, and J.S. Kutner. 2009. Providing massage therapy for people with advanced cancer: What to expect. *J Altern Complem Med* 15(4): 367-371.

Stange, K. 2004. Multimethod research. *Ann Fam Med* 2(1): 2-3.

Tashakkori, A., and C. Teddlie. 2003. *Handbook of mixed methods in social & behavioral research*. Thousand Oaks: Sage.

Tashakkori, A., and C. Teddlie. 1998. *Mixed methodology: Combining qualitative and quantitative approaches*. Thousand Oaks, CA: Sage.

Teddlie, C., and F. Yu. 2007. Mixed methods sampling: A typology with examples. In *The mixed methods reader,* eds. V.L. Plano Clark and J.W. Creswell, 199-228. Los Angeles: Sage. Originally published in *J Mix Method Res* 1(1): 77-100, 2007.

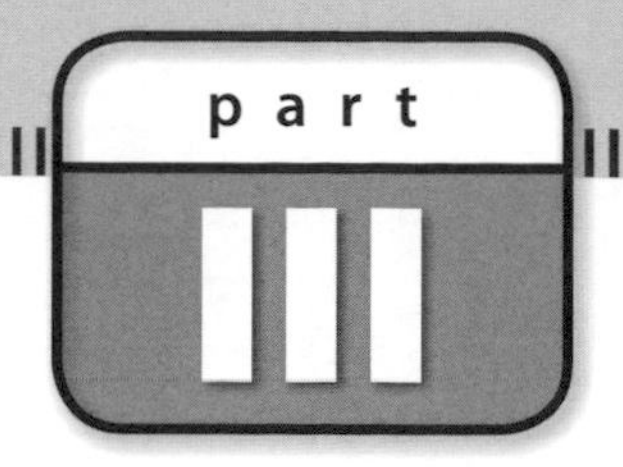

POPULATIONS AND CONDITIONS

These twelve chapters review massage therapy research and present evidence-based practice guidelines for specific populations and conditions likely to be encountered in practice and for which there is sufficient evidence to warrant a full discussion. Together, these chapters cover all stages of human lifespan, and address a wide range of conditions, from physiological and psychological perspectives. Each chapter concludes with a representative case report that provides real-world context for integrating research and practice.

Pediatrics

Stacey Shipwright, BA, RMT

The use of *complementary and alternative medicine* (CAM) as an alternative or adjunct to conventional medicine is increasing in popularity across North America. Current studies suggest that nearly 38% of American adults (Barnes, Bloom, and Nahin 2009) and 54% of Canadian adults (Esmail 2007) used some form of CAM therapy in the preceding year. Of the numerous CAM modalities available, the most commonly used were chiropractic, massage therapy (MT), and relaxation techniques (Barnes, Bloom, and Nahin 2009; Esmail 2007). This trend is also evident in the use of CAM with children (defined here as persons 18 years of age or younger). In Canada, 15% of families with children have used a CAM modality for their child. The most commonly used are chiropractic care, herbal remedies, and MT (Esmail 2007). In the United States, approximately one in nine children have received some form of CAM treatment, the most common being herbal remedies, chiropractic, and deep breathing exercises (Barnes, Bloom, and Nahin 2008).

complementary and alternative medicine

▸ A diverse group of health care systems, practices, and products that are not generally considered part of conventional, allopathic, or Western medicine.

Although MT is not the leading pediatric CAM modality, its popularity is growing. For example, figures from 2006 indicate that 21% of Canadian children had used MT, an increase from 16% in 1997 (Esmail 2007). Massage is being used in this population not only to treat illness or chronic conditions, but also to maintain wellness. This chapter highlights areas of massage therapy research that focus on child populations and pediatric conditions. It also offers treatment guidelines and recommendations for future research.

EFFECTS OF MASSAGE THERAPY ON PEDIATRIC POPULATIONS

As massage therapy for infants and children becomes more widely accepted, consumers, health care practitioners, government agencies, and researchers are asking important questions about the safety and effectiveness of massage for this population. Since Field and colleagues (1986) first published their massage research on weight gain in premature infants, there has been an explosion of interest in the potential of pediatric MT. As with other health care interventions, assumptions about what is safe and effective for adults should not automatically be extended to infants and children. Massage therapy research with a pediatric focus is necessary.

Infants

Notably, some of the most important research pertaining to MT for infants includes the primate studies conducted in the 1950s on the effects of touch, or lack thereof, on the social, cognitive, and emotional development in infant monkeys. The outcomes of those first studies set the groundwork for the importance of touch in healthy development and guided the future direction of research in MT as a form of skilled, conscious touch for human infants.

Infant Development and Touch Communication

Although the importance of touch in infant development was once minimized or even denigrated (Watson and Watson 1928), we now know that touch is an essential component of parent–infant bonding and communication. Numerous studies conducted on humans and mammalian animals, including the famous Harlow primate studies, show that touch is immensely important in social and physical development (Harlow 1958; Harlow and Suomi 1970; Guzzetta et al. 2009). In fact, social isolation and the corresponding absence of touch often lead to agitation, behavioral disturbances, and developmental delays in primates (Suomi, Collins, and Harlow 1973).

While social isolation experiments are not conducted on human infant populations for ethical reasons, research into touch communication is growing within the area of human development. A growing body of literature shows that touch can be used to soothe or arouse infants, regulate their mood, communicate positive and negative emotions, or communicate specific information, such as the presence or absence of a caregiver (Hertenstein 2002; Hertenstein and Campos 2001). Touch has also been found to mediate pain, as demonstrated in a study by Gray, Watt, and Blass (2000), in which infants who were held by their mothers in full ventral skin-to-skin contact during a heel-lance procedure cried and grimaced less and displayed reduced heart rates, compared with control-group infants who were swaddled in their cribs. More research in the regulation of emotional and development wellness, by parents or massage therapists, is needed to determine the long-term effects of touch in infants.

As part of routine health care, infants often undergo painful procedures, such as a heel lance, circumcision, and immunizations. Painful medical procedures during childhood can have negative long-term effects on future responses to pain (Young 2005). Evidence suggests that MT reduces procedural pain in healthy and preterm infants (Gray, Watt, and Blass 2000; Diego, Field, and Hernandez-Reif 2009). Preterm infants who received 15 minutes of moderate-pressure MT prior to the removal of surgical tape exhibited lower heart rates and faster heart-rate recovery following tape removal (Diego, Field, and Hernandez-Reif 2009).

Infants With Low Birth Weight

A Cochrane review of MT for preterm infants or those with low birth weight concluded that massage interventions improved daily weight gain, reduced the length of their hospital stay, and had a positive effect on postnatal complications. However, the review authors also had concerns about the quality of the primary studies, which could not clearly support MT as cost-effective for this specific population (Vickers et al. 2004). Since this review, a number of improved studies focused on infant growth and development do support the effectiveness of MT to increase weight gain (Gonzalez et al. 2009; Massaro et al. 2009; Diego et al. 2007), shorten hospital stays for low-birth-weight infants (Gonzalez et al. 2009), improve their quality of sleep (Kelmanson and Adulas 2006), and reduce their stress behaviors

(Hernandez-Reif, Diego, and Field 2007). In addition, most of these studies examined massage administered by a parent, which potentially maximizes cost effectiveness.

Of particular note is a study that assessed developmental outcomes long after MT was introduced as an intervention. Over 2 years, Procianoy and colleagues (2010) followed low-birth-weight infants who had been randomly assigned to either an intervention group that received MT by their mother in addition to regular skin-to-skin contact or one that received regular skin-to-skin contact only. At the 2-year assessment, growth was similar between the groups, but the MT group exhibited significantly higher scores on the mental development index, as well as borderline increases on the psychomotor development index. The authors concluded that MT by the mother improved neurodevelopment outcomes.

Children and Adolescents

Massage therapy research with children and adolescents covers a wide variety of conditions, including cancer, mental disorders, behavioral and developmental disorders, and respiratory conditions, such as asthma and cystic fibrosis. Although the total number of studies is small, promising outcomes warrant further research for this population.

Cancer

Pediatric cancers are relatively rare. In 2007, in the United States, 10,400 children under age 15 were newly diagnosed with cancer (National Cancer Institute 2008). Figures from Canada indicate that the number of new cancer cases from 2001 to 2005 was, on average, 836 children per year for a total of 4,181 children over a 5-year period (Canadian Cancer Society's Steering Committee 2009). Despite the low incidence rate, having a child diagnosed with cancer is devastating for families. Parents of children with cancer can experience severe emotional distress, including anxiety and depression (Moore 2004). Families require support to reduce their own anxiety and distress and skills to help alleviate suffering in their children. Many families find the support and skills within CAM modalities, including massage.

Much of the available literature on MT for pediatric oncology focuses on the examination of symptom relief in the child (see chapter 17). Findings show that MT reduces anxiety and depression in children with cancer. However, opinion is mixed on whether symptoms, such as nausea, pain, or fatigue, can be influenced significantly by massage (Post-White et al. 2009; Haun, Graham-Pole, and Shortley 2009; Hughes et al. 2008).

Psychosocial

Interest in massage therapy as an adjunct to medical treatment of childhood mental, behavior, and attachment disorders is growing. Concern about the use of antidepressant medications in pediatric populations (Temple 2004) and growing recognition of the importance of sleep (which MT may promote) in improving children's health and well-being (Owens and Jones 2011) are two developments that are helping drive interest in pediatric MT research.

Anxiety and Depression

Research shows that MT consistently reduces *anxiety* and *depression* (see chapter 13). However, most studies have been done with adult populations. Only a small amount of evidence is specific to pediatrics. It should also be noted that much MT research has examined depression or anxiety as a symptom, side effect, or comorbidity of another condition, rather than as the focus of treatment.

anxiety

▸ A mood state, generally experienced as negative and often accompanied by bodily symptoms of tension, in which people think, feel, or behave in ways that indicate they are apprehensive about possible misfortune.

depression

▸ A negative mood state characterized by thoughts, feelings, or behaviors indicative of sadness, despair, low energy, or a reduced capacity for experiencing pleasure.

Of the pediatric-specific depression and anxiety literature available, most studies have occurred within psychiatric inpatient units. A pilot program introduced to a young adult psychiatric inpatient unit in Australia examined the effectiveness of a MT program in reducing stress, anxiety, and aggression. Results of the small study suggested that MT reduced anxiety, resting heart rate, and cortisol levels, as well as hostility and depression (Garner et al. 2008). A similar study of 52 children hospitalized for depression and adjustment disorders reported that MT therapy reduced depression, anxiety, and salivary cortisol levels. The participants also became more compliant to instruction and showed improved sleep (Field et al. 1992).

Some studies have also examined MT as an intervention for reducing children's anxiety in response to invasive procedures. Vannorsdall and colleagues (2004) examined the use of nonessential touch as a means of reducing child distress during lumbar punctures. They concluded that this reduced anxiety and distress, especially among younger children. Similarly, a study of 24 children receiving treatment for severe burns found that MT reduced distress behaviors, such as facial grimacing, crying, and torso movement (Hernandez-Reif et al. 2001).

Autism Spectrum Disorders

autism spectrum disorders

▸ A category of related developmental disorders, such as autistic disorder and Asperger's syndrome, that are typified by restricted or unusual behaviors and impaired social functioning.

As diagnoses of *autism spectrum disorders* rise in the United States and Canada (Centers for Disease Control and Prevention 2010; Norris, Paré, and Starky 2006), new and innovative treatments, including MT, are being sought to manage problematic behaviors and symptoms. Escalona and colleagues (2001) studied 20 autistic children, 3 to 6 years of age, to determine if MT yielded improvements in behavior. The children were randomized to an intervention group, in which a parent delivered massage before bed, or a control group, in which a parent read to them. Attentiveness, playground and classroom behaviors, and sleep were monitored for a 1-month period. The MT group was judged to be more attentive and better rested, and to have experienced a decrease in stereotyped autistic behaviors.

In a qualitative study conducted by Cullen-Powell, Barlow, and Cushway (2005), parents were interviewed concerning what it was like to care for their autistic child, as well as their current experience of touch with their child. Subsequently, the parents were shown how to massage their child. They were then interviewed after having performed massage intervention and again at a 16-week follow-up. Prior to the massage instruction and intervention period, parents reported that touch was often not well received by their children. This was distressing to the parents. After the massage intervention, parents reported that their child responded positively to massage and began to ask for it using nonverbal cues.

ADHD

Parents of children with attention deficit/hyperactivity disorder (ADHD) are increasingly seeking alternative or complementary therapies as an adjunct to pharmacologic intervention or as a monotherapy for their child's disorder (Weber and Newmark 2007), which illustrates the need for research. A study of 30 students with ADHD (Khilnani et al. 2003) found that twice-weekly massage for 1 month resulted in happier mood states and reductions in hyperactivity and daydreaming inattention, as compared to a non-MT control condition. These results are consistent with other studies (Field, Quintino, et al 1998; Maddigan et al. 2003) in which participants who received MT demonstrated less fidgeting and improved classroom behavior.

Aggression

While overall juvenile crime rates in Canada have declined since their peak in 1991, there has been an increase in juvenile violent crime (Taylor-Butts and Bressan

2008). In the United States, youth crime has also decreased with the exception of female juvenile offenders, a group who has seen an increase in violent crime rates (Snyder and Sickmund 2006). The increase in violent crime, typically aggression based (e.g., assaults, homicide, attempted homicide), has led to an emphasis on identifying those youth at risk and implementing appropriate interventions.

Preliminary studies have suggested that MT may decrease aggressive behaviors in children and adolescents (von Knorring et al. 2008; Diego et al. 2002). Von Knorring and colleagues (2008) evaluated the effects of MT in preschool children over a period of 1 year. The results indicated that children with behavioral problems showed decreased aggression after 3 and 6 months, as well as increased levels of attentiveness. Diego and colleagues (2002) studied 17 aggressive adolescents who were randomized into a massage-intervention group or a muscle-relaxation control group. After two 20-minute chair massage sessions over a period of 5 weeks, there was no significant decrease in aggression and anxiety scores as compared to the control group. However, the massaged adolescents reported feeling less hostile, and guardians of the adolescents also noticed a decrease in aggressive behaviors.

Pulmonary Function

Some research has been conducted on juvenile pulmonary function, namely asthma and cystic fibrosis. A study by Field, Henteleff and colleagues (1998) recruited 32 children from a pediatric pulmonary clinic. The children were randomized to a progressive muscle-relaxation control group or an MT intervention group. The massage and muscle-relaxation protocols were performed at home for a period of 30 days. Cortisol levels, anxiety, and pulmonary function were evaluated throughout the study. Researchers found that children in the intervention group showed decreased anxiety and increased pulmonary function, and had a better attitude about their asthma.

In the case of cystic fibrosis, a study randomized 20 children to a massage intervention or a reading control group (Hernandez-Reif et al. 1999). Children in the intervention group received a 20-minute massage from a parent each evening at bedtime, while children in the control group were read to for the same amount of time. Parent and child anxiety were assessed on days 1 and 30 of the study, as were child mood and peak airflow. The study concluded that MT reduced anxiety and improved mood and peak airflow for children with cystic fibrosis.

Safety of Massage Therapy on Infants and Children

While massage therapists believe that MT, in the hands of a qualified practitioner, is safe to perform on infants and children, many pediatric massage studies have failed to (or have chosen not to) report any adverse events. A systematic review on the safety of pediatric massage, currently in progress, has thus far identified some mild adverse events, including local pain or soreness, swelling, mild fevers, and skin rashes. However, very few moderate to serious adverse events have been reported (Adams et al. 2009). Future studies on the safety of pediatric MT are warranted.

EXPLAINING MASSAGE THERAPY EFFECTS

Although some MT effects are established, very little is known about how massage works. Studies of MT mechanisms, including ones that use advanced imaging tools (Sagar, Dryden, and Wong 2007; Sefton et al. 2010) are just beginning to examine how MT produces its beneficial outcomes and how it may relay its effects to so many bodily systems. In addition, theories that attempt to explain MT effects in adults may not be easily extrapolated to a pediatric population.

What follows is a brief summary of theories:

touch communication

▸ The transmission of information, including emotional information, by physical contact.

gate theory

▸ An influential theory that attempts to explain processes of pain transmission and pain reduction as a function of a biological gating mechanism within the spinal cord.

• *Touch communication.* The ability to communicate emotion through touch may influence levels of anxiety and mediate pain (Hertenstein 2002; Gray, Watt, and Blass 2000). Several theories may explain this phenomenon, including learning theories in which children make associations between the type of touch (comforting touch versus abrupt touch) and environmental events, or observe how others react to specific types of touch (Hertenstein 2002).

• *Gate theory.* Melzack and Wall (1965) proposed a theory in which a gate mechanism exists within the dorsal horn of the spinal cord. When large nerve fibers are stimulated, the gate is closed, thus blocking out impulses from smaller nerve fibers that serve as pain receptors. In theory, MT produces stimulation of larger fibers, closing the gate to impulses from smaller nerve fiber, therefore reducing pain. The gate theory has faced criticism over the years as studies have discovered that pain reduction can also result from activity within the cerebral cortex (Inui, Tsuji, and Kakigi 2006).

• *Reduction of cortisol.* Cortisol is a hormone secreted by the adrenal glands in response to stress that produces a number of biochemical reactions within the body. If stress is chronic, the overproduction of cortisol can have a negative effect on the body. Massage therapy has long been thought to reduce levels of cortisol (Field et al. 2005). However, a recent quantitative review indicates that massage therapy's effect on cortisol levels is very small in adults, if the effect exists at all. Nevertheless, the same review found that multiple doses of MT did significantly reduce the cortisol levels of children, though it must be noted that only three studies contributed to this specific effect (Moyer et al. 2011). More research is required to see why there might be such a difference between adults and children in their response to MT.

RECOMMENDATIONS FOR MASSAGE THERAPY PRACTICE

Working with pediatric populations can be challenging, but rewarding. It is in the best interest of everyone involved (the child, parents, and therapist) to work together as a team to support the child. This involves a number of important steps:

1. Educate the parent on the strengths and limits of MT based on the current available evidence.
2. Include the child as part of the process and address any questions and concerns.
3. Ensure that parents feel connected to the process, especially if their child is ill.
4. Instruct parents on how to give their child a massage at home, empowering them and allowing them to feel more bonded to their child and less anxious about their condition (Cullen-Powell, Barlow, and Cushway 2005).

When treating a pediatric client or when instructing parents on how to massage their child, it is important to keep the following in mind:

• *Appropriate treatment length.* Be aware of the amount of time spent treating pediatric patients. In many of the infant studies, treatment time was no more than 15 minutes, while child and adolescent treatments ranged from 20 to 60 minutes.

• *Treatment.* Reflect on the developmental stage of the pediatric patient being treated when considering treatment options. In studies with adolescents, the massage interventions tended to be performed on clothed and seated recipients (Diego et al. 2002). In studies that focused on infants, the subjects were often unclothed (Gonzalez et al. 2009). Practitioners should also be cognizant of the age of the pediatric patient. Younger children may prefer to be massaged by a parent, while an adolescent may prefer not to have a parent present.

• *Consent.* Children, regardless of age, should be asked if they would like to be massaged. Touch is highly personal, and a child, like an adult, may simply not be in the mood to be touched.

consent

▸ The provision of approval or agreement.

• *Delayed medical treatment for serious illness.* Care must be taken that parents and care providers have considered best possible treatment choices. Parents should not delay getting their child the most effective treatment possible, especially for serious illnesses. In some cases, this will mean choosing a proven, conventional, life-saving intervention over an unproven CAM treatment.

DIRECTIONS FOR FUTURE RESEARCH

Compared with some other CAM modalities and with conventional medicine, well-conducted, robust MT research is scarce, especially in regard to pediatric populations. Although current data suggest that MT benefits children, many of the pediatric studies have significant limitations, including small samples, incomplete reporting of statistics, and results and conclusions that are inconsistent with the original study design (Beider and Moyer 2007). Future pediatric MT studies must be conducted with larger participant numbers to increase statistical power, provide sufficient detail on study protocols, and present results and conclusions that acknowledge both the strengths and weaknesses of the study design that was selected.

Further, pediatric research has tended to focus on the realm of the psychosocial outcomes (e.g., anxiety and depression), MT for infants, and MT for specific conditions (e.g., cancer). While these are important areas to pursue, research attention must also be paid to other significant areas, such as examination of dosage, safety, therapist- versus parent-delivered MT, and pediatric MT for wellness.

Case Study

Saleema G. makes an appointment for her 6-year-old son Khalid with a massage therapist on the advice of his oncologist. Khalid has been experiencing a number of symptoms related to his cancer treatments, including nausea, pain, and insomnia. He is also feeling anxious about his illness and depressed that he cannot play outside with friends, since he feels too ill from chemotherapy treatments. Khalid's oncologist thinks that he would benefit from MT.

When they arrive at the MT clinic, Saleema and Khalid are greeted by Vineet, a registered massage therapist. Vineet asks Saleema to complete a written health history for Khalid, and then leads them to the treatment area where he interviews Saleema to obtain more detailed information on Khalid's condition. He learns that Khalid has been undergoing extensive chemotherapy for leukemia. Vineet also asks Khalid how he has been feeling, and where his aches and pains are. All three discuss the possible benefits of massage, along with treatment options and goals. Vineet takes extra time and pays careful attention to ensure that Khalid understands what is being discussed.

(continued)

Case Study *(continued)*

Khalid agrees that he would like to be massaged because he thinks it will make him feel better, but he doesn't want Vineet to give him the massage. Vineet shows Saleema how to give her son a massage and encourages her to give Khalid massage at home or when he is in the hospital receiving treatment. Vineet also educates her on when she should abstain from massaging Khalid (e.g., fever higher than 38 °C [100.4 °F]), and areas to avoid (e.g., medical devices such as PICC lines).

Two weeks later, Vineet contacts Saleema to see how the massage sessions are progressing and to see if she has any questions. Saleema reports that she has been giving Khalid massages before bed and that the time is relaxing for both of them. She has noticed that Khalid falls asleep much more easily than before and that he seems less anxious. In addition, Saleema says she feels empowered because she is able to comfort her son and contribute to his health care needs.

One month from the initial follow-up, Vineet calls Saleema to see how Khalid is doing. Saleema reports that Khalid is doing very well. He no longer requires chemotherapy and the doctors have indicated that he is in remission, but he will have to be monitored over the next several years. Khalid is playing with his friends again and has returned to school. Vineet asks Saleema if she is still massaging Khalid. She reports that as Khalid started feeling better, he wanted fewer and fewer massages until they were not doing any more massage. Saleema thanked Vineet for teaching her how to massage Khalid and for being so supportive.

SUMMARY

Massage therapy is being increasingly used for infants, children, and adolescents, not only to treat illness or chronic conditions, but also to maintain wellness. Given contemporary recognition of the importance of healthy lifestyle choices for children to their future health and well-being and concerns about the use of some medications in this population, there is increasing need for clear guidelines for pediatric MT practice based on best available research evidence.

Infant massage research, which is historically and conceptually linked with primate studies that illustrated the importance of touch for social and cognitive development, generally supports this form of treatment to promote weight gain in premature infants, improve attachment, and reduce pain. For children and adolescents, MT research shows promise for symptom reduction of cancer treatment, reduction of anxiety and depression, promotion of optimal respiratory function, and improvement of emotion and behavior with some developmental disorders. However, further research is needed. In all cases, it is very important to respect children's rights to participate in their care and to identify and be responsive to their preferences about massage.

REFERENCES

Adams, D., A. Whidden, K. Smith, S. Sikora, T. Dryden, and S. Vohra. 2009. Safety of pediatric massage: A systematic review. *Altern Ther Med* 15(3): s135.

Barnes, P.M., B. Bloom, and R.L. Nahin. 2008. Complementary and alternative medicine use among adults and children: United States, 2007. *Natl Health Stat Report* 12: 1-23.

Beider, S., and C.A. Moyer. 2007. Randomized controlled trials of pediatric massage: A review. *Evid-Based Compl Alt* 4(1): 23-34.

Canadian Cancer Society's Steering Committee. 2009. *Canadian cancer statistics 2009.* Toronto, ON: Canadian Cancer Society.

Centers for Disease Control and Prevention. 2010. Autism spectrum disorders (ASDs). www.cdc.gov/ncbddd/autism/research.html.

Cullen-Powell, L.A., J.H. Barlow, and D. Cushway. 2005. Exploring a massage intervention for parents and their children with autism: The implications for bonding and attachment. *J Child Health Care* 9(4): 245-55.

Diego, M.A., T. Field, M. Hernandez-Reif, J.A. Shaw, E.M. Rothe, D. Castellanos, and L. Mesner. 2002. Aggressive adolescents benefit from massage therapy. *Adolescence* 37(147): 597-607.

Diego, M.A., T. Field, M. Hernandez-Reif, O. Deeds, A. Ascencio, and G. Begert. 2007. Preterm infant massage elicits consistent increases in vagal activity and gastric motility that are associated with greater weight gain. *Acta Paediatr* 96(11): 1588-1591.

Diego, M.A., T. Field, and M. Hernandez-Reif. 2009. Procedural pain heart rate responses in massaged preterm infants. *Infant Behav Dev* 32(2): 226-229.

Escalona, A., T. Field, R. Singer-Strunck, C. Cullen, and K. Hartshorn. 2001. Brief report: Improvements in the behavior of children with autism following massage therapy. *J Autism Dev Disord* 31(5): 513-516.

Esmail, N. 2007. Complementary and alternative medicine in Canada: Trends in use and public attitudes, 1997-2006. In *Public Policy Sources,* ed. K. McCahon. Vancouver, BC: Fraser Institute.

Field, T. M., A. Schanberg, F. Scafidi, C. R. Bauer, N. Vega-Lahr, R. Garcia, J. Nystrom and C. M. Kuhn. 1986. Tactile/kinesthetic stimulation effects on preterm neonates. *Pediatrics* 77(5):654-658

Field, T., C. Morrow, C. Valdeon, S. Larson, C. Kuhn, and S. Schanberg. 1992. Massage reduces anxiety in child and adolescent psychiatric patients. *J Am Acad Child Adolesc Psychiatry* 31(1): 125-131.

Field, T., O. Quintino, M. Hernandez-Reif, and G. Koslovsky. 1998. Adolescents with attention deficit hyperactivity disorder benefit from massage therapy. *Adolescence* 33(129):103-108.

Field, T., T. Henteleff, M. Hernandez-Reif, E. Martinez, K. Mavunda, C. Kuhn, and S. Schanberg. 1998. Children with asthma have improved pulmonary functions after massage therapy. *J Pediatr* 132(5): 854-858.

Field, T., M. Hernandez-Reif, M. Diego, S. Schanberg, and C. Kuhn. 2005. Cortisol decreases and serotonin and dopamine increase following massage therapy. *Int J Neurosci* 115(10): 1397-1413.

Garner, B., L.J. Phillips, H.M. Schmidt, C. Markulev, J. O'Connor, S.J. Wood, G.E. Berger, P. Burnett, and P.D. McGorry. 2008. Pilot study evaluating the effect of massage therapy on stress, anxiety and aggression in a young adult psychiatric inpatient unit. *Aust N Z J Psychiatry* 42(5): 414-422.

Gonzalez, A.P., G. Vasquez-Mendoza, A. Garcia-Vela, A. Guzman-Ramirez, M. Salazar-Torres, and G. Romero-Gutierrez. 2009. Weight gain in preterm infants following parent-administered Vimala massage: A randomized controlled trial. *Am J Perinatol* 26(4): 247-252.

Gray, L., L. Watt, and E.M. Blass. 2000. Skin-to-skin contact is analgesic in healthy newborns. *Pediatrics* 105(1): e14.

Guzzetta, A., S. Baldini, A. Bancale, L. Baroncelli, F. Ciucci, P. Ghirri, E. Putignano, A. Sale, A. Viegi, N. Berardi, A. Boldrini, G. Cioni, and L. Maffei. 2009. Massage accelerates brain development and the maturation of visual function. *J Neurosci* 29(18): 6042-6051.

Harlow, H.F. 1958. The nature of love. *Am Psychol* 13(12): 673-685.

Harlow, H.F., and S.J. Suomi. 1970. Nature of love—Simplified. *Am Psychol* 25(2): 161-168.

Haun, J., J. Graham-Pole, and B. Shortley. 2009. Children with cancer and blood diseases experience positive physical and psychological effects from massage therapy. *Int J Ther Massage Bodywork* 2(2): 7-14.

Hernandez-Reif, M., T. Field, J. Krasnegor, E. Martinez, M. Schwartzman, and K. Mavunda. 1999. Children with cystic fibrosis benefit from massage therapy. *J Pediatr Psychol* 24(2): 175-181.

Hernandez-Reif, M., T. Field, S. Largie, S. Hart, M. Redzepi, B. Nierenberg, and T.M. Peck. 2001. Childrens' distress during burn treatment is reduced by massage therapy. *J Burn Care Rehabil* 22(2):191-195; discussion 190.

Hernandez-Reif, M., M. Diego, and T. Field. 2007. Preterm infants show reduced stress behaviors and activity after 5 days of massage therapy. *Infant Behav Dev* 30(4): 557-561.

Hertenstein, M. 2002. Touch: Its communicative functions in infancy. *Hum Dev* 45(2): 70-94.

Hertenstein, M., and J. Campos. 2001. Emotion regulation via maternal touch. *Infancy* 2(4): 549-566.

Hughes, D., E. Ladas, D. Rooney, and K. Kelly. 2008. Massage therapy as a supportive care intervention for children with cancer. *Oncol Nurs Forum* 35(3): 431-442.

Inui, K., T. Tsuji, and R. Kakigi. 2006. Temporal analysis of cortical mechanisms for pain relief by tactile stimuli in humans. *Cereb Cortex* 16(3): 355-365.

Kelmanson, I.A., and E.I. Adulas. 2006. Massage therapy and sleep behaviour in infants born with low birth weight. *Complement Ther Clin Pract* 12(3): 200-205.

Khilnani, S., T. Field, M. Hernandez-Reif, and S. Schanberg. 2003. Massage therapy improves mood and behavior of students with attention-deficit/hyperactivity disorder. *Adolescence* 38(152): 623-638.

Maddigan, B., P. Hodgson, S. Heath, B. Dick, K. St. John, T. McWilliam-Burton, C. Snelgrove, and H. White. 2003. The effects of massage therapy and exercise therapy on children/adolescents with attention deficit hyperactivity disorder. *Can Child Adolesc Psychiatr Rev* 12(2): 40-43.

Massaro, A.N., T.A. Hammad, B. Jazzo, and H. Aly. 2009. Massage with kinesthetic stimulation improves weight gain in preterm infants. *J Perinatol* 29(5): 352-357.

Melzack, R., and P. Wall. 1965. Pain mechanisms: A new theory. *Science* 150(699): 971-979.

Moore, I. 2004. Advancing biobehavioral research in childhood cancer. *JPON* 21(3): 128-131.

Moyer, C.A., L. Seefeldt, E.S. Mann, and L.M. Jackley. 2011. Does massage therapy reduce cortisol? A comprehensive quantitative review. *J Bodyw Mov Ther* 15: 3-14.

National Cancer Institute. 2008. Childhood cancers. www.cancer.gov/cancertopics/factsheet/Sites-Types/childhood.

Norris, S., J. Paré, and S. Starky. 2006. *Childhood autism in Canada: Some issues relating to behavioural intervention.* Ottawa, ON: Library of Parliament.

Owens, J., and C. Jones. 2011. Parental knowledge of healthy sleep in young children: Results of a primary care clinic survey. *J Dev Behav Pediatr* 32(6): 447-453.

Post-White, J., M. Fitzgerald, K. Savik, M.C. Hooke, A.B. Hannahan, and S.F. Sencer. 2009. Massage therapy for children with cancer. *J Pediatr Oncol Nurs* 26(1): 16-28.

Procianoy, R.S., E.W. Mendes, and R.C. Silveira. 2010. Massage therapy improves neurodevelopment outcome at two years corrected age for very low birth weight infants. *Early Hum Dev* 86(1): 7-11.

Sagar, S.M., T. Dryden, and R.K. Wong. 2007. Massage therapy for cancer patients: A reciprocal relationship between body and mind. *Curr Oncol* 14(2): 45-56.

Sefton, J. M., C. Yarar, J. W. Berry, and D. D. Pascoe. 2010. Therapeutic massage of the neck and shoulders produces changes in peripheral blood flow when assessed with dynamic infrared thermography. *J Altern Complement Med* 16(7): 723-732.

Snyder, H., and M. Sickmund. 2006. *Juvenile offenders and victims: 2006 National Report,* ed. Office of Juvenile Justice and Delinquency Prevention. Washington, DC: Office of Juvenile Justice and Delinquency Prevention.

Suomi, S.J., M.L. Collins, and H.F. Harlow. 1973. Effects of permanent separation from mother on infant monkeys. *Dev Psychol* 9(3): 376-384.

Taylor-Butts, A., and A. Bressan. 2008. *Youth crime in Canada, 2006,* ed. Statistics Canada. Ottawa, ON: Minister of Industry.

Temple, R. 2004. Anti-depressant drug use in pediatric populations. Statement before the Senate Subcommittee on Oversight and Investigations, Committee on Energy and Commerce. Accessed July 19, 2011. www.fda.gov/NewsEvents/Testimony/ucm113265.htm.

Vannorsdall, T., L. Dahlquist, J. Pendley, and T. Power. 2004. The relation between nonessential touch and children's distress during lumbar punctures. *Child Health Care* 33(4): 299-315.

Vickers, A., A. Ohlsson, J.B. Lacy, and A. Horsley. 2004. Massage for promoting growth and development of preterm and/or low birth-weight infants. *Cochrane Db Syst Rev* (2): CD000390.

von Knorring, A.L., A. Soderberg, L. Austin, and K. Uvnas-Moberg. 2008. Massage decreases aggression in preschool children: A long-term study. *Acta Paediatr* 97(9): 1265-1269.

Watson, J. and R.A.R. Watson. 1928. *Psychological care of infant and child.*New York: W. W. Norton.

Weber, W., and S. Newmark. 2007. Complementary and alternative medical therapies for attention-deficit/hyperactivity disorder and autism. *Pediatr Clin North Am* 54(6): 983-1006; xii.

Young, K. 2005. Pediatric Procedural Pain. *Ann Emerg Med* 45:160-171.

chapter 7

Pregnancy and Labor

Amanda Baskwill, BEd, RMT

In much of the world, increasing numbers of people are seeking alternative forms of health care to address a myriad of health and wellness concerns. A 2007 U.S. survey indicated that almost 40% of adults had used some form of complementary or alternative therapy (Barnes, Bloom, and Nahin 2008). An even larger proportion of women (69%) in a similar survey indicated they had used complementary therapies. Of those women, almost 44% had used massage (Pettigrew et al. 2004).

Massage therapy (MT) was the most frequently recommended complementary treatment for low back pain during pregnancy (61.4%) in a study conducted in New Haven, Connecticut (Wang et al. 2002). Based on current knowledge, the effects of massage therapy during pregnancy include decreased pain in the back and legs, relaxation, and decreased anxiety and depression (Field et al. 1999; Agren and Berg 2006; Field et al. 2004). Evidence also shows that infant outcomes are improved, including decreased fetal activity, lower incidence of prematurity, and increased birth weight (Field et al. 1999, 2004). Massage therapy is also used during labor and delivery, with emphasis on stress reduction and relaxation, as well as on pain reduction (Huntley, Thompson Coon, and Ernst 2004).

Although massage therapists have been treating women for pregnancy-related symptoms and labor pain for many years, and though many women are interested in receiving massage during pregnancy and labor, this robust practice and healthy enthusiasm is not yet balanced by an equivalent amount of research on pregnancy massage. As such, it must be pointed out that the evidence presented in this chapter is perhaps better considered suggestive than conclusive. Nevertheless, studies exist that carefully examine the value of massage during pregnancy and labor.

EFFECTS OF MASSAGE THERAPY ON PREGNANCY

A study of nondepressed pregnant women found that 10 sessions of massage, each 20 minutes in duration and administered twice per week, resulted in the massage group (n = 13) experiencing less anxiety, improved mood, less back pain, and better sleep on the last day of the study. Levels of norepinephrine, a stress hormone that was assessed in the urine, were also lowered. The women who received massage therapy also had fewer complications during labor and decreased incidence of premature birth (Field et al. 1999).

A phenomenological study of hospitalized pregnant women examined their experiences of massage connected to pregnancy-related nausea (Agren and Berg 2006). Although this type of study cannot determine if massage therapy causes a decrease in pregnancy-related nausea, it did demonstrate that women appreciated the experience of massage and found it to be a moment of relaxation and a distraction from nauseous feelings. Combined with positive findings from other research on massage therapy for nausea during cancer (Billhult, Bergbom, and Stener-Victorin 2004), it seems likely that massage therapy does reduce pregnancy-related nausea. However, additional research is necessary to confirm this.

Currently, there are three studies that examine the effects of MT on depressed pregnant women (Field et al. 2004; Field et al. 2008; Field et al. 2009), each of which investigated partner-delivered MT during pregnancy. The pregnant women who received massage showed reduced depression and anxiety. Some evidence suggests that an elevation of mood continued postpartum (Field et al. 2009). One study (Field et al. 2008) also saw an improvement in the relationship between the woman and her partner, who delivered the massage. Reductions of leg and back pain were also observed.

In relation to the emerging link between maternal mood and fetal development, there may be a significant role for MT in promoting the health and well-being of both pregnant women and their developing children (Van der Bergh et al. 2004; Diego et al. 2009). For example, some childhood conditions, such as asthma, are being linked to maternal mood during pregnancy (Cookson et al. 2009). If MT can reduce maternal stress, it is reasonable to suggest that fetal development could be improved by means of pregnancy massage. Some findings now indicate that MT effects do extend to the fetus *in utero.* Several studies show fewer complications during labor, reduced prematurity, and increased birth weight as a result of pregnancy massage (Field et al. 2004; Field et al. 2008; Field et al. 2009). However, once again, it must be said that more research, including replication studies, is needed.

in utero

▸ Latin for in the uterus; used to refer to the period between an infant's conception and birth.

EFFECTS OF MASSAGE THERAPY ON LABOR

Massage therapy to decrease anxiety and pain during labor has also been investigated. Two studies conducted in Taiwan (Chang, Wang, and Chen 2002; Chang, Wang, and Chen 2006) indicate that partner-delivered MT decreased anxiety and pain during labor, which suggests that massage during labor might be an option for women who desire a noninvasive and nonpharmacological form of pain management. A study conducted by Field and others (1997) also demonstrated that women who received massage during labor reported less pain and anxiety. This study also found that those who received massage had shorter labor, spent a shorter time in the hospital, and experienced less postpartum depression than those who did not receive massage.

Currently, there is no evidence that MT is unsafe for pregnant women or women in labor, since none of the studies just reviewed report any adverse effects. In addition, few MT studies concerned with any condition report adverse or side effects as a result of treatment. On the rare occasions that adverse effects are reported, they are usually associated with treatment administered by an untrained person (Ernst 2003).

EXPLAINING MASSAGE THERAPY EFFECTS

Very few studies have explored the mechanisms by which MT produces its beneficial effects. However, there are several theories. Those most relevant to pregnancy and labor massage include the gate theory of pain reduction, promotion of increased levels of *oxytocin,* and alteration of stress hormone and *neurotransmitter* levels. For example, physical and emotional benefits may be attributable

oxytocin

▸ A hormone, released by the pituitary gland, that can stimulate the uterus to contract and the mammary glands to release milk. Oxytocin is also associated with caregiving behavior in men and women.

to reduced stress hormone levels and increased levels of the neurotransmitters serotonin and dopamine brought about by MT. However, additional research that uses more advanced study designs will be needed to test this and other theories.

The gate theory of pain reduction (Melzack and Wall 1965) suggests that pain signals in a peripheral nerve can be interfered with by competing stimuli prior to their arrival at and perception by the brain. In this way, by applying a mechanical sensation, MT might interfere with pain transmission. An alternate theory for pain reduction is that massage therapy increases levels of oxytocin, a hormone that regulates our ability to trust, bond with, and relate to others (Kosfeld et al. 2005). Increased oxytocin produced in response to MT could explain why mood and even relationships improve following treatment.

Massage therapy significantly decreases anxiety and depression in a variety of populations (Moyer, Rounds, and Hannum 2004). However, it is still not known how these effects are created. Field and colleagues (2004) propose a model in which MT increases levels of the neurotransmitters *serotonin* and *dopamine* and decreases levels of the stress hormones cortisol and norepinephrine. These physiological mechanisms then bring about reduction of negative mood, anxiety, and depression, as well as improving fetal outcomes. However, this theory is challenged by the most recent research on the effect of MT on stress hormones, which shows this effect to be much smaller than previously claimed (Moyer et al. 2011). Clearly, further research on underlying mechanisms is needed.

neurotransmitters

▸ Chemicals that neurons, individual cells of the nervous system, use to rapidly communicate with each other.

serotonin

▸ A neurotransmitter that plays important roles in sleep, memory, and feelings of well-being.

dopamine

▸ A neurotransmitter that plays important roles in movement, motivation, mood, sleep, and learning.

RECOMMENDATIONS FOR MASSAGE THERAPY PRACTICE

Based on available evidence, MT appears to be a safe treatment during pregnancy and labor that can be used to address pain, reduce anxiety and depression, and improve neonatal outcomes. However, it must be acknowledged that this conclusion is based on a small number of studies. Therefore, practicing massage therapists are encouraged to monitor the research literature for emerging studies on safety and efficacy.

Although some of the relevant studies describe a specific protocol for MT treatment, keep in mind that MT protocols in research are done under particular conditions. In practice, massage therapists may find it necessary to modify treatment based on the health and preferences of the client. In addition, note that the studies reviewed have been conducted using relatively healthy research participants. Massage therapists in the field must always conduct a thorough health intake and assessment to determine the appropriateness of treatment, and should modify treatment or refer patients for additional care when necessary.

Evidence-Based Treatment Guidelines

- Based on the current evidence, massage therapy (MT) is believed to be a safe and effective treatment option for pregnant women to address pain, depression, and anxiety. During labor, MT can be used to decrease pain and anxiety. Proper training and education is required before delivering massage therapy to pregnant women.
- Massage therapy during pregnancy has positive effect on the woman receiving massage, and it may also benefit her infant *in utero.*
- The mechanisms of the action responsible for MT benefits are not well understood. Massage therapists should use caution when explaining to patients how effects might be achieved.

DIRECTIONS FOR FUTURE RESEARCH

Continued investigation is the nature of scientific research. With this in mind, the following recommendations for future research are offered.

As has been the case in most MT research, MT studies concerned with pregnancy and labor have relatively small sample sizes. Studies using larger samples will have increased statistical power to elucidate effects. Nevertheless, the value of small- and medium-sized studies should not be entirely discounted.

MT research with high-risk pregnancies would be valuable and informative. During a high-risk pregnancy, anxiety is heightened (McCain and Deatrick 1994), which suggests that MT, with its proven anxiety-reducing effect, might be especially valuable for this population. Further, when high risk is associated with a multiple pregnancy, mothers can experience increased pain due to the additional weight (Mens et al. 1996). This is another instance where MT could be of particular value.

Little is known about the minimum or optimal dosage of MT for any specific condition. In most of the studies cited, measurements were taken before a course of MT treatment began and again after the course of treatment ended. A measurement schedule of this type cannot delineate whether large effects occurred after the first treatment or suddenly at or near the last treatment, or if they were steadily cumulative. Greater frequency of assessment is now needed in clinical MT studies along with MT studies designed expressly for the purposes of uncovering dosage effects.

Future studies should also explore whether differences in outcomes exist when massage is delivered by a massage therapist, trained nurse, or layperson, such as a spouse or partner. Some within massage therapy might argue that such studies could affect the profession negatively if nurses, spouses, or partners were shown to be consistently capable of delivering optimal benefits, but such concerns must not be allowed to stand in the way of progress in the health sciences. It is also important to determine whether outcomes are affected by factors such as familiarity, prior relationship, and training.

Further investigation is needed on the safety of MT for both pregnancy and labor. Based on available evidence, MT is safe for pregnant women. However, it is not perfectly clear that all studies have had a plan for reporting adverse effects, which leaves open the possibility that some unreported cases might have occurred. Future studies should include transparent reporting procedures for any adverse effects experienced by participants.

Finally, mechanism-of-action studies are also needed to uncover how MT delivers its clinical benefits to expectant mothers and their children. An improved understanding of how MT works will inevitably lead to improvements and refinements in how it is administered and in how it can be of the greatest benefit to patients.

Case Study

Beatrix (Bea) L., a 40-year-old elementary school teacher, has been experiencing back pain associated with her pregnancy. On a friend's advice, she makes an appointment at the Downtown Massage Therapy Clinic for her first appointment, where she is met by Rhonda S., her massage therapist. Rhonda conducts a health history interview and assessment to determine whether massage therapy is appropriate for Bea and, if it is, to set goals for the treatment plan. In addition, Bea has some questions about massage and how it might help. She also wants to determine if some or all of MT will be covered by her health insurance.

As Rhonda interviews Bea about her overall health, pregnancy, and treatment expectations, she learns that this is Bea's first pregnancy and that she is due in 3 months. Bea experienced severe morning sickness in the first trimester that has since subsided. She currently experiences indigestion, swelling in her feet and ankles, and low back pain. Otherwise, she indicates she has had no other complications with her pregnancy. Rhonda inquires about Bea's health care in support of her pregnancy and learns that Bea has regular visits with an obstetrician. She is working with a doula who will support her during labor. She has also been seeing a psychotherapist since the third month of her pregnancy.

On further inquiry, Bea informs Rhonda that she has been experiencing some depressed mood since the beginning of her pregnancy, but she ruled out the possibility of antidepressant medication because she was very concerned about possible side effects on the baby. Bea sees the psychotherapist once every 2 weeks for treatment of depression and to help her cope with abandonment by her boyfriend, who left her when she decided to keep the baby against his wishes. She is also coping with a lack of family support, but she has several friends who have been helpful and supportive. Bea admits that she worries about the effect her depression might have on her baby.

Rhonda takes time to talk with Bea about the proposed treatment plan and to address Bea's concerns. Rhonda explains the treatment modifications she will make, such as the use of side-lying positions and supportive pillows and bolsters, to ensure safety and increase Bea's comfort as she enters her third trimester. In addition, Rhonda explains to Bea that while there has so far only been some research on massage, pregnancy, and depression, the results have been good. Rhonda explains that it is important for Bea to continue to see her psychotherapist during the MT treatments. She adds that she will continue to assess Bea's pain and mood to guide care. She also explains to Bea that massage treatment is increasingly covered by third-party insurance. However, Bea will need a formal referral from her primary health care provider for this. Rhonda suggests that Bea contact her insurer to inquire about coverage. Rhonda also reassures Bea that she can provide documentation, such as a treatment plan and details of the treatments provided, which Bea's insurer may require for coverage.

SUMMARY

Even though massage therapists have been treating pregnant women for many years, the research evidence currently available is more suggestive than conclusive. The available studies show promising results for pregnant women, including lessened anxiety, improved mood, reduced back pain, better sleep, and fewer complications during labor and delivery. In addition, women who received massage during labor experienced less pain and anxiety, shorter duration of labor, less time in the hospital, and fewer episodes of postpartum depression. Reduced maternal anxiety and depression likely also benefit *in utero* development. Further, massage therapy is safe. Although a few adverse effects from massage therapy have been reported in other populations, the available research literature does not document any problems for pregnant women. Finally, future research, including replication of existing studies as well as studies of cost-effectiveness and optimal dosage, will extend our knowledge of massage therapy for this important population.

REFERENCES

Agren, A., and M. Berg. 2006. Tactile massage and severe nausea and vomiting during pregnancy: Women's experiences. *Scand J Caring Sci* 20: 169-176.

Barnes, P.M., B. Bloom, and R.L. Nahin. 2008. Complementary and alternative medicine use among adults and children: United States, 2007. *Natl Health Stat Report* 12: 1-24.

Billhult, A., I. Bergbom, and E. Stener-Victorin. 2004. Massage relieves nausea in women with breast cancer who are undergoing chemotherapy. *J Altern Complem Med* 13: 53-57.

Chang, M., S. Wang, and C. Chen. 2002. Effects of massage on pain and anxiety during labor: A randomized controlled trial in Taiwan. *J Adv Nurs* 38: 68-73.

______. 2006. A comparison of massage effects on labor pain using the McGill pain questionnaire. *J Nurs Res* 14: 190-196.

Cookson, H., R. Granell, C. Joinson, Y. Ben-Shlomo, and A.J. Henderson. 2009. Mother's anxiety during pregnancy is associated with asthma in their children. *J Allergy Clin Immun* 123: 847-853.

Diego, M.A., T. Field, M. Hernandez-Reif, S. Schanberg, C. Kuhn, and V.H. Gonzalez-Quintero. 2009. Prenatal depression restricts fetal growth. *Early Hum Dev* 85: 65-70.

Ernst, E. 2003. The safety of massage therapy. *Rheumatol* 42: 1101-1106.

Field, T., M. Hernandez-Reif, S. Taylor, O. Quintino, and I. Burman. 1997. Labor pain is reduced by massage therapy. *J Psychosom Obst Gyn* 18: 286-91.

Field, T., M. Hernandez-Reif, S. Hart, H. Theakston, S. Schanberg, and C. Kuhn. 1999. Pregnant women benefit from massage therapy. *J Psychosom Obst Gyn* 20: 31-38.

Field, T., M. Diego, M. Hernandez-Reif, S. Schanberg, and C. Kuhn. 2004. Massage therapy effects on depressed pregnant women. *J Psychosom Obst Gyn* 15: 115-122.

Field, T., B. Figueiredo, M. Hernandez-Reif, M. Diego, O. Deeds, and A. Ascencio. 2008. Massage therapy reduces pain in pregnant women, alleviates prenatal depression in both parents and improves their relationship. *J Bodyw Mov Ther* 12: 146-50.

Field, T., M. Diego, M. Hernandez-Reif, O. Deeds, and B. Figueiredo. 2009. Pregnancy massage reduces prematurity, low birthweight and postpartum depression. *Infant Behav Dev*: Epublication.

Huntley, A.L., J. Thompson Coon, and E. Ernst. 2004. Complementary and alternative medicine for labor pain: A systematic review. *Am J Obstet Gynecol* 191: 36-44.

Kosfeld, M., M. Heinrichs, P.J. Zak, U. Fischbacher, and E. Fehr. 2005. Oxytocin increases trust in humans. *Nature* 435: 673-676.

McCain, G.C., and J.A. Deatrick. 1994. The experience of high-risk pregnancy. *JOGNN* 23: 421-427.

Melzack, R., and P.D. Wall. 1965. Pain mechanisms: A new theory. *Science* 150: 971-979.

Mens, J.M., A. Vleeming, R. Stoeckart, H. Stam, and C.J. Snijders. 1996. Understanding peripartum pelvic pain: Implications of a patient survey. *Spine* 21: 1363-1369.

Moyer, C.A., J. Rounds, and J.W. Hannum. 2004. A meta-analysis of massage therapy research. *Psych Bull* 130: 3-18.

Moyer, C.A., L. Seefeldt, E.S. Mann, and L.M. Jackley. 2011. Does massage therapy reduce cortisol? A comprehensive quantitative review. *J Bodyw Mov Ther* 15: 3-14.

Pettigrew, A.C., M. O'Brien King, K.K. McGee, and C. Rudolph. 2004. Complementary therapy use by women's health clinic clients. *Altern Ther* 10: 50-55.

Ven den Bergh, B.R.H., E.J.H. Mulder, M. Mennes, and V. Glover. 2005. Antenatal maternal anxiety and stress and the neurobehavioural development of the fetus and child: Links and possible mechanisms: A review. *Neurosci Biobehav R* 29: 237-258.

Wang, S.M., P. DeZinno, L. Fermo, K. William, A.A. Caldwell-Andrews, F. Bravemen, and Z.N. Kain. 2002. Complementary and alternative medicine for low-back pain in pregnancy: A cross-sectional survey. *J Altern Complem Med* 11: 459-464.

chapter 8

Athletes

Stuart Galloway, PhD
Angus Hunter, PhD
Joan M. Watt, MA, MCSP, MSMA

Massage has been used in sport since the times of ancient Rome, but demand has increased hugely in the past 20 to 30 years. According to the National Certification Board for Therapeutic Massage and Bodywork (NCBTMB), the 1996 Atlanta Olympic Games were the first to officially offer massage as part of the core medical service to athletes. In the UK, increasing demand for athletic massage led to the 2002 formation of the Sports Massage Association (www.sportsmassageassociation.org) as a governing body for sport massage practitioners and helped to provide suitably qualified practitioners for that year's Commonwealth Games. Given the popularity of massage therapy (MT) among athletes, it is interesting to note that limited evidence exists for its effectiveness on physiological and psychological responses in this particular population. This chapter explores some of the controversies and issues that may contribute to the conflicting nature of evidence and outlines some areas ripe for future research.

THE VARIED NATURE OF SPORT MASSAGE

Although some sports, such as cycling and track and field, tend to use massage more frequently than others, there has been a distinct increase in the requests for MT from both competitors and coaches in many sports over recent years (Galloway and Watt 2004). Nevertheless, a review by Callaghan (1993) indicated that "the lack of comparable instrumentation and different research designs have led to little agreement amongst researchers over the type of massage to be employed or the length of time needed to be effective." Notably, this statement still holds true for sport massage more than 17 years after it was made. Different reasons exist for using massage with athletes. It is also common for sport massage to be combined with different forms of assisted movement and stretching. This is one of the reasons for the recent suggestion to rename the treatment modality as massage and soft-tissue therapy.

One major problem in the use of sport massage is the varied terminology across countries. Sport massage terminology in the UK and Europe is based on Swedish massage. It continues to use classical French nomenclature, such as *effleurage* (gliding strokes), *petrissage* (kneading strokes), and *tapotement* (tapping strokes). The development of many newer techniques

effleurage

▸ A smooth, gliding massage manipulation that can be performed with a range of pressure.

petrissage

▸ A massage manipulation consisting of kneading.

tapotement

▸ A massage manipulation consisting of rhythmic tapping or percussion of tissues.

adds to the complexity and may lead to potential confusion with terms such as *connective-tissue massage, lymphatic drainage, myofascial release, trigger-point massage,* and others now being adopted by massage therapists. Adding further confusion is the fact that terminology for identical techniques can be completely different in other countries (Sherman et al. 2006). This confusion is more frequently a problem as sport becomes increasingly international.

connective-tissue massage

▸ The broad category of massage techniques directed to and intended to affect connective tissues such as fascia.

myofascial release

▸ A connective tissue massage technique in which sustained pressure and stretching manipulations are applied to connective tissues with the aim of reducing restriction.

lymphatic drainage

▸ A massage approach consisting of gentle pumping manipulations intended to stimulate the lymphatic system and enhance lymphatic return.

trigger-point massage

▸ A massage approach consisting of compression or muscle stripping techniques applied to trigger points, which are hypersensitive spots of taut fibers in skeletal muscle, to reduce their painful effects.

lactate

▸ An acidic metabolic product that accumulates in skeletal muscles when glucose is broken down for energy anaerobically.

EFFECTS OF MASSAGE THERAPY ON ATHLETES

Many studies have attempted to examine the physiological effects of massage by investigating alterations in blood flow to limbs, recovery of muscular force and power production, and muscle fatigue following massage treatments. These mechanisms focus on the potential for massage to aid the recovery of athletes after work of high intensity or long duration, but they could also be considered in evaluating the role of massage in preparation of athletes for competition. It is worth noting that the previous two decades have produced many good reviews on the physiological effects of massage (Barnett 2006; Cafarelli and Flint 1992; Goats 1994; Moraska 2005; Reilly and Ekblom 2005; Tiidus 1999; Weerapong, Hume, and Kolt 2005; Moyer et al. 2011). These highlight the many problems and controversies that exist in the sport massage literature. The purpose of this chapter is not to reexamine all of the evidence contained in these reviews, but to highlight some of their key findings.

Effects on Blood Flow and Lactate Clearance

In many sports, performance is limited by the amount of blood, and the oxygen and nutrients that it carries, that the athlete's body can deliver to the muscles. Consequently, the possibility that massage might be able to improve blood flow, and thereby increase performance, is of great interest to athletes. Similarly, the possibility that massage might facilitate the processing or removal of metabolic wastes, such as *lactate,* from the muscles following intense training or competition, thereby speeding recovery, has also been investigated.

Despite the strong case for effects of massage on blood flow presented by Goats (1994) in his review of therapeutic effects of massage, there are methodological concerns regarding the measurements used. Later evaluations of massage's effect on blood flow assessed using valid and reliable measurement techniques reveal no clear evidence for any influence of massage on blood flow. The studies by Tiidus and Shoemaker (1995) and Shoemaker, Tiidus, and Mader (1997) exemplify this lack of evidence, for they clearly demonstrate that neither muscle mass nor type of massage appear to affect arterial blood flow when measured by Doppler ultrasound. Hinds and colleagues (2004) examined this further, taking into consideration the possibility that Doppler ultrasound used in this way does not distinguish blood flow in skin versus blood flow in muscle.

These authors observed an increase in skin blood flow without an increase in arterial flow following 12 minutes of massage as compared with the control group. They concluded that the increase in skin blood flow might be diverting blood from muscle during recovery. It should therefore come as no surprise that studies examining lactate clearance during recovery from exercise also fail to demonstrate a difference between massage and passive rest. For example, Gupta and others (1996) and Martin and colleagues (1998) reported that 10 to 20 minutes of massage did not improve lactate clearance over passive rest. Furthermore, current understanding of key factors that affect lactate clearance include optimal intensity of exercise recovery, skeletal muscle–fiber content, and lactate transporter expression (Bonen et al. 1979; Thomas et al. 2005), which are unlikely to be directly affected by massage therapy. However, even without improved lactate recovery, some studies have observed subsequent improvements in exercise capacity, exercise performance, or fatigue profile when massage is added to an active recovery period (Monedero and Donne 2000; Ogai et al. 2008; Robertson, Watt, and Galloway 2004).

Effects on Muscle Force and Power Production

Increased muscular performance is desired by virtually every athlete. Stronger, more efficient muscles translate into higher jumps, longer throws, more accurate shots, and greater endurance. Because muscular performance probably influences performance in an important way in almost every sport, the possibility that massage could increase muscular force and power is worth examining.

Fowles, Sale, and MacDougall (2000) examined the effects of 30 minutes of maximal passive stretch on force loss in human skeletal muscle and observed a 28% decline in voluntary force production immediately after the sustained stretching. Thereafter, voluntary force production improved, but it was still significantly lower than prestretch values after 60 minutes. The early force loss (up to 15 minutes poststretch) was explained by reduced neural activation of the muscle as well as by reduced capacity of muscles to generate force (linked to reduced muscle stiffness).

Given that maximal power is a combination of force output of the muscle and the speed at which the force can be generated, Hunter, Watt, and colleagues (2006) examined force production of the knee extensor muscles prior to and following passive rest or massage interventions (using a relaxing massage protocol). Force output at different muscle contraction speeds (60°, 120°, 180°, and 240°/s) declined immediately following massage, but only declined significantly at the slowest contraction velocity (60°/s). The reason for decline in force at slow velocities likely reflects a reduction in muscle stiffness.

Indeed, studies have demonstrated that massage causes improved range of motion (as reviewed in subsequent sections of this chapter) and, thus, greater slack in the system, which would delay rate-of-force development. This response to a relaxing massage could, theoretically, have a negative effect on an athlete's ability to perform slower velocity contractions in sports demanding strength and in some power-based sports, such as Alpine skiing. The knee extends at relatively low speeds of approximately 30° to 70°/s in turns during giant slalom and slalom Alpine skiing, respectively (Berg and Eiken 1999). Higher speed contractions, such as during a football kick, which can be more than 500°/s, would likely be unaffected. Furthermore, studies on stretching have noted that force loss is also velocity specific, primarily affecting slow-velocity contractions (Nelson et al. 2001). Therefore, it appears that massage has a similar effect on muscle to that seen with passive stretching. Thus, the acute effects of massage on production of muscle force and power are likely to depend on the resting muscle length and tension status (i.e., muscle architecture) and the type of massage administered.

Architectural and Neural Effects of Massage

The short-term reductions in force production immediately following massage and the similar response produced by stretching of muscle point toward an architectural explanation for the changes that occur through an increased lengthening or reduced tension of the muscle. Considering the well-documented length–tension relationship of skeletal muscle (Edman and Reggiani 1984; Gordon, Huxley, and

Julian 1966; Marginson and Eston 2001; Rassier, MacIntosh, and Herzog 1999), it is clear that an optimal muscle-fiber length will predictably generate maximum contractile force. Short- and long-term effects of massage directly alter muscle-fiber length and, thus, the force of contraction (Hernandez-Reif et al. 2001; Wiktorsson-Moller et al. 1983). Therefore, depending on the length of the muscle prior to treatment, a massage may either improve or reduce its capacity to generate force. Lengthening of the muscle will increase range of motion (ROM) of a limb. This has been shown following massage interventions (Bell 2008; Hopper et al. 2005; Morien, Garrison, and Smith 2008). Logically, a change in muscle length and ROM could benefit certain sporting performances that require flexibility, such as hurdling. Conversely, preevent massage may hamper performance by altering the length–tension relationship in an undesirable way when maximal force production is of prime importance, as in powerlifting or sprint cycling.

It is worth considering that different massage protocols for sport preparation or recovery may have very different effects on muscle length and tension and subsequent force-generating capacity, which may contribute to the equivocal nature of study findings. A relaxing recovery massage prior to high-intensity activity impairs force. This is likely due to reduced muscle tension as opposed to any alterations in neuromuscular recruitment (Hunter, Watt, et al. 2006). We have recently explored architectural changes from recording skeletal muscle tension alongside force-generating capacity following massage treatment. We observed a decrement in force following massage and we also showed an increase in displacement of the muscle belly, suggesting that a lengthening in the muscle and reduction in stiffness had occurred following massage (Hunter, Smith, et al. 2006).

However, neural alterations cannot be completely discounted, since it has been clearly demonstrated that the neural input required to maintain resting tone of the muscle becomes impaired following massage (Dishman and Bulbulian 2001; Goldberg, Sullivan, and Seaborne 1992; Goldberg et al. 1994; Morelli, Seaborne, and Sullivan 1991; Sullivan et al. 1991). This process occurs from acute lengthening of the muscle (Hernandez-Reif et al. 2001; Wiktorsson-Moller et al. 1983), which in turn stimulates the intrafusal fibers of muscle spindles to discharge an altered signal to the central nervous system (CNS). This then results in reduced resting tension of the skeletal-muscle tendon unit. Clearly, this effect may have clinical benefits for patients who suffer from regular muscle spasms that could be reduced by massage treatment. However, in athletes, this mechanism may only be beneficial in a postexercise recovery period, and it could even be detrimental to performance if administered prior to certain events.

Massage and Pain Sensation

One of the most common symptoms athletes experience is delayed-onset muscle soreness (DOMS) (Ernst 1998). DOMS can range from minor muscle stiffness that dissipates rapidly during daily activities to debilitating pain that impairs movement (Armstrong, Warren, and Warren 1991; Cheung, Hume, and Maxwell 2003). Massage is often used as a treatment to reduce DOMS in the belief that the accumulation of intramuscular fluid (Friden, Sfakianos, and Hargens 1986) will be moved away from the affected area. Although previous evidence is inconclusive (Tiidus 1999), more recent literature reviewed by Howatson and van Someren (2008) indicates that massage is beneficial in alleviating DOMS-related pain. Given that DOMS will result in temporary shortening of the muscle (Paschalis et al. 2007), it is reasonable to speculate that treatment of DOMS with massage could return the muscle closer to its optimal length for maximal force production. However, it is unlikely that the shortening of the muscle during DOMS is the main cause for a decline in force production, since disturbance in the excitation–contraction coupling process has been identified as a prime mechanism (Warren et al. 2001). Nevertheless, the value in treating DOMS with massage is evident, if only to reduce pain.

Psychological Effects of Massage

The most commonly cited study reporting any psychological benefits from sport massage is that of Hemmings and colleagues (2000), who reported an increase in perceived recovery in boxers who received massage versus those who did not. Other work, such as that by Arroyo-Morales and colleagues (2008), also lends some support to psychological effects including a decrease in vigor and increased relaxation following massage when compared with control conditions. Furthermore, popular press articles (Jones 2007) support the view that athletes perceive recovery following massage. Taking these observations alongside those from more clinical literature, which report reductions of trait anxiety and depression following massage therapy (Moyer, Rounds, and Hannum 2004; Moyer 2008), it seems highly probable that psychological effects of massage are driving demand for massage therapy in athlete populations. Given this possibility, future research on massage therapy for athletes should pay particular attention to the psychological effects of massage.

EXPLAINING MASSAGE THERAPY EFFECTS

The beneficial effects of massage for athletes, which seem to be consistently supported by clinical experience but less consistently supported by research evidence, can be divided into two categories: preparation and recovery. Broadly speaking, the aim of preparatory athletic massage is to maximize performance in an imminent event. In many cases, this goal may be inconsistent with a state of relaxation. The muscle-lengthening effect of massage may reduce muscular force, which is undesirable for certain sports or events. However, the ability of massage to increase muscle-fiber length and range of motion may be desirable shortly before events that prioritize flexibility. The ability of massage to reduce anxiety may also be useful on a case-by-case basis for athletes who experience high anxiety prior to competition, though no research has examined this specifically.

During recovery from training or competition, the goals of sport massage shift to speeding recovery and the promotion of relaxation and feelings of well-being. While it has long been asserted that massage promotes blood flow and lactate clearance, mechanisms expected to promote muscular performance following exertion, no clear research evidence exists that massage has these effects. Nevertheless, some studies have observed improved capacity for further exercise when massage is added to active recovery. Similarly, some studies have concluded that massage reduces the pain of DOMS, which would enable a more rapid and successful return to training and competition. However, other studies have failed to find an effect on DOMS. Even the studies that have found such an effect do not clearly indicate its mechanism.

Simply put, the effects of massage for athletes are not adequately explained by the available evidence. The potential of massage to reduce resting muscle tension may underlie several massage benefits. This mechanism should be investigated further.

RECOMMENDATIONS FOR MASSAGE THERAPY PRACTICE

Little scientific evidence exists to support the direct benefits of massage for athletes. In general, massage may be beneficial as part of a warm-up process by increasing ROM, and may assist recovery from intense or prolonged fatiguing exercise. More specifically, what seems to be emerging from the published literature is the importance of resting muscle tension, not only on the outcome of a massage intervention, but also potentially on the choice of massage to administer before or after exercise. Further research is needed that explores the interaction among massage type, duration, and outcomes in relation to changes in resting muscle tension in order to fully identify the optimal massage intervention strategy. Consideration also needs to be given to the specific sport and the optimal ROM or muscle tension required for achieving peak performance. This is because some athletes, according to their sport, benefit from moderate muscle stiffness, while others may benefit from increased laxity in specific muscle groups.

Evidence-Based Treatment Guidelines

Massage in athlete populations can be divided into several specific contexts:

1. Pretraining or precompetition
2. Intertraining or intercompetition
3. Posttraining or postcompetition
4. Massage for treatment of a specific problem
5. Massage to satisfy psychological need

Despite studies on the more general effects of sport massage, a few studies still support the efficacy of massage as it pertains to these specific contexts (though there is no shortage of anecdotal evidence). Essentially, pretraining or precompetition massage should help preparation for activity and competition and should enhance (but never replace) warm-up routines. Depending on the activity to be undertaken and the outcome most desired (e.g., increased muscle power or greater flexibility, help with tissue repair, increased relaxation, or greater concentration and alertness), massage strokes can vary from very stimulating to fairly gentle but flowing. Intertraining or intercompetition therapy may well use ice massage, and practitioners must always be aware that at this stage, sport-induced tissue damage can be present, which will obviously affect the choice of techniques. Posttraining or postcompetition massage can be used in place of cool-down if the competitor is too exhausted to perform this actively. It must be noted, however, that there is no clear-cut evidence of the true effect of massage on DOMS.

Massage for the treatment of a specific problem can cover a huge range of issues. Among the most common in athletes are tension areas in muscle and fascia, scar tissue, long-standing tendon pathology, and circulation problems. Specific massage interventions must always be carefully planned to fit in with the training and competition diary, and they are best administered during the lay-off or rest period.

Massage for psychological needs is requested by athletes, not to address a specific physiological problem or outcome, but to provide a perceived benefit. Provided it does not interfere with training and competition, this type of massage administration can be useful. However, great care must be taken to ensure an athlete does not become massage dependent. Such dependency has been observed firsthand in a sprint athlete for whom a specific tightness in the shoulders was relieved through massage in the preevent period. Immediately after the massage, the athlete won a major championship medal. From then on, this athlete requested massage at every event as part of his essential precompetition routine, despite having no tightness in the shoulders. Of course, this type of therapy may be part of a psychological benefit to the athlete, but it can be time consuming for practitioners who are already hard pressed to deal with many demands for treatment at major events. In addition, the dependent athlete may begin to believe that a good performance is impossible if massage is unavailable.

DIRECTIONS FOR FUTURE RESEARCH

Given that athletes and sport massage therapists believe that massage has an important role to play in the sport preparation and recovery processes, it is surprising that the scientific literature has only clearly demonstrated a few physiological, neurological, biomechanical, or psychological benefits. A therapy so widely demanded yet with such a small body of positive evidence should surely stimulate the interest to undertake further research work in this area among the communities of exercise scientists, massage therapists, and physical therapists. Unfortunately, on close examination of the available literature, it becomes apparent that the lack of positive findings may be related to common design issues that make many study outcomes equivocal or impossible to compare. In short, research in the field of sport massage has been hampered by many methodological variations and by poor experimental control during the intervention phases of most trials.

All of the factors indicated in table 8.1 may influence the sensitivity of detecting massage effects on sport performance. This chapter previously notes that the literature does, to some extent, support short-term changes in muscle tension and psychological benefits from massage, but sustained physiological and performance benefits have not always been consistently observed across studies. Given that the beneficial effects of active recovery following intense exercise are well established (Ahmaidi et al. 1996, Dodd et al. 1984; Weltman, Stamford, and Fulco 1979), research examining massage interventions on recovery of muscle function must include active recovery of some sort in all phases of the experimental design.

It would be prudent to suggest that all research focused on the role of massage in recovery adopt a standardized exercise task prior to any intervention. For example,

Table 8.1 Common Research Design Limitations in Sport Massage Studies

Variable	Range observed in studies	Outcome variable affected
Massage duration	2-30 minutes	Could affect all outcome variables
Massage type	Relaxing to stimulatory	May reverse findings on speed, strength, and power measures
Warm up	None to completely standardized warm up	Could affect all outcome variables
Active recovery	None to 15 minutes	Any recovery measures
Stretching	None to 5 minutes of standardized static stretching	Mainly impacts speed, strength, and power measures
Prior activity or diet	None, or self-standardized to completely controlled standardized	Could affect all outcome variables

if the exercise mode was running, it would be to run for a set period of time at a prescribed intensity or a prescribed distance in a set period of time to ensure that pretreatment stress is identical. However, in many studies, the intensity of the initial exercise bout is not controlled, which leads to difficulty in interpreting the data. In addition, studies should control for dietary intake throughout the experimental period, since diet can clearly influence performance and recovery (Maughan, King, and Lea 2004). Therefore, by improving the methodological aspects of massage studies, researchers will be better able to document reliable and valid outcomes and to yield a more complete interpretation of the potential benefits of massage.

In summary, most of the research literature on sport massage has so far uncovered little evidence for physiological or psychological mechanisms that support recovery and restoration of muscle function. However, more recent massage research findings and their parallels with the literature on stretching raise interesting possibilities about the physiological effects of sport massage and the role it may play in the preparation and recovery processes in athletes. Clearly, further laboratory and field work are needed to evaluate resting muscle tension and the effects of sport massage, given its popularity among athletes.

Key issues ripe for investigation include determining optimal timing and duration of massage and optimal intensity or type of massage, contrasting acute (hours) and chronic (days) effects of massage, elucidating the effects of resting muscle tension on massage outcome, and revealing other physiological mechanisms associated with massage therapy. However, it should be emphasized that careful study design and implementation of tight controls are required to detect meaningful differences in key outcome variables. In addition, well-controlled studies should aim to systematically evaluate the effects of different massage interventions and durations on physiological and psychological outcome variables in all massage use phases (pretraining or precompetition, intertraining or intercompetition, posttraining or postcompetition, massage for treatment of a specific problem, and massage to satisfy psychological need). Furthermore, a key area for development of international understanding and for interpretation of future research work on massage in sport would be to develop an internationally recognized handbook of terminology. To do this, an international body would need to be formed and a consensus reached regarding terminology.

Case Study

Ivan, a 23-year-old male decathlete, presented on the evening before the start of a national decathlon. He reported that he was unable to achieve full range of movement in his right hamstring. A subjective assessment revealed that he was in excellent general health and very fit, and that he had no known allergies. He originally tore his right hamstring at age 17, and has experienced problems with it since then. He had physical therapy at the time of the injury, but has had no follow-up care or advice. He was not taking any medication and did not report any other health problems.

Objective assessment revealed that he disliked doing flexibility exercises and that he used inadequate warm-up and cool-down procedures. Observations of Ivan and movement assessments indicated that while he was very fit, he exhibited a stiff movement pattern. His right hip flexion was 20° less than his left, and his lower musculotendinous junction of the biceps femoris showed scarring and lacked elasticity. All other ranges of movement of both joints were limited at end range. Medial rotation of both hips was reduced by 20% of normal. Ivan had no low back problems. His sensation and skin temperature were normal, and he showed no evidence of allergy, cuts, or skin abrasions.

An acute treatment plan was implemented to gain sufficient range of movement to allow safe participation in the decathlon and to increase range of movement. A long-term plan to improve flexibility and optimize joint range of motion was devised. Massage intervention for day 1 was implemented as follows:

Before the event, MT included stroking, effleurage with grade-1 or grade-2 pressure (Watt 1999), petrissage with pressure ranging from grades 1 through 3 (Watt 1999), and trigger pointing and acupressure to specific problem areas with grade-1 or grade-2 pressure. Myofascial and soft-tissue release were performed. Massage was administered between competitions (intercompetition massage). These steps were preceded with ice massage between events 4 and 5. After the event, muscle rolling and non–weight bearing stretches were introduced.

Massage treatment for day 2 was implemented as on day 1. The outcome of this treatment was that Ivan completed the event with no further damage. He continued with regular massage and specific stretching with the aim of increasing range of motion. A final assessment revealed that he had an equal range of motion in the hamstrings of both legs, with a general improvement in flexibility and retention of a small, nonsymptomatic scarred area in the right biceps femoris.

SUMMARY

Massage for athletes has a long history. In modern times, its use is growing as athletes, trainers, and clinicians increasingly explore ways to promote recovery and performance. However, in contrast to its longevity and popularity, the scientific research in support of sport massage is limited and conflicting in its findings. Ample opportunities exist for extending our knowledge of this intervention with research on sport-massage mechanisms and outcomes. Research to delineate the types and patterns of massage that optimally correspond to the varied needs of different athletes and specific sport contexts is also needed.

Even with the limited state of current evidence, some guidelines for evidence-based practice can be specified. In particular, a recognition that massage can reduce resting muscle tension can inform when and how massage should be used, and not used, in relation to the specific demands of athletes' sports and whether they are approaching or recovering from a competition. Massage therapists need to attend to emerging research in this area, since the potential for performance gains from evidence-based practice is substantial.

REFERENCES

Ahmaidi, S., P. Granier, Z. Taoutaou, J. Mercier, H. Dubouchaud, and C. Prefaut. 1996. Effects of active recovery on plasma lactate and anaerobic power following repeated intensive exercise. *Med Sci Sports Exerc* 28: 450-456.

Armstrong, R.B., G.L. Warren, and J.A. Warren. 1991. Mechanisms of exercise-induced muscle fibre injury. *Sports Med* 12: 184-207.

Arroyo-Morales, M., N. Olea, M. Martinez, A. Hidalgo-Lozano, C. Ruiz-Rodriguez, and L. Rodriguez. 2008. Psychophysiological effects of massage-myofascial release after exercise: A randomized sham-control study. *J Altern Complement Med* 14: 1223-1229.

Barnett, A. 2006. Using recovery modalities between training sessions in elite athletes: Does it help? *Sports Med* 36: 781-796.

Bell, J. 2008. Massage therapy helps to increase range of motion, decrease pain and assist in healing a client with low back pain and sciatica symptoms. *J Bodyw Mov Ther* 12: 281-289.

Berg, H.E., and O. Eiken. 1999. Muscle control in elite alpine skiing. *Med Sci Sports Exerc* 31: 1065-1067.

Bonen, A., C. Campbell, R. Kirby, and A. Belcastro. 1979. A multiple regression model for blood lactate removal in man. *Pflugers Arch* 380: 205-210.

Cafarelli, E., and F. Flint. 1992. The role of massage in preparation for and recovery from exercise. An overview. *Sports Med* 14: 1-9.

Callaghan, M.J. 1993. The role of massage in the management of the athlete: A review. *Br J Sports Med* 27: 28-33.

Cheung, K., P. Hume, and L. Maxwell. 2003. Delayed onset muscle soreness: Treatment strategies and performance factors. *Sports Med* 33: 145-164.

Dishman, J.D., and R. Bulbulian. 2001. Comparison of effects of spinal manipulation and massage on motorneuron excitability. *Electromyogr Clin Neurophysiol* 41: 97-106.

Dodd, S., S.K. Powers, T. Callender, and E. Brooks. 1984. Blood lactate disappearance at various intensities of recovery exercise. *J Appl Physiol* 57: 1462-1465.

Edman, K.A., and C. Reggiani. 1984. Redistribution of sarcomere length during isometric contraction of frog muscle fibres and its relation to tension creep. *J Physiol* 351: 169-198.

Ernst, E. 1998. Does post-exercise massage treatment reduce delayed onset muscle soreness? A systematic review. *Br J Sports Med* 32: 212-214.

Fowles, J.R., D.G. Sale, and J.D. MacDougall. 2000. Reduced strength after passive stretch of the human plantarflexors. *J Appl Physiol* 89: 1179-1188.

Friden, J., P.N. Sfakianos, and A.R. Hargens. 1986. Muscle soreness and intramuscular fluid pressure: Comparison between eccentric and concentric load. *J Appl Physiol* 61: 2175-2179.

Galloway, S.D., and J.M. Watt. 2004. Massage provision by physiotherapists at major athletics events between 1987 and 1998. *Br J Sports Med* 38: 235-236.

Goats, G.C. 1994. Massage—The scientific basis of an ancient art: Part 2. Physiological and therapeutic effects. *Br J Sports Med* 28: 153-156.

Goldberg, J., S.J. Sullivan, and D.E. Seaborne. 1992. The effect of two intensities of massage on H-reflex amplitude. *Phys Ther* 72: 449-457.

Goldberg, J., D.E. Seaborne, S.J. Sullivan, and B.E. Leduc. 1994. The effect of therapeutic massage on H-reflex amplitude in persons with a spinal cord injury. *Phys Ther* 74: 728-737.

Gordon, A.M., A.F. Huxley, and F.J. Julian. 1966. The variation in isometric tension with sarcomere length in vertebrate muscle fibres. *J Physiol* 184: 170-192.

Gupta, S., A. Goswami, A.K. Sadhukhan, and D.N. Mathur. 1996. Comparative study of lactate removal in short term massage of extremities, active recovery and a passive recovery period after supramaximal exercise sessions. *Int J Sports Med* 17: 106-110.

Hemmings, B., M. Smith, J. Graydon, and R. Dyson. 2000. Effects of massage on physiological restoration, perceived recovery, and repeated sports performance. *Br J Sports Med* 34: 109-114.

Hernandez-Reif, M., T. Field, J. Krasnegor, and H. Theakston. 2001. Lower back pain is reduced and range of motion increased after massage therapy. *Int J Neurosci* 106: 131-145.

Hinds, T., I. McEwan, J. Perkes, E. Dawson, D. Ball, and K. George. 2004. Effects of massage on limb and skin blood flow after quadriceps exercise. *Med Sci Sports Exerc* 36: 1308-1313.

Hopper, D., S. Deacon, S. Das, A. Jain, D. Riddell, T. Hall, and K. Briffa. 2005. Dynamic soft tissue mobilisation increases hamstring flexibility in healthy male subjects. *Br J Sports Med* 39: 594-598.

Howatson, G., and K.A. van Someren. 2008. The prevention and treatment of exercise-induced muscle damage. *Sports Med* 38: 483-503.

Hunter, A.M., I.J. Smith, J.M. Watt, C. Yirrell, and S.D. Galloway. 2006. The effect of massage on force production and tensiomyography. *Med Sci Sports Exerc.* 38: S27-S27.

Hunter, A.M., J.M. Watt, V. Watt, and S.D. Galloway. 2006. Effect of lower limb massage on electromyography and force production of the knee extensors. *Br J Sports ed* 40: 114-118.

Jones, G. 2007. Massaging the figures. *Cycling Weekly*, August 2. www.cyclingweekly.co.uk.

Marginson, V., and R. Eston. 2001. The relationship between torque and joint angle during knee extension in boys and men. *J Sports Sci* 19: 875-880.

Martin, N.A., R.F. Zoeller, R.J. Robertson, and S.M. Lephart. 1998. The comparative effects of sports massage, active recovery, and rest in promoting blood lactate clearance after supramaximal leg exercise. *J Athl Train* 33: 30-35.

Maughan, R.J., D.S. King, and T. Lea. 2004. Dietary supplements. *J Sports Sci* 22: 95-113.

Monedero, J., and B. Donne. 2000. Effect of recovery interventions on lactate removal and subsequent performance. *Int J Sports Med* 21: 593-597.

Moraska, A. 2005. Sports massage. A comprehensive review. *J Sports Med Phys Fitness* 45: 370-380.

Morelli, M., D.E. Seaborne, and S.J. Sullivan. 1991. H-reflex modulation during manual muscle massage of human triceps surae. *Arch Phys Med Rehabil* 72: 915-919.

Morien, A., D. Garrison, and N.K. Smith. 2008. Range of motion improves after massage in children with burns: A pilot study. *J Bodyw Mov Ther* 12: 67-71.

Moyer, C.A. 2008. Affective massage therapy. *Int J Ther Massage and Bodyw* 1: 3-5.

Moyer, C.A., J. Rounds, and J.W. Hannum. 2004. A meta-analysis of massage therapy research. *Psych Bull* 130: 3-18.

Moyer, C.A., L. Seefeldt, E.S. Mann, and L.M. Jackley. 2011. Does massage therapy reduce cortisol? A comprehensive quantitative review. *J Bodyw Mov Ther* 15: 3-14.

NCBTMB.Consumers' massage facts. www.ncbtmb.org/consumers_massage_facts.php.

Nelson, A.G., I.K. Guillory, C. Cornwell, and J. Kokkonen. 2001. Inhibition of maximal voluntary isokinetic torque production following stretching is velocity-specific. *J Strength Cond Res* 15: 241-246.

Ogai, R., M. Yamane, T. Matsumoto, and M. Kosaka. 2008. Effects of petrissage massage on fatigue and exercise performance following intensive cycle pedalling. *Br J Sports Med* 42: 534-538.

Paschalis,V., M.G. Nikolaidis, G. Giakas, A.Z. Jamurtas, A. Pappas, and Y. Koutedakis. 2007. The effect of eccentric exercise on position sense and joint reaction angle of the lower limbs. *Muscle Nerve* 35: 496-503.

Rassier, D.E., B.R. MacIntosh, and W. Herzog. 1999. Length dependence of active force production in skeletal muscle. *J Appl Physiol* 86: 1445-1457.

Reilly, T., and B. Ekblom. 2005. The use of recovery methods post-exercise. *J Sports Sci* 23: 619-627.

Robertson, A., J.M. Watt, and S.D. Galloway. 2004. Effects of leg massage on recovery from high intensity cycling exercise. *Br J Sports Med* 38: 173-176.

Sherman, K.J., M.W. Dixon, D. Thompson, and D.C. Cherkin. 2006. Development of a taxonomy to describe massage treatments for musculoskeletal pain. *BMC Complem Alter M* 6(24). www.biomedcentral.com/1472-6882/6/24.

Shoemaker, J.K., P.M. Tiidus, and R. Mader. 1997. Failure of manual massage to alter limb blood flow: Measures by Doppler ultrasound. *Med Sci Sports Exerc* 29: 610-614.

Sullivan, S.J., Williams, L.R., Seaborne, D.E., and Morelli, M. 1991. Effects of massage on alpha motoneuron excitability. *Phys Ther* 71(8): 555-560.

Thomas, C., S. Perrey, K. Lambert, G. Hugon, D. Mornet, and J. Mercier. 2005. Monocarboxylate transporters, blood lactate removal after supramaximal exercise, and fatigue indexes in humans. *J Appl Physiol* 98: 804-809.

Tiidus, P.M. 1999. Massage and ultrasound as therapeutic modalities in exercise-induced muscle damage. *Can J Appl Physiol* 24: 267-278.

Tiidus, P.M., and J.K. Shoemaker. 1995. Effleurage massage, muscle blood flow and long-term post-exercise strength recovery. *Int J Sports Med* 16: 478-483.

Warren, G.L., C.P. Ingalls, D.A. Lowe, and R.B. Armstrong. 2001. Excitation-contraction uncoupling: Major role in contraction-induced muscle injury. *Exerc Sport Sci Rev* 29: 82-87.

Watt, J. 1999. *Massage for sport.* Wiltshire, England: Crowood Press.

Weerapong, P., P.A. Hume, and G.S. Kolt. 2005. The mechanisms of massage and effects on performance, muscle recovery and injury prevention. *Sports Med* 35: 235-256.

Weltman, A., B.A. Stamford, and C. Fulco. 1979. Recovery from maximal effort exercise: Lactate disappearance and subsequent performance. *J Appl Physiol* 47: 677-682.

Wiktorsson-Moller, M., B. Oberg, J. Ekstrand, and J. Gillquist. 1983. Effects of warming up, massage, and stretching on range of motion and muscle strength in the lower extremity. *Am J Sports Med* 11: 249-252.

chapter 9

Massage and Older Adults

Diana L. Thompson, LMP

The demographics of aging are changing as life expectancy increases. The number of older adults (aged 65 and older) in the United States is expected to peak at 71.5 million in 2030, up from 35 million in 2000, at which time they will constitute 20% of the total population (Greenberg 2008). Compared to previous generations, older Americans will be more racially diverse and better educated, and will have a higher median income (Federal Interagency Forum on Aging-Related Statistics 2008). Given that the use of complementary and alternative medicine (CAM) is more predominant among people with higher income and more education (Barnes, Bloom, and Nahin 2008; AARP and NCCAM 2007), and that massage therapy (MT) is the most popular practitioner-based CAM modality that people pay to receive (Barnes, Bloom, and Nahin 2008), it is reasonable to expect that demand for MT from this segment of the population will continue to increase significantly.

The health of older adults varies widely, so it is challenging to identify a typical profile. Massage practitioners, therefore, need to understand the range of health conditions common to this growing population in order to apply safe and effective treatment plans. Approximately 80% of older adults have at least one chronic health condition and 50% have at least two chronic conditions, the most common being hypertension, arthritis, heart disease, cancer, and diabetes (Greenberg 2008; Federal Interagency Forum on Aging-Related Statistics 2008). Despite this diversity in the health status of older adults, it is useful to identify three broad categories of health status that can guide care and treatment. These are healthy, active elders, elders living with chronic conditions, and elders requiring palliative care.

EFFECTS OF MASSAGE THERAPY ON OLDER ADULT POPULATIONS

While consumers identify MT as a favored treatment option (Barnes, Bloom, and Nahin 2008), there is no conclusive evidence supporting any specific MT techniques for the medical conditions common to older adults. This is because study protocols are often not clearly defined. Comparative studies of best practices or dosage have not yet been conducted. In addition, no common taxonomy or nomenclature for techniques has been adopted. That said, the number and kinds of MT studies have been increasing, especially in the past decade. These have provided some evidence that MT is a safe and noninvasive approach to a variety of conditions, such as anxiety and depression (Moyer, Rounds, and Hannum 2004), pain (Tsao 2007), loss of function due to disability (Dryden, Baskwill, and Preyde 2004), and side effects of medical treatments, including constipation (Lämås et al. 2009), fatigue (Currin and Meister 2008), and nausea (Billhult, Bergbom, and Stener-Victorin 2007).

Healthy, Active Older Adults

Thirty-nine percent of noninstitutionalized older adults assessed their health as very good or excellent (AARP and NCCAM 2007). However, aging involves common physiological and psychological changes that affect digestion, vision, balance, mobility, and mood, among others (Davis and Srivastiva 2003). Therefore, even healthy and active older adults may require treatment for commonly occurring functional concerns in these areas. Conditions for which MT has been researched likely to occur in this population include pain, loss of balance, decreased flexibility, and constipation.

Even healthy and active older adults can experience normal symptoms related to aging, including pain, reduced balance, decreased flexibility, and constipation. This section outlines the research literature that examines MT treatment of these symptoms.

Pain

Pain, which is present in 45% to 85% of older adults, might be the most prevalent, complex, and undertreated condition facing this population. Pain is influenced by a variety of factors, including depression, diminished activities and social engagements, sleep disturbances, malnutrition, sensory impairment, numerous medical conditions, and disabilities. Pain reduction has positive effects on a host of conditions, but physicians may be reluctant to refer to CAM treatments, such as massage for pain, due to limited knowledge of these modalities (Davis and Srivastava 2003).

Notably, the pain treatments most commonly prescribed by physicians, including medications, physical therapy, and exercise, are those that are least preferred by older adults. Older adults are more likely to prefer massage, topical analgesics, hot and cold packs, relaxation education, and movement classes (Davis and Srivastava 2003; Reid et al. 2008). In addition, self-care techniques that are easily incorporated into a MT session can also be useful, since they are low-cost and are not associated with side effects. They may also translate into improved self-management of other common chronic conditions (Reid et al. 2008). Massage therapists should be mindful of what older adults consider helpful remedies and should consider adding self-care to treatment plans.

Several randomized controlled trials have examined MT for low back pain (LBP) (Walach, Guthlin, and M. Konig 2005; Hasson et al. 2004; Cherkin et al. 2001; Hernandez-Reif et al. 2001; Preyde 2000), which is the most common painful condition across all ages (Barnes, Bloom, and Nahin 2008). However, there have been no studies on MT for LBP specifically in older adults. It is likely that the protocols with demonstrated effectiveness for treating pain in adults should also be applicable to older adults (see chapter 12), but research with older adults is needed.

Loss of Balance, Decreased Flexibility

Aging brings a progressive decrease in muscle strength and joint flexibility, visual perception, vestibular function, and somatosensory sensitivity. All of these contribute to balance impairments, which increase the risk of falling and affect older adults' safety and ability to live independently. Balance impairments can also be caused or exacerbated by lack of exercise, neurological disorders, arthritis, or other medical conditions and their treatments (Davis and Srivastava 2003; Vaillant et al. 2009). Maintaining strength, flexibility, and endurance limits the risk of falling and helps older adults to stay active and maintain physical health (Berger, Klein, and Commandeur 2007).

Vaillant and colleagues (2009) found significant improvement in elders' performance in two out of three balance tests after a single session of MT, including the application of friction, static and glide pressure, and mobilization techniques focused on the foot and ankle, combined with mobilization. In other studies, mobility increased and pain decreased when MT was combined with water-based mobilization therapy (Forestier et al. 2009). The reduced muscular loads associated with movement in water may reinforce proprioceptive input, thereby leading to improvement (Berger, Klein, and Commandeur 2008). Massage therapists who work in a spa environment or have access to warm pools should consider MT and mobilizations done underwater or in combination with water therapy.

Constipation

Older adults are five times more likely than younger adults to report constipation, which accounts for more than 2.5 million physician visits per year in the United States (Lämås et al. 2009). The increased prevalence in this population may be partly attributable to pain, medications, decreased mobility, decreased bowel motility, illnesses such as strokes, decrease in fluid intake (often due to self-management of incontinence), and poor diet (Davis and Srivastava 2003). A randomized controlled trial of abdominal massage for the management of constipation found that this treatment decreased the severity of gastrointestinal symptoms, especially symptoms associated with constipation and pain syndrome (Lämås et al. 2009; Lämås et al. 2010), which are outcomes that may represent particular value for older adults.

Older Adults Living With Chronic Conditions

Though 39% of noninstitutionalized older adults self-report excellent to very good health, it is simultaneously true that 80% of older adults have one or more chronic health conditions (AARP and NCCAM 2007; Greenberg 2008; Federal Interagency Forum on Aging-Related Statistics 2008). Although older adults may present with a positive outlook on their health, massage therapists must be mindful of possible underlying or undiagnosed conditions, such as insomnia, arthritis, cancer (see chapter 17), and anxiety or depression (see chapter 13). Chronic conditions for which there is specific MT research that are likely to be encountered with this population include arthritis, dementia, and insomnia.

Arthritis

The term *arthritis* refers to joint inflammation, and is used to describe more than 100 rheumatic conditions that affect the joints, the tissues surrounding the joints, and other connective tissue. The most common form of arthritis is osteoarthritis, a disease characterized by degeneration of cartilage and its underlying bone within a joint, as well as bony overgrowth. The breakdown of these tissues leads to pain and joint stiffness. An estimated 27 million American adults have osteoarthritis, 17 million of whom are older adults. In fact, 50% of older adults report having arthritis. Other common rheumatic conditions include gout, fibromyalgia (see chapter 16), and rheumatoid arthritis (CDC 2006).

Currently, no cure exists for osteoarthritis. Treatment focuses on relieving symptoms and improving function. Recent studies have investigated the effects of MT on osteoarthritis, though none has focused exclusively on older adults. In a randomized controlled trial investigating MT for osteoarthritis of the knee, Swedish massage techniques were administered to 68 adults with osteoarthritis. One-hour sessions were provided twice weekly for the first 4 weeks, then weekly for the next 4 weeks. Results suggest that MT is efficacious in the treatment of osteoarthritis of the knee, with beneficial results persisting for weeks following treatment. Massage therapy was well tolerated by people with painful osteoarthritis, and it decreased pain and improved function in participants who were allowed to maintain their usual treatment (Perlman et al. 2006). Spa therapies, including mud and paraffin application, shower massage, and manual massage and exercises under water, also have a positive effect on osteoarthritis by reducing pain and improving health status in patients suffering from osteoarthritis (Vaht, Birkenfeldt, and Ubner 2008; Forestier et al. 2009).

Dementia

Loss of memory and decline in cognitive functioning are some of the most tragic consequences of aging. Although no research exists on the effects of MT on improving memory or cognitive function, the effect of MT on agitation, which is associated with the advanced stages of dementia and affects up to 80% of adults with Alzheimer's disease (Woods, Craven, and Whitney 2005; Gerdner, Hart, and Zimmerman 2008), has been studied. In a recent study titled "Massage in the Management of Agitation in Nursing Home Residents with Cognitive Impairment," five dimensions of agitation were assessed. These were wandering, being verbally agitated or abusive, acting physically agitated or abusive, being socially inappropriate or disruptive, and resisting care. Fifty-four elders with moderate to severe dementia were given six massage therapy sessions, consisting primarily of gentle effleurage, over a 2-week intervention period. Decreases in agitation were significant both during and following massage intervention for all dimensions except for socially inappropriate or disruptive behavior (Holliday-Welsh, Gessert, and Renier 2009). Finally, it should be noted that because persons with dementia are less able to adapt to common environment and mental changes, consistency and a predictable treatment routine may be especially important components of MT with this population.

Insomnia

Sleep patterns change with age. The elderly sleep less than when they were younger and many have difficulty falling asleep. They may also wake more easily and often and may spend less time in deep sleep. In some cases, these changes may be related to anxiety, pain associated with a chronic illness, or an increased need to urinate at night. Sleep deprivation can lead to confusion and other mental deficits. Treatment of insomnia in older adults is made more difficult by the fact that use of sedatives is discouraged because of the added risks of delirium and falls for this population (Flaherty 2008)

Acupressure, which can be a component of MT, has been shown to have a positive effect on insomnia in patients with cancer who were previously nonresponsive to pharmacological interventions (Cerrone et al. 2008). In studies of measures on pain and quality of life (QOL), statistically significant results were noted improvement in sleep and depression after massage therapy, even when few results were noted for pain and QOL (Soden, Vincent, and Craske 2004). In a study comparing massage to the use of relaxation recordings, older adults preferred massage therapy, even though both interventions showed significant results (Hanley, Stirling, and Brown 2003).

Older Adults Requiring End-of-Life Care or Palliative Care

Palliative care seeks to improve the quality of life for people with a terminal illness, as opposed to focusing on curing the illness. Hospice care, a specific form of palliative care, is especially valuable when the end of life is imminent (Beider 2005). An estimated 1.45 million people received hospice services in 2008, and approximately 38.5% of all U.S. deaths occurred under hospice care. Thirty-eight percent of these were due to cancer, followed in frequency by heart disease, dementia, and lung disease (NHPCO 2009). Massage therapy is a popular palliative care treatment in Canadian and U.S. hospices, since it is capable of offering support and comfort to those at the end of their lives and to their families (Oneschuk et al. 2007; Kozak et al. 2009). In this setting, MT treatment goals do not vary greatly, given that the primary goal is providing comfort. For example, since long-term benefits are not the priority for a hospice resident whose condition is advanced, MT practitioners may not focus on reducing fibrous adhesions.

palliative care

▸ Care or treatment that focuses on relieving the symptoms of a terminal illness and maximizing patient comfort and dignity, in contrast to focusing on maximal extension of life.

Massage therapy is one of the most commonly offered complementary therapies in U.S. and Canadian hospices, although researchers note that lack of funding and insufficient staff knowledge limit its wider use (Oneschuk et al. 2007; Kozak et al. 2009).

A study that illustrates the value of qualitative research captured the experience of persons in palliative care who received MT. It found that MT generated physical well-being and mental relaxation, as well as feelings of inner respite, freedom, and liberation from illness. Individual participants remarked that they "felt uplifted and happy," experienced "relaxation without the illness because [they] did not think about it at all," and "felt strengthened in some way" (Cronfalk et al. 2009).

Similarly, patients in a study that combined MT and meditation showed significant improvement in overall and spiritual quality of life. These benefits may not have occurred with meditation alone, since meditation effects may be blunted unless the patients' need for physical contact is also addressed (Williams et al. 2005). Touch is a valuable component of end-of-life care, both for symptoms like pain, anxiety, and sleep, and for QOL concerns, including communication, comfort, and spiritual care. Although evidence exists that MT may have immediate benefits on pain and mood in end-of-life care, simple touch is also an effective intervention for this population, with documented benefits for QOL (Kutner et al. 2008). MT can also be used to address end-of-life patients' need for human contact, comfort, and communication (Russell, Beinhorn, and Frenkel 2008; Kolcaba, Schirm, and Steiner 2006).

EXPLAINING MASSAGE THERAPY EFFECTS

Little is known about the specific causes of massage therapy benefits. Given the range and complexity of the experience and symptoms of aging in both healthy and fragile older adults and the wide range of effects outlined in the MT research cited for conditions as diverse as dementia, arthritis, constipation, and insomnia, it is likely that the causal mechanisms of massage therapy vary across the specific symptoms and conditions. Mechanism-of-action studies are needed that will more specifically determine how massage therapy influences cognition, communication, balance, and other important outcomes for this population. See chapter 23 for further discussion of this issue.

RECOMMENDATIONS FOR MASSAGE THERAPY PRACTICE

Providing massage therapy to older adults can be challenging, given the wide range of conditions and the rapidly changing health status older adults may exhibit. That said, it can be very rewarding to deliver attention, comfort, and relief to an often isolated population with massage therapy.

Massage therapy must be modified for older adults to account for changes in sensation and physical abilities, and for psychosocial issues associated with aging (Rose 2010). Effective communication is an especially important aspect of treatment, to ensure that attention is given to areas of need and to avoid the possibility of overtreatment, which could increase pain or other symptoms. Guidelines for MT with older adults, which are based on our current understanding of the complexity of their health and wellness, combined with the small amount of MT research with this growing population, are summarized in the following sections.

Healthy, Active Elders

- Assess for common conditions, such as pain, loss of flexibility or balance, and constipation.
- Determine the client's goals in receiving MT.
- Identify medications, possible contraindications, or reasons for caution concerning treatment.
- Assess severity of symptoms before and after sessions to allow tracking of progress. This may include the following:
  - Use of 0-10 visual analog scale for pain or functioning.
  - Use of a goniometer for range of motion.
  - Record of bowel movements, including perceived strain.
- Administer MT techniques consistent with the treatment goals of the client and therapist. Approaches might include the following:
  - Slow-stoke effleurage or trigger-point therapy for pain reduction.
  - Static and glide friction and active assisted and passive stretching for increasing mobility of feet and ankles (intended to improve balance).
  - Abdominal massage in the direction of motility to reduce constipation.

Older Adults With Chronic Conditions

- Determine presence of a chronic condition and investigate possible contraindications or reasons for caution concerning treatment. Chronic conditions with this population may include arthritis, dementia, or insomnia, among others.
- Determine the client's goals in receiving MT.
- Work interprofessionally with the client's primary health care provider to address progress and concerns.
- Identify symptoms associated with the client's expression of the condition.

- Identify conditions of aging that may be complicating the chronic condition. These may include loss of balance, reduction of sensation, or change in cognitive abilities.
- Assess regularly for changes in health status or medication intake.
- Assess symptom severity before and after sessions to allow tracking of progress. This may include the following:
  - Use of 0-10 visual analog scale for arthritis pain.
  - Observation of relaxation or reduction in agitation in persons with dementia.
  - Record of sleep duration and quality in persons with insomnia.
- Administer MT techniques consistent with the treatment goals of the client and therapist. Approaches might include the following:
  - *Arthritis.* Treatment includes slow-stroke MT or trigger-point therapy for reduction of pain; passive and active assisted movement and stretching, or static and glide friction for improvement of balance and flexibility; and manual lymph drainage for reduction of swelling.
  - *Dementia.* Treatment to reduce agitation and promote relaxation includes craniosacral therapy, reflexology, acupressure, and soothing, gentle, and attentive strokes.
  - *Insomnia.* Treatment to promote relaxation includes aromatherapy, reflexology, acupressure, comforting touch, and soothing, gentle, and attentive strokes.

Older Adults in Need of Palliative Care

- Create a safe and comfortable environment.
- Observe institution's strict protocols for hygiene and communication with staff, family, and the older adult.
- Attend to safety and comfort of the older adult. Be aware of medical equipment, position of the bed and pillows, and lighting.
- Avoid deep touch, large joint movements, surgical sites, lesions, or rashes.
- Attend to the safety and comfort of yourself and the staff with regard to working around beds, wheel chairs, and medical equipment.
- Identify specific clinical considerations and the contraindications associated with specific conditions.
- Provide massage techniques that will accomplish the client's goals for the session and your goals for care. Techniques might include comfort touch, reflexology, acupressure, and an emphasis on MT techniques that are gentle, slow, comforting, attentive, and respectful.

Based on Rose 2010; MacDonald 2005; Thompson 2006.

DIRECTIONS FOR FUTURE RESEARCH

First and foremost, more MT research needs to be conducted for this growing population. This includes studies with larger samples that are capable of verifying, or possibly overturning, our existing knowledge. In addition, dosing, the effectiveness of various MT modalities, and the effectiveness of MT in combination with adjunct therapies all need to be researched with older adults. The effectiveness of self-massage and self-massage education should also be studied with this population.

Given the observation that funding is often lacking for complementary therapies such as MT, research for older adults should also include measures of cost-effectiveness. Long-term studies should explore whether older adults who receive MT make fewer physician visits, show reduced occurrence of chronic health conditions, or rely less on medications.

Finally, we need to better understand the effect of practitioner education, training, and experience on outcomes. Many studies have been done using family members or nursing staff to provide MT, so little is known concerning the importance of training, including whether licensed massage therapists are generally more effective than other persons pressed into service to provide MT for this population.

Case Study

Grace, a healthy and active woman of 74 years with a positive outlook on her health and her life, decided to try massage for her chronic low back pain (CLBP). After further exploration from massage therapist Rick, a history of a pulmonary embolism, diagnosed 15 years prior, was revealed. This limits her ability to do cardiorespiratory exercise, though Grace still does Pilates and some resistance training guided by a trainer. In addition, Rick learned that Grace underwent low back surgery 2 years prior to remove a cyst on her lumbar spine. Previously, Grace was an enthusiastic equestrian, but she has not been on a horse in several years due to her CLBP and a small but significant decline in her sense of balance. Her ultimate goal in receiving MT was to get back on a horse.

Grace received twice-monthly MT sessions from Rick for 2 years. Massage therapy focused on working the deep external rotators of her hip, hip flexors, lumbosacral muscles and fascia, as well as on mobilization of the feet and ankles. In addition, she also received MT to her neck, shoulders, and back. Rick paid particular attention to her ribs, using fascial unwinding techniques to mobilize them. Her LBP improved considerably, only becoming problematic during and after a few long trips to attend horse shows. She decided to attempt horseback riding again.

Her return to riding was successful, and she felt strong and exuberant with the joy of reuniting with her passion. Three years after her return to riding, she suffered a fall in her home and injured her back. She sought additional help from Rick. After several months of MT, she was once again sleeping normally and was able to return to most activities of daily living without pain. However, at this time, she reevaluated the importance of horseback riding in her life. She decided that although she was thrilled to have accomplished her return to riding 3 years earlier, she would now be content with her current level of activity. Grace continues to use regular MT and exercise to stay flexible and strong and continues to comfortably travel considerable distances to enjoy horse shows.

SUMMARY

For the diverse, growing, and steadily changing population of older adults, massage therapy offers a variety of evidence-informed treatment options for maintenance of health and relief from symptoms associated with specific conditions. Promising results have been obtained for conditions associated with aging, including anxiety, depression, insomnia, constipation, arthritis pain, and reduced flexibility and balance. In addition, massage and simple touch are valuable components of end-of-life care, both for symptoms including pain, anxiety, and sleep, and for quality-of-life concerns, including enhancement of communication, comfort, and dignity. Specialized training in massage therapy for older adults is an essential part of successful treatment.

REFERENCES

American Association of Retired Persons (AARP), and National Centre for Complementary and Alternative Medicine (NCCAM). 2007. *Complementary and alternative medicine: What people 50 and older are using and discussing with their physicians.* http://assets.aarp.org/rgcenter/health/cam_2007.pdf.

Barnes, P.M., B. Bloom, and R.L. Nahin. 2008. Complementary and alternative medicine use among adults and children: United States, 2007. *Nat Health Stat Rep* 12: 1-23.

Berger, L., C. Klein, and M. Commandeur. 2008. Evaluation of the immediate and midterm effects of mobilization in hot spa water on static and dynamic balance in elderly subjects. *Ann Readapt Med Phys* 51: 90-95.

Beider, S. 2005. An ethical argument for integrated palliative care. http://ecam.oxfordjournals.org/cgi/reprint/neh089v1.pdf.

Billhult, A., I. Bergbom, and E. Stener-Victorin. 2007. Massage relieves nausea in women with breast cancer who are undergoing chemotherapy. *J Altern Complement Med* 13(1): 53-57.

Centers for Disease Control and Prevention (CDC). 2006. Prevalence of doctor-diagnosed arthritis and arthritis-attributable activity limitation: United States, 2003-2005. *MMWR Weekly* 55(40): 1089-1092.

Cerrone, R., L. Giani, B. Galbiati, G. Messina, M. Casiraghi, E. Proserpio, M. Meregalli, P. Trabattoni, P. Lissoni, and G. Gardani. 2008. Efficacy of HT7 point acupressure stimulation in the treatment of insomnia in cancer patients and in patients suffering from disorders other than cancer. *Minerva Medica* 99(6): 535-537.

Cherkin, D.C., D. Eisenberg, K.J. Sherman, W. Barlow, T.J. Kaptchuk, J. Street, and R.A. Deyo. 2001. Randomized trial comparing traditional Chinese medical acupuncture, therapeutic massage, and self-care education for chronic low back pain. *Arch Intern Med* 161: 1081-1088.

Cronfalk, B.S., P. Strang, B.M. Ternestedt, and M. Friedrichsen. 2009. The existential experiences of receiving soft tissue massage in palliative home care—An intervention. *Support Care Cancer* 17: 1203-1211.

Currin, J., and E.A. Meister. 2008. A hospital-based intervention using massage to reduce distress among oncology patients. *Cancer Nurs* 31(3): 214-221.

Davis, M., and M. Srivastava. 2003. Demographics, assessment and management of pain in elderly. *Drug Aging* 20(1): 23-57.

Dryden, T., A. Baskwill, and M. Preyde. 2004. Massage therapy for the orthopaedic patient: A review. *Orthop Nurs* 23(5): 327-332.

Federal Interagency Forum on Aging-Related Statistics. 2008. *Older Americans 2008: Key indicators of well-being.* Federal Interagency Forum on Aging-Related Statistics. Washington, DC: U. S. Government Printing Office.

Flaherty, J.H. 2008. Insomnia among hospitalized older persons. *Clin Geriatr Med* 24: 51-67.

Forestier, R., H. Desfour, J.M. Tessier, A. Francon, A.M. Foote, C. Genty, C. Rolland, C.F. Roques, and J.L. Bosson. 2009. Spa therapy in the treatment of knee osteoarthritis, a large randomized multicentre trial. *Ann Rheum Dis.* 69(4): 660-665.

Gerdner, L.A., L.K. Hart, and M.B. Zimmerman. 2008. Craniosacral still point technique: Exploring its effect in individuals with dementia. *J Gerontol Nurs* 34(3): 36-45.

Greenberg, S. 2008. A profile of older Americans: 2008 administration on aging. U.S. Department of Health and Human Services. www.aoa.gov/aoaroot/aging_statistics/Profile/index.aspx.

Hanley, J., O. Stirling, and C. Brown. 2003. Randomized controlled trial of therapeutic massage in the management of stress. *Br J Gen Pract* 53(486): 20-25.

Hasson, D., B. Arnetz, L. Jeliveus, and B. Edelstam. 2004. A randomized clinical trial of the treatment effects of massage compared to relaxation tape recordings on diffuse long-term pain. *Psychother Psychosom* 73: 17-24.

Hernandez-Reif, M., T. Field, J. Krasnegor, and H. Theakston. 2001. Lower back pain is reduced and range of motion increased after massage therapy. *Int J Neurosci* 106: 131-145.

Hodgson, N. A., and S. Anderson. 2008. The clinical efficacy of reflexology in nursing home residents with dementia. *J Altern Complem Med* 14(3): 269-275.

Holliday-Welsh, D.M., C.E. Gessert, and C.M. Renier. 2009. Massage in the management of agitation in nursing home residents with cognitive impairment. *Geriatr Nurs* 30: 108-117.

Kolcaba, K., V. Schirm, and R. Steiner. 2006. Effects of hand massage on comfort of nursing home residents. *Geriatr Nurs* 27: 85-91.

Kozak, L.E., L. Kayes, R. McCarty, C. Walkinshaw, S. Congdon, J. Kleinberger, V. Hartman, and L.J. Standish. 2009. Use of complementary and alternative medicine (CAM) by Washington State hospices. *Am J Hosp Palliat Me* 5(6): 463-468.

Kutner, J.S., M.C. Smith, L. Corbin, L. Hemphill, K. Benton, B.K. Mellis, B. Beaty, S. Felton, T.E. Yamashita, L.L. Bryant, and D.L. Fairclough. 2008. Massage therapy verses simple touch to improve pain and mood in patients with advanced cancer: A randomized trial. *Ann Intern Med* 149: 369-379.

Lämås, K., L. Lindholm, H. Stenlund, B. Engstrom, and C. Jacobsson. 2009. Effects of abdominal massage in management of constipation—A randomized controlled trial. *Int J Nurs Stud* 46: 759-767.

Lämås, K., L. Lindholm, B. Engström, and C. Jacobsson. 2010. Abdominal massage for people with constipation: A cost utility analysis. *J Adv Nurs* 66(8): 1719-1729.

MacDonald, G. 2005. *Massage for the hospital patient and medically frail client.* Hagerstown, MD: Lippincott, Williams and Wilkins.

Moyer, C.A., J. Rounds, and J.W. Hannum. 2004. A meta-analysis of massage therapy research. *Psychol Bull* 130(1): 3-18.

National Hospice and Palliative Care Organization (NHPCO). 2009. NHPCO facts and figures: Hospice care in America." www.nhpco.org/files/public/Statistics_Research/NHPCO_facts_and_figures.pdf.

Oneschuk, D., L. Balneaves, M. Verhoef, H. Boon, C. Demmer, and L. Chiu. 2007. The status of complementary therapy services in Canadian palliative care settings. *Support Care Cancer* 15: 939-947.

Perlman, A.I., A. Sabina, A.L. Williams, V.Y. Njike, and D.L. Katz. 2006. Massage therapy for osteoarthritis of the knee: A randomized controlled trial. *Arch Intern Med* 166(22): 2533-2538.

Preyde, M. 2000. Effectiveness of massage therapy for sub-acute low back pain: A randomized controlled trial. *CMAJ* 162: 1815-1820.

Reid, M.C., M. Papaleontiou, A. Ong, R. Breckman, E. Wethington, and K. Pillemer. 2008. Self-management strategies to reduce pain and improve function among older adults in community settings: A review of the evidence. *Pain Med* 9(4): 409-424.

Rose, M.K. 2010. *Comfort touch: Massage for the elderly and the ill.* Hagerstown, MD: Lippincott, Williams, and Wilkins.

Russell, N.C., C.M. Beinhorn, and M.A. Frenkel. 2008. Role of massage therapy in cancer care. *J Altern Complem Med* 4(2): 209-214.

Soden, K., K. Vincent, and S. Craske. 2004. A randomized controlled trial of aromatherapy massage in a hospice setting. *Palliative Med* 18(2): 87-92.

Thompson, D. L. 2006. *Hands heal: Communication, documentation, and insurance billing for manual therapists.* 3rd ed. Hagerstown, MD: Lippincott, Williams, and Wilkins.

Tsao, J.C. 2007. Effectiveness of massage therapy for chronic, non-malignant pain: A review. *Evid-Based Complement Altern Med* 4(2): 165-179.

Vaht, M., R. Birkenfeldt, and M. Ubner. 2008. An evaluation of the effect of differing lengths of spa therapy upon patients with osteoarthritis. *Complement Ther Clin Pract* 14: 60-64.

Vaillant, J., A. Rouland, P. Martigne, R. Braujou, M.J. Nissen, J.L. Caillat-Miousse, N. Vuillerme, V. Nougier, and R. Juvin. 2009. Massage and mobilization of the feet and ankles in elderly adults: Effect on clinical balance performance. *Manual Ther* 14(6): 661-664.

Walach, H., C. Guthlin, and M. Konig. 2005. Efficacy of massage therapy in chronic pain: A pragmatic randomized trial. *J Altern Complem Med* 9: 837-846.

Williams, A.L., P.A. Selwyn, L. Liberti, S. Molde, V.Y. Njike, R. McCorkle, F.D. Zelterman, and D.L. Katz. 2005. A randomized controlled trial of meditation and massage effects on quality of life in people with late stage disease: A pilot study. *J Palliat Med* 8(5): 939-952.

Woods, D.L., and M. Dimond. 2002. The effect of therapeutic touch on agitated behavior and cortisol on persons with Alzheimer's disease. *Biol Res Nur* 4(2): 104-114.

Woods, D.L., R.F. Craven, and J. Whitney. 2005. The effects of therapeutic touch on behavioral symptoms of persons with dementia. *Altern Ther* 11(1): 66-74.

Headache

Albert Moraska, PhD

Headache, identified by pain located above a plane formed from the outer corner of the eyes to the center of the external auditory canals, is a common and sometimes debilitating health condition. More than 90% of the population has experienced a headache (Barna and Hashmi 2004). The associated pain not only affects personal well-being and quality of life (Holroyd et al. 1999; Holroyd et al. 2000; Rasmussen 1993), but also poses a significant socioeconomic burden in the form of lost workdays and decreased productivity. With the onset of recurrent headaches typically occurring in young adulthood, those who suffer from headaches can be affected for much of their productive lives (Rasmussen 1999). In a typical year, 12% of those with headache miss up to four work days (Rasmussen 1999; Schwartz, Stewart, and Lipton 1997), which accounts for 20% of absences due to sickness (Rasmussen, Jensen, and Olesen 1992). When all types are considered, the amount of disability that they cause would rank headache within the top 10 health concerns worldwide (Stovner et al. 2007).

The use of complementary and alternative medicine (CAM) and therapies to address complaints is common among headache sufferers. Data reported from clinic sites throughout the world note that between 30% and 84% of sufferers use at least one CAM modality to specifically address their headaches (Gaul et al. 2009). Most patients who seek CAM therapies use treatments that are body oriented rather than biologically oriented (e.g., herbs, nutritional supplements). They cite massage therapy (MT) as the first or second most popular treatment modality, with up to 46.1% employing MT (Gaul et al. 2009; Rossi et al. 2006). Although the number of studies examining MT as a treatment for headache is not large, the available studies show promising results for both tension-type and migraine headaches. Given the prevalence of headache and the increasing use of MT for the treatment of associated symptoms (e.g., pain, function, mood, stress relief), this chapter reviews the research on types of headaches and the evidence on MT effectiveness, and suggests clinical guidelines.

HEADACHE TYPES

The International Classification of Headache Disorders (ICHD-II) identifies 13 main categories of headache (Olesen et al. 2004). However, present purposes are best served by distinguishing tension-type headache (TTH), migraine headache, and secondary headache. Commonalities among TTH and migraine, which are potentially important to understand in clinical settings, are also noted.

Tension-Type Headache (TTH)

tension-type headache

▸ The most common type of headache, usually experienced as a dull ache, which resolves with time or pain medication.

Tension-type headache is experienced as a dull ache that typically resolves with time or in response to nonprescription analgesics. Specific TTH symptoms are listed in figure 10.1. Duration varies, but commonly is shorter than 8 hours. For many, headaches first occur between 25 and 30 years of age. They are most frequent between 30 and 40 years of age, with minimally decreased incidence in successive decades. Prevalence of TTH is about 25% greater in women (Jensen and Stovner 2008). Though a single TTH may be minimally disruptive, frequent TTHs represent a clinical condition.

The ICHD-II characterizes TTH as episodic or chronic, based on the frequency of headache occurrence.

Episodic Tension-Type Headache

episodic tension-type headaches (ETTH)

▸ A system for categorizing tension-type headaches based on frequency. Infrequent ETTH consists of 12 or fewer episodes in a year, while frequent ETTH is more than 12 and as many as 180 episodes in a year.

Episodic tension-type headaches (ETTH) can be further separated into infrequent and frequent forms. Infrequent ETTH is characterized by headaches occurring on fewer than 12 days per year, whereas frequent ETTH occurs 12 to 180 days per year. Additionally, for frequent ETTH, this pattern must have been in place for at least 3 months. At any given time, the episodic form of TTH affects between 20% and 42% of adults (Schwartz et al. 1998; Stovner et al. 2007).

Chronic Tension-Type Headache

chronic tension-type headache

▸ A pattern of 15 or more headache episodes per month for at least 3 months.

A person may progress from ETTH to a more serious variant identified as *chronic tension-type headache* (CTTH). Someone with CTTH experiences headaches 15 or more days per month for at least 3 months. These frequent and extended periods of pain increase the likelihood of detrimental neurological changes compared with ETTH (Herren-Gerber et al. 2004; Lipchik et al. 1996). Such changes make CTTH more difficult to treat effectively (Holroyd 2002). They can even lead to migraine-like symptoms, which may prevent accurate diagnosis. CTTH affects about 3% of the population (Pascual, Colas, and Castillo 2001; Stovner et al. 2007).

Migraine Headache

migraine headache

▸ A type of moderate to severe headache, sometimes preceded by visual disturbances, that results from the hyperexcitability of nociceptors.

Migraine headaches result from a structurally normal nervous system that responds abnormally to a range of nonnoxious stimuli, which can include foods or their ingredients (e.g., wine, cheese, caffeine), hormonal changes, or environmental stressors, such as stressful situations, changes in sleep, or changes in barometric pressure (Hauge, Kirchmann, and Olesen 2010; Fukui et al. 2008). The migraine originates within brain structures, but the resultant pain comes from hyperexcitability of nociceptors located in the peripheral vasculature (Olesen et al. 2009). Pain from migraine headache can last between 30 minutes and 72 hours. It is of moderate to severe intensity. Characteristics of migraine headache are presented in figure 10.1.

About 12% of adults and between 5% and 10% of children have suffered a migraine. They are more likely to fall in the age range of 15 to 55 years and to have a family history of migraine. Migraine is three times more common in women than in men (Lipton, Stewart, et al. 2001), but is less common in the elderly. Frequency often decreases after menopause (Rasmussen 1993). In 20% to 30% of cases, the ordinary migraine symptoms are accompanied by aura, a slow onset of neurological symptoms prior to the actual headache. An aura most often takes the form of a visual disturbance, but may also be sensed as a tingling sensation in the face or as difficulty speaking. The aura occurs before headache pain begins and usually lasts less than an hour. Box 10.1 describes a case example of someone experiencing a migraine with aura.

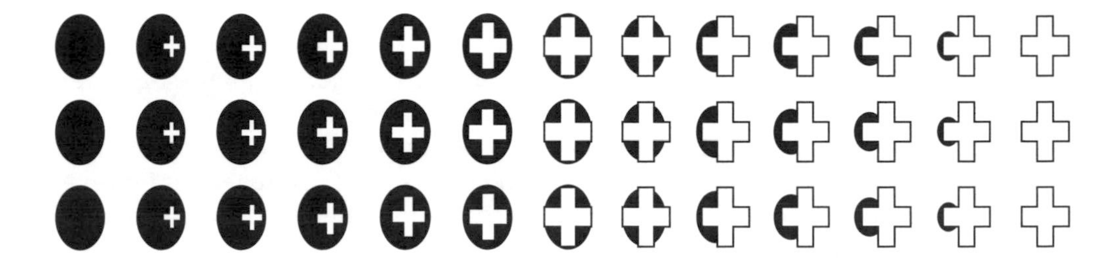

Migraine symptoms

- Unilateral or bilateral location
- Pulsating pain
- Moderate to severe intensity
- Aggravated by routine physical activity
- Nausea or vomiting

Tension-type headache symptoms

- Bilateral location
- Pressing or tightening pain
- Mild to moderate intensity
- Not aggravated by routine physical activity
- No nausea or vomiting

Figure 10.1 Characteristics of migraine and tension-type headaches.

BOX 10.1
Case Example of Migraine

About 88% of the population has not experienced a migraine; therefore, it can be helpful to have migraine attack described in detail. Below is the depiction of the experiences of a woman during her typical migraine attack.

"My first symptom is usually blurred vision that makes it difficult to discern fine details, such as reading, although larger objects are reasonably clear. I typically have no headache pain during this aura phase, which usually lasts 30 to 60 minutes. If I am able to find a dark room and force myself to sleep at this point, there is a good chance that I can sleep through the worst of the headache pain."

"If I can't sleep, a headache will start slowly, with a heavy sensation in the frontal region of my head and increasing nausea. After 15 minutes, the pain will escalate rapidly and reach an excruciating level (9 or 10 on a 10-point scale) within a few minutes. Exposure to light makes the headache worse. Pain is usually on one side of my head and throbbing. It is aggravated by physical effort. Even mild activities, such as walking, can worsen the pain. The sensation of nausea and the need to vomit increase over the next few hours. I have found that vomiting provides temporary relief of headache pain, but the effect is short lived and sometimes leads to dehydration. I am unable to do any activity during this phase and time seems to pass very slowly. Even thinking is difficult, and I feel frustrated that this time is so unproductive. I close my eyes and try to think about nothing, almost as if I am in a meditative state. The worst of the pain dissipates in about 3 to 4 hours."

"Over the final hour, my headache pain begins to decrease and reaches a moderate level (4 or 5 out of 10). Pain continues to decrease over the next 24 hours, but I still have a low-level headache and sensory effects. During this period, I am able to function somewhat normally, although sudden head movement immediately causes a severe headache for a few minutes. Eventually, the headache dissipates and I can return to all of my usual activities."

Secondary Headaches

TTH and migraine cover the majority of the primary headaches a massage therapist will encounter in practice. Other forms of headache that relate to injury, substance abuse, medication overuse, or disease processes are considered secondary headache. Given the breadth of causes and the general lack of research involving massage therapy for these conditions, they are not specifically addressed here.

Commonalities Among TTH and Migraine

Although TTH and migraine are different entities, it is now recognized that headache severity, rather than specific symptoms, is of key importance. It is common for people diagnosed with TTH to also experience migraine-like symptoms, and vice versa (Turkdogan et al. 2006). As such, a continuum of headache may exist where definite TTH and migraine anchor their respective ends (figure 10.1). It is likely that a person seeking massage therapy for treatment of headache will have elements of both TTH and migraine.

SECONDARY ISSUES FOR HEADACHE SUFFERERS

Affective and emotional factors figure prominently in chronic pain disorders, including headache (Andrasik et al. 2005). With this in mind, treatment for such conditions should address these factors in addition to addressing pain (Holroyd et al. 2000). A recent study of TTH sufferers demonstrates the viability of this approach. Patients who received a series of 12 MT sessions reported significant reductions of depression, anxiety, and daily stress, in addition to decreased headache pain (Moraska and Chandler 2009).

Anxiety and Depression

Anxiety, depression, and headache are all frequently comorbid. Anxiety disorders and depression are five times more prevalent in headache sufferers than they are in matched samples of people without headaches (Holroyd et al. 2000; Juang et al. 2000; Zwart et al. 2003). Because of the frequency with which anxiety, depression, and headache occur together, and of MT's promising effects on anxiety and depression (see chapter 13), this form of treatment may be of special value to headache sufferers.

Stress

Stressful life events are implicated in the onset, exacerbation, and maintenance of headache (De Benedittis, Lorenzetti, and Pieri 1990). This factor can increase the frequency of headaches (Houle and Nash 2008). Stress is the most common headache trigger for both migraine and CTTH (Rasmussen 1993; De Benedittis, Lorenzetti, and Pieri 1990), with 88% of TTH patients reporting it as a precipitating factor (Holroyd et al. 2000). Small but recurrent stressful events are considered more problematic than major events (De Benedittis and Lorenzetti 1992). CTTH sufferers not only report a greater number of daily stresses than healthy control subjects, but they also view similar events as more stressful (Holroyd et al. 2000).

CAUSES OF HEADACHE

Headache is a symptom of an underlying pathology, rather than a disease itself. For most people with primary TTH, the underlying pathology is myofascial pain syndrome (Kuan 2009), in which headache pain originates in skeletal muscle and fascia and possibly in conjunction with myofascial trigger points (MTrPs). For migraine headache, the underlying pathology is less clear.

Muscular

The ICHD-II identifies a skeletal-muscle component associated with TTH (Olesen et al. 2004). TTH sufferers report elevation in skeletal muscle tenderness, increased presence of active MTrPs, and physical abnormalities in cervical and cranial muscles (Fernández-de-las-Peñas, Alonso-Blanco, Cuadrado, et al. 2006b, Fernández-de-las-Peñas, Alonso-Blanco, Fernández-Carnero, et al. 2006). Pain originating from an MTrP can refer to other body regions and can exactly reproduce a headache patients' pain complaint (Fernández-de-las-Peñas, et al. 2007). In one study, MTrPs were identified in the suboccipital muscles of all CTTH subjects, but were only identified in 30% of a healthy control group (Fernández-de-las-Peñas, Alonso-Blanco, Cuadrado, et al. 2006a).

A forward head position requires prolonged contraction of cervical musculature and is a contributing factor in TTH. The amount of forward head posture correlates with headache frequency and duration, and the presence of MTrPs in the suboccipital muscles (Fernández-de-las-Peñas, Alonso-Blanco, Cuadrado, et al. 2006a). Poor workplace ergonomics or jaw clenching lead to increased presence of MTrPs in the trapezius muscle, which may predispose people to headache (Treaster et al. 2006).

With regard to migraine headache, a bilateral increase in tenderness of the temporalis muscle is noted, even though the headaches typically occur on only one side (Fernández-de-las-Peñas et al. 2009). Cervical muscles in migraine patients also exhibit greater tenderness (Leistad et al. 2006; Mongini et al. 2004) and an increased presence of MTrPs (Calandre et al. 2006). These may sensitize the central nervous system, increase vulnerability to migraine triggers, or heighten the pain response during migraine. However, the exact relationship between muscle tenderness and migraine pain is not well understood, and more research is needed.

Neurological

For migraine with or without aura, the initiating event occurs in the occipital lobe of the brain, with subsequent effects in the peripheral vasculature that lead to pain (Chakravarty and Sen 2010). The occipital lobe is where vision is interpreted, and disruption in this region accounts for the visual abnormalities associated with aura. Efferent impulses from the trigeminal nerve signal chemicals to be released at peripheral arteries and arterioles, causing vasodilation and a pulsating effect in the temporal artery. Stretching of the blood vessel walls sensitizes nerve endings, and nociceptive chemicals are released that initiate pain sensation. Much of the pain experienced during a migraine headache is a response from peripheral nociceptors located in the meninges and meningeal arteries. Notably, experimental stimulation of cerebral arteries in people without a history of migraine produces referred pain to retro-orbital and temporal regions, which are common areas of migraine pain. This result suggests that such nociceptor signaling and neuronal activity play an important role in generating migraine pain (Olesen et al. 2009).

While most neurological headache research has focused on migraine, it should be noted that neuronal changes also occur in people with chronic pain, such as CTTH. Such neurological changes are difficult to reverse, making treatment more difficult when headache frequency increases for a prolonged period, as is the case when episodic TTH progresses to chronic TTH (Bendtsen 2000; Fernández-de-las-Peñas, Cuadrado, et al. 2007).

EFFECTS OF MASSAGE THERAPY ON HEADACHE

Although the number of studies examining massage therapy as a treatment for headache is not large, the available studies show promising results for both tension-type and migraine headaches. Specific studies have also separately examined massage therapy as the sole form of treatment, and as a component of a multimodal treatment approach.

Tension-Type Headache

Studies of massage for TTH have either used massage as one component of a treatment program or as the sole form of treatment.

Massage as a Component of TTH Treatment

Two clinical trials have included massage as part of a physical therapy program for treating TTH, which included treatments to correct posture, induce relaxation, and reduce daily stressors (Hammill, Cook, and Rosecrance 1996; Torelli, Jensen, and Olesen 2004). Both studies report a significant reduction in headache frequency, the single most important headache measure, with effects persisting 12 weeks past cessation of treatment. However, massage is only a small portion of the treatment programs in these studies. Also, secondary headache measures of intensity and duration were only minimally affected.

Massage as the Sole Treatment for TTH

Three studies using within-group design have examined massage therapy as the sole treatment for TTH. The massage administered in each of these studies emphasized reduction of MTrP activity in cervical and cranial muscles. Each study provided a relatively high number of massage treatment sessions (8-12), administered with high regularity (2-5 massage sessions per week). Duration of sessions ranged across studies from 30 to 50 minutes.

All three studies found a reduction in the frequency of headaches, which was as high as 50% in two of the studies (Puustjarvi, Airaksinen, and Pontinen 1990; Quinn, Chandler, and Moraska 2002). Secondary measures of headache pain, intensity, and duration were reduced by at least 30% in the two studies that assessed those variables (Moraska and Chandler 2008; Quinn, Chandler, and Moraska 2002). Further, treatment effects were seen to persist beyond the treatment period at 3 weeks (Moraska and Chandler 2008) and at 6 months (Puustjarvi, Airaksinen, and Pontinen 1990) compared to baseline. Nevertheless, it must be noted that this is a small number of studies with a relatively small number of total subjects, and that the limitations of within-group design leave open the possibility that the observed effects were due to causes other than massage.

No peer-reviewed studies have examined the immediate effect of massage on a current headache, but a single 40-minute massage session, also designed to reduce trigger points in the head, neck and shoulder regions, did reduce self-reported headache pain 24 hours after the session in 11 patients with CTTH (Toro-Velasco et al. 2009). In addition, self-massage of cranial musculature is regularly employed by 25% of TTH patients to reduce pain, even though the benefit wanes within 5 minutes, and only 8% report good or excellent pain relief (Zanchin et al. 2001).

Migraine

Preemption of migraine pain with massage, consisting of vigorous bilateral compression and massage to the frontal branches of the temporal artery, was reported in 81% of cases when treatment was administered at the first sign of aura and continued until aura dissipated, which may take as long as 1 hour (Lipton 1986). When massage therapy was administered after the headache phase had begun, the treatment was ineffective at aborting pain. However, another study reports that such treatment may still provide some relief if it is applied over the greater occipital nerve field (Piovesan et al. 2007).

Massage therapy for prevention of migraine has been successful in some studies. However, it may take as much as 5 weeks of weekly or twice-weekly massage before improvement is noted. When massage treatment is directed toward the occipital region with various stroking, mobilization, and rhythmic techniques, a reduction in headache frequency is found. However, the effect appears to be greater for mild headaches, since this treatment did not change the number of moderate and severe migraines (Hernandez-Reif et al. 1998). In another study, massage applied to the muscles of the back, shoulders, head, and neck using neuromuscular techniques and trigger-point therapy reduced the frequency of migraine by 33%, but did not affect headache intensity (Lawler and Cameron 2006).

EXPLAINING MASSAGE THERAPY EFFECTS

Several mechanisms may underlie the effect of massage therapy on headache. These include the reduction of MTrP activity, compression of the temporal artery, vibration of occipital or trigeminal nerves, and reduction of stress. However, before expanding on these, it must be noted that each of these mechanisms is speculative. Further research on MT mechanisms of action is needed.

Treatment of MTrPs may alleviate TTH because the regions of referred pain patterns often overlap the regions of headache pain. The use of massage for pain reduction associated with MTrPs is supported in pain patients more generally (Fernández-de-las-Peñas, Alonso-Blanco, Fernández-Carnero, et al. 2006; Fryer and Hodgson 2005) and in TTH patients who report a reduction in both local and referred pain following treatment (Toro-Velasco et al. 2009). Furthermore, CTTH patients with headaches shorter than 8.5 hours in duration and fewer than 5 days per week in frequency respond well to MTrP treatment (Fernández-de-las-Peñas et al. 2008). On the other hand, it must also be noted that MTrP treatments may initiate or worsen headache, including migraines, in some cases (Calandre et al. 2006).

Vigorous bilateral compression and massage to the frontal branches of the temporal artery is a successful technique for preventing a migraine if administered at the start of aura (Lipton 1986). If a migraine has already begun, compression on the temporal artery is much less successful, but an estimated 30% of persons still benefit (Drummond and Lance 1983). Conversely, compression on jugular veins, resulting in venous distention, can aggravate migraine headache, particularly if patients are lying down or have a long-lasting (>30h) headache (Chou et al. 2004; Doepp et al. 2003). In a single-subject study, massage stimulation over the greater occipital nerve territory reduced migraine pain intensity, but it was insufficient to terminate headache. However, this may be an area for future research, since electrical stimulation and acupuncture in the suboccipital region have been successful at addressing migraine (Linde et al. 2009). Possibly, these techniques stimulate large-diameter nerve fibers that are sensitive to touch, pressure, and vibration, which then inhibit the transmission of the thinner pain fibers at the spinal cord (Melzack 1999).

While it is possible that trigger-point therapy is effective on patients with migraine headache, it is also possible that massage acts in a different, less specific manner. Stress is a trigger for both TTH and migraine and is implicated in perpetuating headache. Treatment strategies that help reduce patient stress, including massage, may provide an indirect mechanism to reduce headache over the long term.

RECOMMENDATIONS FOR MASSAGE THERAPY PRACTICE

Judging from the available studies, massage delivered by a trained massage therapist, with a focus on trigger points and muscle tension in the head, neck, and shoulders, can reduce the frequency and intensity of headaches. More specifically, massage therapy for both tension-type and migraine-type headaches should focus on the reduction of trigger points in cervical and cranial muscles. Treatment during the aura phase of migraine-type headaches should also include bilateral compression and massage to the frontal branches of the temporal artery. Massage for general relaxation is also of value to this population. It should be applied to reduce chronic pain, anxiety, and depression, which may also be present in headache sufferers. In addition, care should be taken to limit their exposure to light, sound, odors, and other common headache triggers during treatment. Massage therapists should also educate clients about posture, exercise, relaxation methods, and identification of headache triggers.

Evidence supports immediate benefits from a single session of massage and longer-term benefits from a series of MT treatments. However, immediate reduction of pain may be limited when massage is applied during a headache. Additional research is needed to determine the length and number of sessions, MT techniques, and approaches that are most effective for headache sufferers.

DIRECTIONS FOR FUTURE RESEARCH

Although all categories of headache need further research to clearly identify whether massage is an effective complementary treatment, several areas would particularly benefit from additional focus. Clarification regarding whether massage is effective for ETTH and CTTH is needed, since adaptations of the central nervous system occur in patients with chronic pain. Also, the question of whether massage therapy used in combination with other treatments, such as medication or biofeedback, may yield benefit beyond either treatment alone has not been addressed. The lack of a clear separation between migraine and TTH makes research into massage for headache particularly challenging, since different bodywork techniques may benefit one condition more than the other. A concerted research effort is needed to determine which types of massage in which dosages are the most effective for directly or indirectly reducing the pain and suffering of headaches,

Case Study

Robert T. and Julie R., a couple, both suffered frequent headaches for nearly 18 years. Robert's problem was a recurring daily headache of low but persistent pain that usually began in the morning and was often still present by evening. His physician speculated that his headaches were of neurological origin. Julie's headaches were less frequent, but still occurred three or four times per week. They were of moderate intensity. In recent years, they were increasingly interfering with her work and social life. Julie assumed that her headaches were caused by muscle tension, since she was frequently tense at work and because rubbing her temples was sometimes effective at providing relief. Julie and Robert had both visited several headache specialists and had tried many over-the-counter and prescription medications, but were dissatisfied with the results since their effectiveness was limited. Both were also concerned about side effects of medication.

Robert and Julie were intrigued by a bulletin for a headache treatment study investigating the use of massage, and they both enrolled. The study provided eight 30-minute massage sessions by a trained massage therapist, Stephan D. Following thorough individual health histories and physical assessments, Stephan explained that he would primarily follow a specific MT protocol designed for the study. He added that he was permitted to adapt some aspects of the protocol, such as the amount of time devoted to certain muscles, to focus on their unique needs. He further explained that MT treatment would focus on the reduction of muscle tension and trigger points in the shoulder, neck, and face. Robert and Julie were shown how to rate their pain on a scale so their responses to treatment could be quantified. They were informed that at the end of the study, they would be provided with information on self-massage and exercises for reducing and treating headaches.

Midway through the study, Julie confidently reported a dramatic improvement in her condition, even though her headache log indicated only a slight improvement in headache frequency, duration, and intensity. Curiously, the quantitative data seemed to underestimate the value of MT for Julie. By the end of the study, Julie was convinced of MT's positive effects, since she was now experiencing no more than one headache per week. Further, when she did have a headache, it seemed to be less intense and shorter in duration than before.

By contrast, at the end of the study, Robert reported that his headache pain had marginally improved. He now had occasional headache-free days, and the intensity of his headaches seemed to have decreased slightly. More evident, however, was that his attitude seemed improved; he felt happier and more relaxed, and Julie thought that he seemed more enthusiastic about participating in social activities. Based on these results, Julie and Robert both regularly used the self-massage techniques that they had been taught, and supplemented these with regular MT appointments aimed at managing their headaches and improving their quality of life more generally.

SUMMARY

Headaches are a common health complaint, and headache sufferers are already using massage therapy as an approach to treatment. Though the amount of research examining massage therapy for headache reduction and prevention is small, the results are promising and do provide some guidelines for treatment. Therapists working with this condition need to be able to differentiate tension-type headache from migraine headache; provide treatment that focuses on the reduction of trigger points in the head, neck, and shoulders; and educate their patients about posture, exercise, relaxation methods, and avoidance of headache triggers. They should also be prepared to offer evidence-based advice for minimizing headache. Future research should take care to differentiate the effect of massage on chronic versus episodic tension-type headaches, since different underlying adaptations of the central nervous system among these conditions may affect outcomes. Additional research is also needed to determine the length and number of MT sessions and the techniques and approaches that are most effective.

REFERENCES

Andrasik, F., G.L. Lipchik, D.C. McCrory, and D.A. Wittrock. 2005. Outcome measurement in behavioral headache research: Headache parameters and psychosocial outcomes. *Headache* 45 (5): 429-437.

Barna, S., and M. Hashmi. 2004. Occipital neuralgia. *Pain Manag Rounds* 1(7): 1-6.

Bendtsen, L. 2000. Central sensitization in tension-type headache—Possible pathophysiological mechanisms. *Cephalalgia* 20(5): 486-508.

Calandre, E.P., J. Hidalgo, J.M. Garcia-Leiva, and F. Rico-Villademoros. 2006. Trigger point evaluation in migraine patients: An indication of peripheral sensitization linked to migraine predisposition? *Eur J Neurol* 13(3): 244-249.

Chakravarty, A., and A. Sen. 2010. Migraine, neuropathic pain and nociceptive pain: Towards a unifying concept. *Med Hypotheses* 74(2): 225-231.

Chou, C.H., A.C. Chao, S.R. Lu, H.H. Hu, and S.J. Wang. 2004. Cephalic venous congestion aggravates only migraine-type headaches. *Cephalalgia* 24(11): 973-979.

De Benedittis, G., and A. Lorenzetti. 1992. The role of stressful life events in the persistence of primary headache: Major events vs. daily hassles. *Pain* 51(1): 35-42.

De Benedittis, G., A. Lorenzetti, and A. Pieri. 1990. The role of stressful life events in the onset of chronic primary headache. *Pain* 40(1): 65-75.

Doepp, F., S.J. Schreiber, J.P. Dreier, K.M. Einhaupl, and J.M. Valdueza. 2003. Migraine aggravation caused by cephalic venous congestion. *Headache* 43(2): 96-98.

Drummond, P.D., and J.W. Lance. 1983. Extracranial vascular changes and the source of pain in migraine headache. *Ann Neurol* 13(1): 32-37.

Fernández-de-las-Peñas, C., C. Alonso-Blanco, M.L. Cuadrado, R.D. Gerwin, and J.A. Pareja. 2006a. Trigger points in the suboccipital muscles and forward head posture in tension-type headache. *Headache* 46 (3):454-60.

———. 2006b. Myofascial trigger points and their relationship to headache clinical parameters in chronic tension-type headache. *Headache* 46(8): 1264-1272.

Fernández-de-las-Peñas, C., C. Alonso-Blanco, J. Fernández-Carnero, and J.C. Miangolarra-Page. 2006. The immediate effect of ischemic compression technique and transverse friction massage on tenderness of active and latent myofascial trigger points: A pilot study. *J Bodyw Mov Ther* 10(1): 3-9.

Fernández-de-las-Peñas, C., M.L. Cuadrado, L. Arendt-Nielsen, D.G. Simons, and J.A. Pareja. 2007. Myofascial trigger points and sensitization: An updated pain model for tension-type headache. *Cephalalgia* 27(5): 383-393.

Fernández-de-las-Peñas, C., H. Y. Ge, L. Arendt-Nielsen, M. L. Cuadrado, and J. A. Pareja. 2007. "The local and referred pain from myofascial trigger points in the temporalis muscle contributes to pain profile in chronic tension-type headache." *CJP* 23(9): 786-792.

Fernández-de-las-Peñas, C., J.A. Cleland, M.L. Cuadrado, and J.A. Pareja. 2008. Predictor variables for identifying patients with chronic tension-type headache who are likely to achieve short-term success with muscle trigger point therapy. *Cephalalgia* 28(3): 264-275.

Fernández-de-las-Peñas, C., P. Madeleine, M.L. Cuadrado, H.Y. Ge, L. Arendt-Nielsen, and J.A. Pareja. 2009. Pressure pain sensitivity mapping of the temporalis muscle revealed bilateral pressure hyperalgesia in patients with strictly unilateral migraine. *Cephalalgia* 29(6): 670-676.

Fryer, G., and L. Hodgson. 2005. The effect of manual pressure release on myofascial trigger points in the upper trapezius muscle. *J Bodyw Mov Ther* 9: 248-255.

Fukui, P.T., T.R. Goncalves, C.G. Strabelli, N.M. Lucchino, F.C. Matos, J.P. Santos, E. Zukerman, V. Zukerman-Guendler, J.P. Mercante, M.R. Masruha, D.S. Vieira, and M.F. Peres. 2008. Trigger factors in migraine patients. *Arq Neuro-psiquiatr* 66(3A): 494-499.

Gaul, C., R. Eismann, T. Schmidt, A. May, E. Leinisch, T. Wieser, S. Evers, K. Henkel, G. Franz, and S. Zierz. 2009. Use of complementary and alternative medicine in patients suffering from primary headache disorders. *Cephalalgia* 29(10): 1069-1078

Hammill, J.M., T.M. Cook, and J.C. Rosecrance. 1996. Effectiveness of a physical therapy regimen in the treatment of tension-type headache. *Headache* 36(3): 149-153.

Hauge, A., M. Kirchmann, and J. Olesen. 2010. Trigger factors in migraine with aura. *Cephalalgia* 30(3): 346-353.

Hernandez-Reif, M., J. Dieter, T. Field, B. Swerdlow, and M. Diego. 1998. Migraine headaches are reduced by massage therapy. *Int J Neurosci* 96: 1-11.

Herren-Gerber, R., S. Weiss, L. Arendt-Nielsen, S. Petersen-Felix, G. Di Stefano, B.P. Radanov, and M. Curatolo. 2004. Modulation of central hypersensitivity by nociceptive input in chronic pain after whiplash injury. *Pain Med* 5(4): 366-376.

Holroyd, K.A. 2002. Behavioral and psychologic aspects of the pathophysiology and management of tension-type headache. *Curr Pain Headache Rep* 6(5): 401-407.

Holroyd, K.A., P. Malinoski, M.K. Davis, and G.L. Lipchik. 1999. The three dimensions of headache impact: Pain, disability and affective distress. *Pain* 83(3): 571-578.

Holroyd, K.A., M. Stensland, G.L. Lipchik, K.R. Hill, F.S. O'Donnell, and G. Cordingley. 2000. Psychosocial correlates and impact of chronic tension-type headaches. *Headache* 40(1): 3-16.

Houle, T., and J.M. Nash. 2008. Stress and headache chronification. *Headache* 48(1): 40-44.

Jensen, R., and L.J. Stovner. 2008. Epidemiology and comorbidity of headache. *Lancet Neurol* 7(4): 354-361.

Juang, K.D., S.J. Wang, J.L. Fuh, S.R. Lu, and T.P. Su. 2000. Comorbidity of depressive and anxiety disorders in chronic daily headache and its subtypes. *Headache* 40(10): 818-823.

Kuan, T.S. 2009. Current studies on myofascial pain syndrome. *Curr Pain Headache Rep* 13(5): 365-369.

Lawler, S.P., and L.D. Cameron. 2006. A randomized, controlled trial of massage therapy as a treatment for migraine. *Ann Behav Med* 32(1): 50-59.

Leistad, R.B., T. Sand, R.H. Westgaard, K.B. Nilsen, and L.J. Stovner. 2006. Stress-induced pain and muscle activity in patients with migraine and tension-type headache. *Cephalalgia* 26(1): 64-73.

Linde, K., G. Allais, B. Brinkhaus, E. Manheimer, A. Vickers, and A.R. White. 2009. Acupuncture for migraine prophylaxis. *Cochrane Db Syst Rev* 1: CD001218.

Lipchik, G.L., K.A. Holroyd, C.R. France, S.A. Kvaal, D. Segal, G.E. Cordingley, L.A. Rokicki, and H.R. McCool. 1996. Central and peripheral mechanisms in chronic tension-type headache. *Pain* 64(3): 467-475.

Lipton, R.B., S. Diamond, M. Reed, M.L. Diamond, and W.F. Stewart. 2001. Migraine diagnosis and treatment: Results from the American Migraine Study II. *Headache* 41(7): 638-645.

Lipton, R.B., W.F. Stewart, S. Diamond, M.L. Diamond, and M. Reed. 2001. Prevalence and burden of migraine in the United States: Data from the American Migraine Study II. *Headache* 41(7): 646-657.

Lipton, S.A. 1986. Prevention of classic migraine headache by digital massage of the superficial temporal arteries during visual aura. *Ann Neurol* 19(5): 515-516.

Melzack, R. 1999. From the gate to the neuromatrix. *Pain* 6: S121-S126.

Mongini, F., G. Ciccone, A. Deregibus, L. Ferrero, and T. Mongini. 2004. Muscle tenderness in different headache types and its relation to anxiety and depression. *Pain* 112(1-2): 59-64.

Moraska, A. and C. Chandler. 2009. "Changes in psychological parameters in patients with tension-type headache following massage therapy: a pilot study." *J Man Manip Ther* 17(2): 86-94.

Moraska, A., and C. Chandler. 2008. Changes in clinical parameters in patients with tension-type headache following massage therapy: A pilot study. *J Man Manip Ther* 16(2): 106-112.

Olesen, J., M. Bousser, D. Diener, D. Dodick, M. First, P.J. Goadsby, H. Goebel, M.J. Lainez, J.W. Lance, R. Lipton, G. Nappi, F. Sakai, J. Schoenen, S. Silberstein, and T. Steiner. 2004. The international classification of headache disorders: 2nd edition. *Cephalalgia* 24(1): S9-S160.

Olesen, J., R. Burstein, M. Ashina, and P. Tfelt-Hansen. 2009. Origin of pain in migraine: Evidence for peripheral sensitisation. *Lancet Neurol* 8(7): 679-690.

Pascual, J., R. Colas, and J. Castillo. 2001. Epidemiology of chronic daily headache. *Curr Pain Headache Rep* 5(6): 529-536.

Piovesan, E.J., F. Di Stani, P.A. Kowacs, R.A. Mulinari, V.H. Radunz, M. Utiumi, E.B. Muranka, M.L. Giublin, and L.C. Werneck. 2007. Massaging over the greater occipital nerve reduces the intensity of migraine attacks: Evidence for inhibitory trigemino-cervical convergence mechanisms. *Arq Neuro-psiquiatr* 65(3A): 599-604.

Puustjarvi, K., O. Airaksinen, and P.J. Pontinen. 1990. The effects of massage in patients with chronic tension headache. *Acupunct Electrother Res* 15(2): 159-162.

Quinn, C., C. Chandler, and A. Moraska. 2002. Massage therapy and frequency of chronic tension headaches. *Am J Public Health* 92(10): 1657-1661.

Rasmussen, B.K. 1993. Migraine and tension-type headache in a general population: Precipitating factors, female hormones, sleep pattern and relation to lifestyle. *Pain* 53(1): 65-72.

———. 1999. Epidemiology and socio-economic impact of headache. *Cephalalgia* 19(25): S20-S23.

Rasmussen, B.K., R. Jensen, and J. Olesen. 1992. Impact of headache on sickness absence and utilisation of medical services: A Danish population study. *J Epidemiol Community Health* 46(4): 443-446.

Rossi, P., G. Di Lorenzo, J. Faroni, M.G. Malpezzi, F. Cesarino, and G. Nappi. 2006. Use of complementary and alternative medicine by patients with chronic tension-type headache: Results of a headache clinic survey. *Headache* 46(4): 622-631

Schwartz, B.S., W.F. Stewart, and R.B. Lipton. 1997. Lost workdays and decreased work effectiveness associated with headache in the workplace. *J Occup Environ Med* 39(4): 320-327.

Schwartz, B.S., W.F. Stewart, D. Simon, and R.B. Lipton. 1998. Epidemiology of tension-type headache. *JAMA* 279(5): 381-383.

Stovner, L.J., K. Hagen, R. Jensen, Z. Katsarava, R. Lipton, A. Scher, T. Steiner, and J.A. Zwart. 2007. The global burden of headache: A documentation of headache prevalence and disability worldwide. *Cephalalgia* 27(3): 193-210.

Torelli, P., R. Jensen, and J. Olesen. 2004. Physiotherapy for tension-type headache: A controlled study. *Cephalalgia* 24(1): 29-36.

Toro-Velasco, C., M. Arroyo-Morales, C. Fernández-de-las-Peñas, J.A. Cleland, and F.J. Barrero-Hernandez. 2009. Short-term effects of manual therapy on heart rate variability, mood state, and pressure pain sensitivity in patients with chronic tension-type headache: A pilot study. *J Manipulative Physiol Ther* 32(7): 527-535.

Treaster, D., W.S. Marras, D. Burr, J.E. Sheedy, and D. Hart. 2006. Myofascial trigger point development from visual and postural stressors during computer work. *J Electromyogr Kinesiol* 16(2): 115-124.

Turkdogan, D., S. Cagirici, D. Soylemez, H. Sur, C. Bilge, and U. Turk. 2006. Characteristic and overlapping features of migraine and tension-type headache. *Headache* 46(3): 461-468.

Zanchin, G., F. Maggioni, F. Granella, P. Rossi, L. Falco, and G.C. Manzoni. 2001. Self-administered pain-relieving manoeuvres in primary headaches. *Cephalalgia* 21(7): 718-726.

Zwart, J.A., G. Dyb, K. Hagen, K.J. Odegard, A.A. Dahl, G. Bovim, and L.J. Stovner. 2003. Depression and anxiety disorders associated with headache frequency. The Nord-Trondelag Health Study. *Eur J Neurol* 10(2): 147-152.

chapter 11

Neck and Shoulder Pain

Bodhi G. Haraldsson, RMT

Neck and shoulder pain are common, costly, and similar to low back pain in their potential to cause difficulties and resist treatment (Côté, Cassidy, and Carroll 2000; Brosseau et al. 2001). Further, people with spinal problems often have significantly higher medical expenditures than those without (Martin et al. 2008). The closely related condition of shoulder pain is also associated with high costs and client burden (Meislin, Sperling, and Stitik 2005). It is unsurprising, then, that people with these conditions are increasingly seeking massage therapy (MT) for treatment (Sherman et al. 2005; Eisenberg et al. 1998). This chapter outlines some common causes of neck and shoulder pain, reviews the relevant research on the efficacy and safety of MT for these conditions, and suggests directions for future research. Evidence-based treatment guidelines and a case study are also provided.

CLASSIFICATION OF NECK PAIN

The exact origin of neck pain is often difficult to identify, despite efforts to determine its various causes (Borghouts, Koes, and Bouter 1998). This failure to clearly uncover its origins has mandated the use of a classification system for neck pain that is based on pain severity, as opposed to anatomy or *pathophysiology* (Guzman, Hurwitz, et al. 2008). This classification system is outlined in box 11.1.

pathophysiology

▸ The study of disturbance to normal physical, mechanical, or biochemical functions produced by disease or abnormality.

BOX 11.1

Classification System for the Neck-Pain Task Force

Grade-1 neck pain	Neck pain and associated disorders with no signs or symptoms suggestive of major structural pathology and minor to no interference with activities of daily living. Major structural pathologies include (but are not limited to) fracture, vertebral dislocation, and injury to the spinal cord, infection, neoplasm, or systemic disease, including the inflammatory arthropathies.
Grade-2 neck pain	No signs or symptoms of major structural pathology, but major interference with activities of daily living.
Grade-3 neck pain	No signs or symptoms of major structural pathology, but presence of neurological signs, such as decreased deep-tendon reflexes, weakness, or sensory deficits.
Grade-4 neck pain	Signs or symptoms of major structural pathology.

EPIDEMIOLOGY OF NECK AND SHOULDER PAIN

epidemiology

▸ The study of health conditions, including their prevalence and distribution, within a population or society.

Extensive reviews of neck pain prognoses in the *epidemiology* of neck and shoulder pain show that 50% to 85% of people with neck pain do not experience a complete recovery. Less optimal outcomes are associated with increased age, poor overall health, and the existence of prior painful conditions. Reduced mental health and an absence of effective health coping skills also predict poorer outcomes (Carroll, Hogg-Johnson, Côté, et al. 2008; Carroll, Hogg-Johnson, van der Velde, et al. 2008; Carroll, Holm, Hogg-Johnson, et al. 2008).

Whiplash-associated disorders are one of the most common causes of neck pain, making up more than 27% of vehicular injuries in U.S. emergency rooms (Quinlan et al. 2004). Symptoms of this complex musculoskeletal condition include high levels of initial pain and disability, both of which are also predictors of slower recovery for conditions involving neck pain (Williams et al. 2007; Walton et al. 2009).

Painful disorders of the shoulder, including bursitis, tendinitis, rotator cuff tears, adhesive capsulitis, impingement syndrome, avascular necrosis, and degenerative joint disease, are some of the most commonly seen musculoskeletal conditions in primary care settings (Dinnes et al. 2003). Injury and degeneration of the rotator cuff is the leading cause of shoulder pain (Beaudreuil et al. 2009), though it should also be noted that the nature of shoulder disorders varies by age. Instances of traumatic injury and inflammatory and instability processes are more prevalent in younger people, while degenerative conditions are more prevalent in older people (Padeter, Berg, and Thal 2009).

EFFECTS OF MASSAGE THERAPY ON NECK AND SHOULDER PAIN

Since the seminal monograph that redefined whiplash and its treatment was issued (Spitzer et al. 1995), there have been several comprehensive reviews of neck pain treatment that included MT. One of these reviews determined that there is no evidence that conventional medicine is any more effective for treatment of neck pain than alternative and complementary interventions (Hurwitz et al. 2008). Rickards (2006) reviewed the effects of myofascial trigger-point massage for neck pain and found modest support for its efficacy, including the encouraging fact that the highest quality trials showed the most evidence for benefits. Haraldsson and others (2006) conducted a systematic review of 19 individual studies of MT for mechanical neck disorders, 6 of which examined MT as the sole form of treatment. Evidence from 6 MT-only studies was judged to be both limited and inconsistent. Similarly, the studies that combined MT with other approaches did not clearly reveal any optimal form of combination therapy. Verhagen and others (2007) reached similar conclusions in a review of treatments for whiplash. The 29 existing studies provided little evidence that either active or passive treatments were effective in relieving symptoms associated with grade-1 or grade-2 whiplash.

Some individual studies of MT for neck pain are also worthy of mention. Sherman and colleagues (2009) randomized 64 subjects to receive either a combination of MT and self-care instructions or self-care instructions alone. Results indicated that MT was beneficial for treating chronic neck pain, at least in the short term. Vassiliou and colleagues (2006) compared the combination of MT, exercise, and heat to the use of a soft collar in 200 patients, and found that the MT group significantly outperformed the soft collar group at a 6-month follow-up. It is worth noting that the finding in both of these studies, that MT combined with exercise was beneficial, is consistent with the conclusions reached in a Cochrane review of MT for low back pain (Furlan et al. 2009; see chapter 12 for more information).

Currently, no systematic reviews are specifically concerned with MT as treatment for shoulder pain. The Philadelphia Panel (Brosseau et al. 2001) concluded that insufficient studies were available to provide anything more than limited evidence for the effectiveness of MT for this condition. In a review of the broader category of manual therapies for musculoskeletal shoulder disorders, Ho, Sole, and Munn (2009) were able to include one MT-only study and three other studies that combined MT with other manual therapies. They concluded that MT combined with mobilizations and movement was more effective than no treatment for short-term outcomes, and that treatment with MT alone also had short-term benefits for nonspecific shoulder pain.

Given the limited evidence for practice, it is important to keep in mind that insufficient or no available evidence for a particular approach does not necessarily mean that the approach should not be used. An absence of evidence is not evidence of absence. Rather, limited evidence indicates that research is needed to confirm the leading approaches that are most clinically viable. When choosing an approach, the best available evidence is critical to sound clinical decision making.

EXPLAINING MASSAGE THERAPY EFFECTS

The mechanisms of massage therapy effects are not well understood, though the results of research on neck and shoulder pain permit some informed speculation. In contrast to treatments that emphasize immobilization, the gentle motion induced by massage therapy may interrupt defensive or rigid postures and may promote range of motion, which would serve to lessen muscular rigidity, tension, and pain in these regions (Weerapong, Hume, and Kolt 2005). Massage therapy may also interrupt inflammatory processes that contribute to certain cases of shoulder or neck pain, though the evidence for this is currently marginal (Hilbert, Sforzo, and Swensen 2003). In addition, massage therapy's ability to reduce anxiety may underlie several specific effects, including the reduction of pain and muscular tension (Moyer, Rounds, and Hannum 2004).

RECOMMENDATIONS FOR MASSAGE THERAPY PRACTICE

Based on the available data, treatment of neck and shoulder pain should include MT provided by a well-trained therapist, since training reduces the risk of harm. In addition, patients should be informed of the importance of self-care, mobility and strengthening exercises that can benefit these conditions, and patient education to reduce pain and improve function. Massage therapists should assess pain and function as part of record keeping so that progress can be monitored. Patients whose pain or function deteriorates, or those who show signs of nerve compression, should be referred to a physician.

Massage therapists often function as primary health care practitioners, since most clients are self-referred (Sherman et al. 2005), and primary health care practitioners must have sufficient awareness of the medical conditions that can mimic musculoskeletal complaints (Boudreau and Pinto 2001). Therefore, clinical assessment skills, such as the ability to conduct effective physical examinations and accurately interpret clients' behaviors during illness, are vital. Logically, poor clinical assessment skills are likely to lead to poor treatment outcomes (Olaya-Contreras and Styf 2009). Interpretation of clinical assessment data needs to be viewed through the lens of best available research evidence. Four main outcomes derived from the process of clinical physical examination are outlined in box 11.2 (Jull et al. 2008).

BOX 11.2

Clinical Physical Examination: Four Main Outcomes

- First is a physical diagnosis gained from the impairments presenting in the articular and joint systems, abnormal sensory features, and disturbances in sensorimotor control, and their relationship to the patient's symptoms and functional impairments.
- Second is an understanding of how postures, movement, and activity affect the patient's disorder in terms of both aggravating and relieving sensory symptoms.
- Third is a practical understanding of how the work environment and activities, sport, or activities of daily living could be contributing to the disorder.
- Fourth is the application of outcome measures from which to evaluate treatment progress.

Neck Pain Assessment

Physical examination of neck pain is most accurate when it is used to rule out a structural lesion or neurological compression. Further, visual estimation and external measurement devices for assessment of cervical range of motion are equally reliable, though sole reliance on diagnostic imaging is problematic for directing care (Nordin et al. 2008). However, assessment of spinal joint movement, prior to treatment, does not change the outcome of a single therapy session (Haas et al. 2003).

Self-reported client assessment used to evaluate perceived pain, function, disability, and psychosocial status has also been shown to be valuable (Nordin et al. 2008). Radicular pain provocation tests (contralateral neck rotation and extension of the arm and the fingers of the affected side) have been shown to be the most predictive in detecting probable nerve-root compression (Nordin et al. 2008), along with positive Spurling and Valsalva tests, when taken in context with health history and other physical findings (Rubinstein et al. 2007). Magnetic resonance imaging (MRI) is moderately reliable in identifying degenerative changes in the neck, especially when changes in imaging cannot be correlated with neck pain symptoms. In addition, measuring the degree of cervical *lordosis* or *kyphosis* does not indicate cervical muscle spasm or whiplash injuries (Nordin et al. 2008).

lordosis

▸ An excessive inward curvature of the spine.

kyphosis

▸ An excessive outward curvature of the spine.

Shoulder Pain Assessment

Potential sources of referred pain include cervical spondylolysis, cervical arthritis, cervical disc disease, myocardial ischemia, reflex sympathetic dystrophy, diaphragmatic irritation, thoracic outlet syndrome, and gallbladder disease (Stevenson and Trojian 2002). A review of the diagnostic performance of clinical tests for rotator cuff disease did not show any test to be superior in diagnosing rotator cuff disease (Beaudreuil et al. 2009). In fact, the tests reviewed had a significant likelihood of giving the clinician a false positive (indication of injury when one is not actually present) or a false negative (failure to find a present injury) result. Therefore, clinicians are advised to not rely exclusively on clinical testing for assessment of rotator cuff pathologies; it is important to take a more holistic approach. Hughes, Taylor, and Green (2008) recommend palpation; Napoleon test; lift-off test; belly-press test; drop-arm test; or a combination of Hawkins, painful arc, and infraspinatus tests to assess a rotator cuff tear.

Adverse Events

Reporting of adverse events from MT is sorely lacking in the neck and shoulder pain literature. Only 3 of the 19 neck pain studies in a recent review reported on adverse events (Haraldsson et al. 2006). In those 3 studies, the adverse events from MT reported were short lived and benign, mostly pertaining to transient discomfort after treatment. Further research in this area is needed.

Clinical Guidelines

Though the effectiveness of purely educational interventions for neck pain has been challenged (Haines et al. 2008), providing clients with a better understanding of the natural course of their neck pain is likely a key to an effective and holistic approach to treatment (Haldeman, Carroll, and Cassidy 2008). The best available evidence for treatment of neck pain includes a combination of MT, exercise, traction, and client education (Gross et al. 2009).

Symptom progression for grade-3 neck pain should be monitored for signs of nerve compression. If symptom progression occurs, the client should be referred for neurological consultation. Otherwise, clients can be reassured that most neck pain is self-limiting and that the development of spinal instability, neurological injury, or serious ongoing disability is rare. A timely return to work and daily activities should be promoted.

Similarly, for shoulder pain, treatment outcomes should be monitored carefully. This includes patients' ability to resume activities of daily living. Clients whose condition worsens should be referred for medical consultation. Otherwise, a combination of exercise and MT to increase range of motion and muscle strength is advisable. Clients can be reassured that most shoulder pain, like neck pain, is self-limiting in nature.

DIRECTIONS FOR FUTURE RESEARCH

Based on available research, MT combined with exercise is a promising treatment approach that should be targeted for further investigation. Research designs capable of discriminating the specific effective treatment components and combinations, such as factorial study designs, would be especially useful. Fascial massage is another emerging area of MT research that is particularly relevant to the treatment of chronic shoulder pain, and should be emphasized (Day, Stecco, and Stecco 2009). Finally, methodological problems and shortcomings are common in MT research (Ezzo 2007). Particular attention needs to be paid to combination trials, practitioner qualifications, adequate dosage, and appropriate controls.

Case Study

Jim T., a banker and recreational runner in his mid-40s, recently decided, at the urging of some friends, to try MT for his intermittent neck pain. Jim had previously used MT and had found it beneficial for athletic recovery following his training and races. However, he was unsure if it would work as well for his neck pain, which he attributed to the aftereffects of

(continued)

Case Study *(continued)*

two car accidents and to the normal aging process. Prior to trying MT, and on the advice of his medical doctor, Jim has used nonprescription medications and rest for neck pain relief, with inconsistent results.

Mary, Jim's massage therapist, impressed him with her thorough assessment at their first appointment. This includes both physical assessment and the use of a neck-pain questionnaire to track improvement. After performing additional intake interview procedures and carefully recording Jim's range of motion in the neck, upper back, and shoulder regions, Mary initiated a discussion about Jim's prognosis and her proposed treatment plan. Mary informed Jim that the general findings of her overall assessment, combined with his overall good health and history of regular exercise, were encouraging predictors of a likely positive outcome.

Mary recommended a treatment protocol involving three MT sessions in the first week, two in the second week, and one in the third week. She also suggested that Jim avoid other treatments, unless they are medically necessary, since this could be a valuable and informative way for him to assess the effectiveness of MT for his condition. This knowledge may be especially important if he has bouts of neck pain in the future. Mary informed Jim that as part of MT treatment, she would teach him some specific exercises and self-care techniques, such as the use of hydrotherapy and breathing exercises, to help him to manage neck pain himself. Because Jim mentioned that his job is stressful, Mary also provided information on a stress management course that he may want to try in addition to receiving MT.

Following his course of MT treatment, Jim was pleased to experience noticeable improvement, although the complete recovery he had hoped for did not occur. He came to realize that his neck pain is a chronic condition that is likely to flare up from time to time, and that such episodes are often linked to stressful times in his life. Nevertheless, he received a number of effective strategies to help him manage his pain and stress. He plans to continue using MT as needed for treatment of neck pain.

SUMMARY

Neck and shoulder pain are common, costly conditions, and overall, the effectiveness of most treatments appears to be limited in magnitude and duration. Nevertheless, some studies show that MT may benefit these conditions, especially when it is combined with exercise and patient education. Beneficial outcomes from MT may be the result of improved range of motion and increased flexibility, reduction of muscle tension, interruption of inflammatory processes, reduction of anxiety, or increased feelings of well-being, but additional research is needed to confirm the effects and elucidate the underlying mechanisms. Finally, people who have serious neck or shoulder pain, or any case that deteriorates during the course of treatment, should be referred to a physician.

REFERENCES

Beaudreuil, J., R. Nizard, T. Thomas, M. Peyre, J.P. Liotard, P. Boileau, T. Marc, C. Dromardh, E. Steyeri, T. Bardina, P. Orcela, and G. Walch. 2009. Contribution of clinical tests to the diagnosis of rotator cuff disease: A systematic literature review. *Joint, Bone, Spine: Revue du Rhumatisme* 76(1): 15-19.

Borghouts, J.A.J., B.W. Koes, and L.M. Bouter. 1998. The clinical course and prognostic factors of non-specific neck pain: A systematic review. *Pain* 77(1): 1-13.

Boudreau, L.A., and A. Pinto. 2001. Acute lymphangitis mimicking mechanical neck pain. *J Manip Physiol Ther* 24(7): 474-476.

Brosseau, L., P. Tugwell, G.A. Wells, and P. Panel. 2001. Philadelphia Panel evidence-based clinical practice guidelines on selected rehabilitation interventions for neck pain. *Phys Ther* 81(10): 1701-1717.

Carroll, L.J., L.W. Holm, S. Hogg-Johnson, P. Côté, J.D. Cassidy, S. Haldeman, M. Nordin, E.L. Hurwitz, E.J. Carragee, G. van der Velde, P.M. Peloso, and J. Guzman 2008. Course and prognostic factors for neck pain in whiplash-associated disorders (WAD): Results of the bone and joint decade 2000-2010 task force on neck pain and its associated disorders. *Spine* 33(4): S83-S92.

Carroll, L.J., S. Hogg-Johnson, P. Côté, D. Cassidy, S. Haldeman, M. Nordin, E.L. Hurwitz, E.J. Carragee, G. van der Velde, P.M. Peloso, and J. Guzman. 2008. Course and prognostic factors for neck pain in workers: Results of the bone and joint decade 2000-2010 task force on neck pain and its associated disorders. *Spine* 33(4): S93-S100.

Carroll, L.J., S. Hogg-Johnson, G. van der Velde, S. Haldeman, L.W. Holm, E.J. Carragee, E.L. Hurwitz, P. Côté, M. Nordin, P.M. Peloso, J. Guzman, and J. D. Cassidy. 2008. Course and prognostic factors for neck pain in the general population: Results of the bone and joint decade 2000-2010 task force on neck pain and its associated disorders. *Spine* 33(4): S75-S82.

Côté, P., J.D. Cassidy, and L. Carroll. 2000. The factors associated with neck pain and its related disability in the Saskatchewan population. *Spine* 25(9): 1109-1117.

Day, J.A., C. Stecco, and A. Stecco. 2009. Application of fascial manipulation technique in chronic shoulder pain—Anatomical basis and clinical implications. *J Bodyw Mov Ther* 13(2): 128-135.

Dinnes, J., E. Loveman, L. McIntyre, and N. Waugh. 2003. The effectiveness of diagnostic tests for the assessment of shoulder pain due to soft tissue disorders: A systematic review. *Health Technol Asses* 7(29): iii, 1-166.

Eisenberg, D.M., R.B. Davis, S.L. Ettner, S. Appel, S. Wilkey, M. Van Rompay, and R.C. Kessler. 1998. Trends in alternative medicine use in the United States, 1990-1997: Results of a follow-up national survey. *JAMA* 280(18): 1569-1575.

Ezzo, J. 2007. What can be learned from Cochrane systematic reviews of massage that can guide future research? *J Altern Complem Med* 13(2): 291-295.

Furlan, A.D., M. Imamura, T. Dryden, and E. Irvin. 2009. Massage for low back pain. *Spine* 34(16): 1669-1684.

Gross, A., T. Haines, C.H. Goldsmith, L. Santaguida, L.M. McLaughlin, P. Peloso, S. Burnie, J. Hoving, and Cervical Overview Group (COG). 2009. Knowledge to action: A challenge for neck pain treatment. *J Orthop Sport Phys* 39(5): 351-363.

Guzman, J., S. Haldeman, L.J. Carroll, E.J. Carragee, E.L. Hurwitz, P. Peloso, M. Nordin, J.D. Cassidy, L.W. Holm, P. Côté, G. van der Velde, and S. Hogg-Johnson. 2008. Clinical practice implications of the bone and joint decade 2000-2010 task force on neck pain and its associated disorders: From concepts and findings to recommendations. *Spine* 33(4): S199-S213.

Guzman, J., E.L. Hurwitz, L.J. Carroll, S. Haldeman, P. Côté, E.J. Carragee, P.M. Peloso, G. van der Velde, L.W. Holm, S. Hogg-Johnson, M. Nordin, and J. D. Cassidy. 2008. A new conceptual model of neck pain: Linking onset, course, and care: The bone and joint decade 2000-2010 task force on neck pain and its associated disorders. *Spine* 33 (4): S14-S23.

Haas, M., E. Groupp, D. Panzer, L. Partna, S. Lumsden, and M. Aickin. 2003. Efficacy of cervical endplay assessment as an indicator for spinal manipulation. *Spine* 28(11): 1091-1096.

Haines, T., A. Gross, C.H. Goldsmith, and L. Perry. 2008. Patient education for neck pain with or without radiculopathy. *Cochrane Db Syst Rev* 4: CD005106.

Haldeman, S., L.J. Carroll, and J.D. Cassidy. 2008. The empowerment of people with neck pain: Introduction: The bone and joint decade 2000-2010 task force on neck pain and its associated disorders. *Spine* 33(4): S8-S13.

Haraldsson, B.G., A.R. Gross, C.D. Myers, J.M. Ezzo, A. Morien, C. Goldsmith, P.M. Peloso, G. Bronfort, and Cervical Overview Group. 2006. Massage for mechanical neck disorders. *Cochrane Db Syst Rev* 3: CD004871.

Hilbert, J.E., G.A. Sforzo, and T. Swensen. 2003. The effects of massage on delayed onset muscle soreness. *Brit J Sport Med* 37: 72-75.

Ho, C.C., G. Sole, and J. Munn. 2009. The effectiveness of manual therapy in the management of musculoskeletal disorders of the shoulder: A systematic review. *Manual Ther* 14(5): 463-474.

Hughes, P.C., N.F. Taylor, and R.A. Green. 2008. Most clinical tests cannot accurately diagnose rotator cuff pathology: A systematic review. *Aust J Physiother* 54: 159-170.

Hurwitz, E.L., E.J. Carragee, G. van der Velde, L.J. Carroll, M. Nordin, J. Guzman, P.M. Peloso, L.W. Holm, P. Côté, S. Hogg-Johnson, J.D. Cassidy, and S. Haldeman. 2008. Treatment of neck pain: Noninvasive interventions: Results of the bone and joint decade 2000-2010 task force on neck pain and its associated disorders. *Spine* 33(4): S123-S152.

Jull, G., M. Sterling, D. Falla, J. Treleaven, and S. O'Leary. 2008. *Whiplash, headache, and neck pain: Research-based directions for physical therapies*. 1st ed. Edinburgh: Churchill Livingstone.

Martin, B. I., R. A. Deyo, S. K. Mirza, J. A. Turner, B. A. Comstock, W. Hollingworth, and S. D. Sullivan. 2008. "Expenditures and Health Status Among Adults With Back and Neck Problems." JAMA 299(6): 656-664.

Meislin, R.J., J.W. Sperling, and T.P. Stitik. 2005. Persistent shoulder pain: Epidemiology, pathophysiology, and diagnosis. *Am J Orthopedics* 34(12): S5-S9.

Moyer, C.A., J. Rounds, and J.W. Hannum. 2004. A meta-analysis of massage therapy research. *Psychol Bull* 130: 3-18.

Nordin, M., E.J. Carragee, S. Hogg-Johnson, S.S. Weiner, E.L. Hurwitz, P.M. Peloso, J. Guzman, G. van der Velde, L.J. Carroll, L.W. Holm, P. Côté, J.D. Cassidy, and S. Haldeman. 2008. Assessment of neck pain and its associated disorders: Results of the bone and joint decade 2000-2010 task force on neck pain and its associated disorders. *Spine* 33(4): S101-S122.

Olaya-Contreras, P., and J. Styf. 2009. Illness behavior in patients on long-term sick leave due to chronic musculoskeletal pain. *Acta Orthopaedica* 80(3): 380-385.

Pateder, D. B., J. H. Berg, and R. Thal. 2009. "Neck and shoulder pain: differentiating cervical spine pathology from shoulder pathology." *J Surg Orthop Adv* 18(4):170-174.

Quinlan, K.P., J.L. Annest, B. Myers, G. Ryan, and H. Hill. 2004. Neck strains and sprains among motor vehicle occupants: United States, 2000. *Accident Anal Prev* 36(1): 21-27.

Rickards, L.D. 2006. The effectiveness of non-invasive treatments for active myofascial trigger point pain: A systematic review of the literature. *Int J Osteopath Med* 9(4): 120-136.

Rubinstein, S., J. Pool, M. van Tulder, I. Riphagen, and H. de Vet. 2007. A systematic review of the diagnostic accuracy of provocative tests of the neck for diagnosing cervical radiculopathy. *Eur Spine J* 16(3): 307-319.

Sherman, K.J., D.C. Cherkin, R.J. Hawkes, D.L. Miglioretti, and R.A. Deyo. 2009. Randomized trial of therapeutic massage for chronic neck pain. *Clin J Pain* 25(3): 233-238.

Sherman, K.J., D.C. Cherkin, J. Kahn, J. Erro, A. Hrbek, R.A. Deyo, and D.M. Eisenberg. 2005. A survey of training and practice patterns of massage therapists in two U.S. states. *BMC Complem Altern M* 5: 13.

Stevenson, J.H., and T. Trojian. 2002. Evaluation of shoulder pain. *J Fam Practice* 51(7): 605-611.

Spitzer, W.O., M.L. Skovron, L.R. Salmi, J.D. Cassidy, J. Duranceau, S. Suissa, and E. Zeiss. 1995. Scientific monograph of the Quebec task force on whiplash-associated disorder: Redefining 'whiplash' and its management. *Spine* 20(8): S1-S73.

Vassiliou, T., G. Kaluza, C. Putzke, H. Wulf, and M. Schnabel. 2006. Physical therapy and active exercises: An adequate treatment for prevention of late whiplash syndrome? Randomized controlled trial in 200 patients. *Pain* 124(1): 69-76.

Verhagen, A.P., G. Scholten-Peeters, S. van Wijngaarded, R. de Bie, and S. Bierma-Zeinstra. 2007. Conservative treatments for whiplash. *Cochrane Db Syst Rev* 2: CD003338.

Walton, D.M., J. Pretty, J.C. Macdermid, and R.W. Teasell. 2009. Risk factors for persistent problems following whiplash injury: Results of a systematic review and meta-analysis. *J Orthop Sport Phys* 39(5): 334-350.

Weerapong, P., P.A. Hume, and G.S. Kolt. 2005. The mechanisms of massage and effects on performance, muscle recovery and injury prevention. *Sports Med* 35: 235-256.

Williams, M., E. Williamson, S. Gates, S. Lamb, and M. Cooke. 2007. A systematic literature review of physical prognostic factors for the development of late whiplash syndrome. *Spine* 32(25): E764-E780.

Low Back Pain

Trish Dryden, MEd, RMT
Andrea D. Furlan, MD, PhD
Marta Imamura, MD, PhD
Emma L. Irvin, BA

Low back pain (LBP) is a significant health problem in adults. Between 70% and 85% of the population will experience LBP at some time in their lives (Andersson 1999). Almost 90% of all patients with acute LBP get better quite quickly, regardless of the therapy; however, the remaining 10% are at risk of developing chronic low back pain (CLBP) and disability, which account for more than 90% of social costs for back incapacity (Waddell 1998). Given both its prevalence and its potential for causing disability, it is unsurprising that persons with LBP are motivated to find effective treatments, and that an increasing number of LBP sufferers report using massage (Eisenberg et al. 1998).

EFFECTS AND SAFETY OF MASSAGE THERAPY FOR LOW BACK PAIN

This section reviews current research on the effectiveness and safety of massage for low back pain. Table 12.1 examines and summarizes 13 studies. In addition, a review of the research on potential harms concludes that massage therapy (MT) for LPB is a safe therapeutic intervention, especially when conducted by trained practitioners. Some contraindications to treatment, as well as risk of postmassage discomfort, are reported.

Effects

Although LBP is a benign and self-limiting condition, many patients look for some type of therapy to relieve their symptoms and to provide them with hope for a cure. For this reason, it is possible to list more than 50 potential therapies that promise to relieve pain, lessen suffering, or even cure LBP. However, supportive evidence exists for only a minority of these therapies (Chaitow 2004). When experiencing pain or discomfort, it is a natural reaction to rub or hold the affected area to reduce sensation. At the most basic level, massage is a way of easing pain while simultaneously promoting relaxation and well-being and offering an environment of good care.

Nonspecific LBP is defined as low back pain that cannot be reliably attributed to a specific disease or spinal abnormality. More than 85% of patients presenting with back pain have pain that is nonspecific in origin (Chou and Huffman 2007). A recently updated Cochrane systematic review (Furlan et al. 2008) found 13 randomized trials of massage for nonspecific LBP; these are summarized in table 12.1. Seven of the studies were judged to have a high risk of bias (a bias score of 5 or less on an 11-point scale). According to short- and long-term follow-ups from two studies that compared MT to an inert therapy (sham treatment), massage was shown to improve both pain and function significantly more than the inert therapy (Preyde 2000; Geisser et al. 2005). In eight studies, massage was compared to other active treatments. One study showed that reflexology on the feet had no effect on pain and functioning (Quinn, Hughes, and Baxter 2008). In another study, the beneficial effects of MT in patients with chronic low back pain (CLBP) lasted at least 1 year after the end of the treatment (Cherkin et al. 2001). Two studies compared two different techniques of massage. One concluded that acupressure massage produces better results than classic (Swedish) massage (Franke et al. 2000) and another concluded that Thai massage produces similar results to classic (Swedish) massage (Chatchawan, Thinkhamrop, and Kharmwan 2005). Two other trials concerned with LBP also deserve mention here, though they were excluded from the 2008 Cochrane review because they studied patients whose LBP was caused by the specific medical condition of disc protrusion, rather than studying nonspecific LBP. In one of these trials, massage performed better than traction (Zhang and Chen 2004), while in the other, massage therapy achieved the same benefits as spinal mobilization (Liu and Zhang 2000).

Furlan and colleagues (2008) concluded that "massage was superior for pain and function on both short- and long-term follow-ups. Massage was similar to exercise, and it was superior to joint mobilization, relaxation therapy, physical therapy, acupuncture, and self-care education." However, it should also be noted that the studies vary in methodological quality, populations, massage techniques, and comparison groups. The majority of these studies assessed improvements of pain and function immediately after the sessions or in the short term. Few studies measured outcomes at long-term follow-up. In addition, massage was clearly most effective when it was delivered with exercises and education (Preyde 2000; Little et al. 2008; Franke et al. 2000; Geisser et al. 2005).

Most recently, a large-scale (N = 401) longitudinal study by Cherkin and colleagues (2011) took the important step of comparing two different types of massage therapy to each other and to standard care. After 10 weeks of treatment, subjects in the relaxation massage and structural massage groups had fewer symptoms of back pain and experienced less associated disability than those in the standard care group. Most of these gains were still observed at the 52-week follow-up. Concerning the two types of massage that were being compared across the 52-week study, the researchers state that "no clinically meaningful difference between relaxation and structural massage was observed in terms of relieving disability or symptoms."

Safety

Massage is recognized as a safe therapeutic modality, with few risks or adverse effects. However, there are contraindications, such as applying massage to an area with acute inflammation, skin infection, a nonconsolidated fracture, a burn, a deep-vein thrombosis, or tumor (Vickers and Zolman 1999). Precautions (i.e., light pressure only) should be taken when providing massage to patients using anticoagulant therapy and to those diagnosed with hemophilia or myositis ossificans (Rachlin 2002).

Table 12.1 Summary of Individual Studies Included in the Cochrane Review of Massage for Low Back Pain

Study	Bias score (11 = least risk of bias)	Harmful outcomes	Conclusions
Preyde 2000	8	None reported	A series of MT sessions is beneficial for patients with subacute LBP; benefits endure 1 month after cessation of MT sessions.
Franke et al. 2000	5	None reported	Acupuncture massage outperformed Swedish MT for both disability and pain.
Cherkin et al. 2001	8	13% of participants experienced some discomfort or pain during or after a treatment session.	MT is effective for persistent LBP and provides lasting benefits; MT may be an effective alternative to conventional medical care for persistent LBP.
Hernandez-Reif et al. 2001	4	None reported	MT reduced pain and symptoms associated with chronic LBP.
Hsieh et al. 2004	6	None reported	MT in the form of acupressure is effective in reducing LBP.
Yip and Tse 2004	4	None reported	A series of acupoint electrode stimulation followed by MT in the form of acupressure is effective for short-term LBP relief.
Geisser et al. 2005	5	None reported	MT in the form of manual therapy combined with adjuvant exercise may benefit chronic LBP; functioning was unimproved.
Chatchawan, Thinkhamrop, and Kharmwan 2005	8	23% of participants experienced some discomfort or pain during or after a treatment session; 5% exhibited allergic reaction to massage oil.	2 different types of MT were effective for nonspecific LBP associated with trigger points.
Farasyn, Meeusen, and Nijs 2006	4	None reported	MT in the form of deep cross-friction massage increased pain threshold over specific muscles.
Hsieh et al. 2006	7	None reported	MT in the form of acupressure was effective in reducing LBP and was superior to conventional physical therapy.
Field et al. 2007	1	None reported	MT group reported fewer instances of pain, anxiety, depression, and sleep disturbance than relaxation control group.
Mackawan et al. 2007	7	None reported	MT in the form of traditional Thai massage temporarily relieved nonspecific LBP and slightly outperformed joint mobilization.
Poole, Glenn, and Murphy 2007	3	None reported	The addition of MT in the form of reflexology plus standard care was not more effective than standard care alone.

MT = massage therapy, LBP = low back pain.

Adapted from A.D. Furlan et al., 2008, "Massage for low-back pain," *Cochrane Database System Review* 8(4): CD001929. Copyright Cochrane Collaboration, reproduced with permission.

Although adverse effects are rare, some discomfort can result from MT for LBP. The studies of highest quality report a very similar proportion of participants affected in this way. In one study, minor pain or discomfort was experienced by 13% of the 78 massage participants during or shortly after receiving massage for LBP (Cherkin et al. 2001). Similarly, between 11% and 12% of 180 participants in another study reported temporary (10-15 min.) soreness after receiving massage (Chatchawan, Thinkhamrop, and Kharmwan 2005). Specific massage techniques, such as deep friction, compression, or ischemic compression, might result in greater soreness or bruising (Cherkin et al. 2001; Simons, Travell, and Simons 1999). In addition, citing evidence from 16 case reports and 4 case series, Ernst (2003) concluded that "the majority of adverse effects were associated with exotic types of manual massage or massage delivered by laymen, while massage therapists were rarely implicated." This illustrates the important role of training in providing safe practice.

EXPLAINING MASSAGE THERAPY EFFECTS

The mechanisms of action in MT are not well understood, though it seems likely that its results come about through a complex interplay of both physical and mental pathways. Massage therapy to affected soft and connective tissues may induce local biochemical changes that modulate local blood flow and regulate oxygenation in muscles (Sefton et al. 2010; Goats 1994), although the evidence for this is disputed (see chapter 8 on athletes). Local effects may subsequently influence neural activity at the level of spinal cord segments, thereby modulating the activities of subcortical nuclei that influence both mood and pain perception (Sagar, Dryden, and Wong 2007). A recent research finding suggests that MT may lead to an increase of the hormone oxytocin, which stimulates feelings of well-being, prosocial behavior, and maternal bonding (Morhenn et al. 2008). This proposed mechanism of action may help to explain one of the most well-established effects of massage: the reduction of anxiety (Moyer, Rounds, and Hannum 2004).

Massage may increase the recipient's pain threshold by promoting the release of *endorphins* and serotonin (Ernst 1999). The gate-control theory predicts that massaging a particular area stimulates large-diameter nerve fibers. These fibers provide inhibitory input for T cells (which are the first cells that project into the central nervous system within the spinal cord). T-cell activity is depressed (conversely, small-diameter nerve fibers, or nociceptive fibers, have an excitatory input), and pain relief follows (Melzack and Wall 1996).

endorphins

▸ Chemicals produced by the pituitary gland and hypothalamus that reduce pain and induce feelings of well-being.

Another possibility is that massage therapy may provide its benefits by shifting the autonomic nervous system from a state of sympathetic response to a state of parasympathetic response. However, support for this theory is not universal. It has been suggested that MT may promote a sympathetic response of the autonomic nervous system (Moyer, Rounds, and Hannum 2004). Massage therapy has also been proposed to increase local blood circulation, improve muscle flexibility, intensify the movement of lymph, and loosen adherent connective tissue (Lee, Itoh, and Yang 1990). These actions may alternately improve reuptake of local *nociceptive* and *inflammatory mediators,* increase pain-free range of motion, and improve muscle function. Studies that investigate MT mechanisms are needed to delineate underlying biological and psychological effects of massage and their relationship to outcomes. A better understanding of how MT works would clearly help guide future development of clinical trials and, ultimately, clinical practice.

nociceptive mediators

▸ Hormones and neurotransmitters that influence pain perception.

inflammatory mediators

▸ Chemicals released by injured cells that influence inflammation, including swelling, redness, and the perception of heat.

RECOMMENDATIONS FOR MASSAGE THERAPY PRACTICE

Based on the evidence to date, massage delivered by a trained massage therapist for patients with nonspecific, subacute, or chronic LPB, results in pain relief, reduction of swelling or mobilization of adhesive tissues, and increased function. Effects are observed immediately after the MT session. They can persist for months or, as observed in one study, up to 1 year. Better results are obtained when massage therapists educate clients about self-care and exercise. More studies are needed to determine the optimal length and number of sessions needed to produce positive effects and to further examine which specific MT techniques are most effective. Also, no solid research exists on the sequencing and combining of various CAM interventions (e.g., chiropractic, acupuncture, and meditation) with MT for the optimal treatment of pain and function in LBP. In addition, research studies are needed to determine the effect of MT on patients' ability to return to work and on the cost-effectiveness of massage as an intervention for LBP.

The clinical practice guidelines for nonpharmacological treatments for LBP put forth by the American Pain Society and American College of Physicians (Chou and Huffman 2007) found good evidence that cognitive-behavioral therapy, exercise, spinal manipulation, and interdisciplinary rehabilitation are all moderately effective for chronic or subacute (4 weeks in duration) LBP. Benefits over placebo, sham therapy, or no treatment averaged 10 to 20 points on a 100-point visual analogue pain scale, 2 to 4 points on the Roland–Morris disability questionnaire, or standardized mean difference–effect sizes of 0.5 to 0.8. They found fair evidence that acupuncture, massage, yoga (Viniyoga), and functional restoration are also effective for CLBP. For acute LBP (4 weeks in duration), the only nonpharmacological therapies with evidence of efficacy are superficial heat (good evidence for moderate benefits) and spinal manipulation (fair evidence for small to moderate benefits). Although serious harmful outcomes seemed to be rare, data were poorly reported. No trials addressed optimal sequencing of therapies. Methods for tailoring therapy to individual patients are still in early stages of development.

Clinical Guidelines for Massage Therapy and Nonspecific CLBP

The following are based on the best available evidence to date:

- Massage therapy is believed to be a safe and effective treatment choice for patients with nonspecific, subacute LPB, or CLBP, to reduce pain and improve function.
- Results are improved if patient education and exercise are included.
- Massage therapist training reduces risk of harm.
- Massage therapists should assess and record baseline measures of pain and function and should monitor progress throughout the treatment plan.
- Patients whose CLBP or function worsens should be referred to a medical practitioner for reassessment.
- Massage therapists should provide patients with evidence-based information on the natural, self-limiting history of LBP and should advise patients on the importance of self-care and exercise in helping to reduce pain and improve function.
- Massage therapists should be mindful of the positive effects of relaxation on mood, pain, and overall sense of well-being.

- The mechanisms of action for massage therapy are not fully understood. Massage therapists should be able to describe to patients in plain language that massage is thought to achieve its results through a complex interplay of physical and mental modes of action.

DIRECTIONS FOR FUTURE RESEARCH

The conclusions of a workshop report from the 2009 North American Research Conference on Complementary and Integrative Medicine (Moyer, Dryden, and Shipwright 2009) suggest that in spite of the field's late start in research and the inconsistencies in the quality and scope of MT research to date, modern scientific methods and technologies rigorously applied to future studies can lead to impressive progress in the next 20 years (see chapter 23).

Studies addressing questions of efficacy need to be rigorously controlled. Factorial design can be used to assess the effectiveness of treatments alone or in combination (Ezzo 2007). Since most outcomes in LBP are subjective measures, the ideal control group is one that ensures that treatments are equally credible and acceptable to patients to minimize placebo effects and high dropout rates (Fregni et al. 2010; Haraldsson et al. 2006). MT includes numerous techniques, and each one needs to be evaluated for effectiveness and cost-effectiveness. Little is understood about how much massage and what kind of massages are effective for LBP. A much-needed first trial comparing "focused structural massage" and "relaxation massage" is underway (Cherkin et al. 2009). The effect of MT in different settings (private practice, hospital, primary care, pain clinics) and with various populations (acute or chronic pain, presence of other aggravating factors, and different countries with different cultures and different styles of massage) also need to be individually assessed.

Future trials may also examine whether the benefits of massage can be increased if the therapist has many years of experience or is a licensed therapist. They should examine the role of treatment session length by including two (or more) levels of this variable, as well as the experience of the therapist by using massage therapists with different experience and training. Authors should discuss the clinical relevance of the results, including patients' return to work as an outcome and long-term follow-up. They are encouraged to follow the CONSORT (Consolidated Standards of Reporting Trials) Statement for reporting their trials (Moher et al. 2001). The CONSORT Statement provides clear reporting guidelines for a trial's design, conduct, analysis, and interpretation to help readers assess the validity of its results. Studies should also use the standard outcomes for trials of LBP (Deyo et al. 1998) to provide homogenous information for future systematic reviews and meta-analyses. When presenting the results, researchers are encouraged to show the baseline characteristics using point estimates (mean, median) with standard deviations (for continuous variables), as well as the number of patients in each category (for categorical variables) and for every follow-up measure. When researchers present only the difference between the baseline and the follow-up, these data cannot be pooled with studies that report both baseline and follow-up values.

In addition, increased generation of high-quality case reports and qualitative and mixed-method studies will help us more fully understand MT as a complex intervention (Kania, Porcino, and Verhoef 2008). They will also add much needed richness and depth in application to clinical practice. The process and context of treatment and the values and beliefs of both the patient and the therapist can influence the patients' experience and their health outcomes (see chapter 22). As part of collaborative, patient-centered care, the ethical and reflective practitioner carefully evaluates and applies evidence from many sources and across disciplines to enhance clinical decision making, positive patient outcomes, and respectful and meaningful communication with individual patients.

Case Study

Samir P. is a 35-year-old software developer who has been referred to massage therapy (MT) by his family physician for the treatment of nonspecific, chronic low back pain (CLBP). Having spoken briefly with Samir by phone, massage therapist Anna N. then reviews the evidence on LBP and CLBP in advance of her initial meeting with Samir so she can begin to formulate her initial assessment and treatment plan.

Using Pubmed (www.Pubmed.com) and other public access databases, Anna searches using keywords, such as "massage" and "low back pain." She finds several peer-reviewed articles and a recent Cochrane systematic review of the literature. Reading through the materials, Anna notes that current best evidence indicates MT is a safe and moderately effective treatment for CLBP. She also learns that it is important to include appropriate exercises in her recommendations for client self-care. She plans to carefully record her assessments, MT techniques, and client outcomes in order to track her client's progress and to monitor effectiveness and safety.

Anna understands that no research evidence exists about best techniques to use or about optimal session length or number of treatments. Therefore, she will need to rely exclusively on her clinical training and experience, combined with her client's feedback. Anna decides that careful monitoring of her client's progress will be enhanced if she uses standardized and validated measurement tools before and after each treatment. She uses the IN-CAM outcomes database to find the instruments (www.outcomesdatabase.org) and chooses a pain scale measure—the visual analogue pain rating scale (Scott and Huskisson 1976)—and a disability index—the Roland–Morris disability questionnaire (Roland and Fairbank 2000)—to help her objectively monitor Samir's progress.

In their first meeting, Anna discovers that Samir is an otherwise healthy, 35-year-old male who is partnered and has two preschool children. He has a stressful computer programming job that requires a long commute by car. Samir has little time for either exercise or relaxation. Reviewing his health history, Anna notes that Samir has been prescribed over-the-counter ibuprofen for pain by his family physician, but he takes no other form of prescription medication or any natural health products. Samir informs Anna that he has no allergies to oils or lotions.

Samir states that his pain is worse at the end of the day, especially after the long drive home, and that it feels like a dull, constant ache located in a spot he points to in his low back. The pain does not radiate into his legs or his trunk, but he often feels stiff after sitting. He also finds that lifting his children is both difficult and painful. He sometimes wakes up at night from his LBP when he is changing positions in bed. He has noticed that the pain is somewhat relieved after taking a hot shower, resting, or taking ibuprofen, but that it comes back within a few hours. Currently, he describes his pain as a 6 on a 10-point pain scale. He states that his goals are to find relief for the pain and to feel better overall—less stressed and more relaxed. He also states that he will know he has achieved these goals when he is more able to do normal activities of living with his family and friends without pain and when he is able to sleep better.

Anna talks with Samir about the natural, self-limiting history of LBP and the potential benefits and risks of receiving MT treatment. She outlines the physical assessment protocol she will use to help identify which muscles, soft tissues, and joints are most affected. Following her assessment, Anna proposes a conventional treatment of Swedish back massage with the

(continued)

Case Study *(continued)*

addition of specific trigger-point therapy and fascial stretching techniques to various muscles, along with the use of moist heat. She explains that she would also like to teach Samir some specific stretches and strengthening exercises that he can do at home. She reminds him that she will ask him to fill out the pain and disability questionnaires at the end of sessions so that they can monitor his progress.

Based on her initial assessment, Samir's preferences, and her clinical experience, Anna proposes a treatment plan that consists of a series of graduated treatments over a few weeks. She describes how she will progress the depth and pressure of her massage treatments and the kinds of exercises she will introduce. She tells Samir that she will provide him with a more detailed treatment plan when she sees him at his next appointment, based on his response to the first treatment, and that she will continue to reassess, monitor, and adjust the treatment plan accordingly. Samir asks Anna a few questions about his prognosis, which she happily answers based on the evidence she has read and her experience. Samir gives his informed consent to the treatment plan.

Anna proceeds with the massage, being careful to take note of specific areas of muscle tension and pain. She maintains good communication with Samir during the treatment so she can understand his experience and modify the pressure according to Samir's own pain tolerance. She is also mindful that her speech is not verbally intrusive during the massage so that Samir can rest and get the additional benefit of a generalized relaxation response from the massage.

At the end of the massage portion of the session, Anna teaches Samir the first set of exercises through demonstration and practice. She instructs him to do the exercises at home and at his office and gives him a reminder form describing the exercises and the numbers of repetitions. She reminds him that he might feel some increased discomfort in his low back for the first few hours after the massage. Though she thinks it is unlikely, she advises him that if he experiences a flare-up of pain over the next few days, he should call her right away to determine whether it is a symptom requiring further attention. She then books his next appointment and gives him a few additional basic relaxation techniques, including controlled breathing or taking a warm bath, that he can also use at home for self-care and pain management.

At the end of 6 weeks, Samir is discharged from treatment since he is sleeping better and is feeling pain-free, stronger, and more energetic, yet more relaxed. He assures Anna that he will continue his exercise program and that he will return to massage if he feels the need. Anna also lets him know that he is welcome to use massage on a regular basis as part of his overall self-care and relaxation plan.

SUMMARY

Low back pain is a significant problem, especially in an aging population. Although most nonacute low back pain resolves itself over time regardless of treatment, 10% of patients will develop chronic low back pain. Based on the best available evidence, massage therapy is a safe and effective treatment choice to reduce pain and improve function in patients with nonspecific, subacute, or chronic low back pain. Results are improved if patient education and exercise are included. Massage therapists' training further reduces an already low risk of harm.

The mechanisms of action by which massage therapy reduces back pain remain unclear. However, given the myriad effects associated with MT, an interplay of physical and mental mechanisms seems likely. Future clinical trials should be rigorously controlled. They should also examine the role of treatment session length and frequency and further examine both different types of massage manipulations. Authors should discuss the clinical relevance of the results, including cost analysis, and should use patients' return to work as an outcome, including long-term follow-up. Authors are encouraged to follow the CONSORT statement for reporting and to use standard outcomes for trials to provide homogenous information for future systematic reviews and meta-analyses. In addition, qualitative studies are needed to examine the influence of nonspecific effects, including the therapeutic relationship, attitudes, values, and beliefs, in order to more fully understand the results of massage on chronic low back pain.

REFERENCES

Andersson, G.B. 1999. Epidemiological features of chronic low-back pain. *Lancet* 354: 581-585.

Chatchawan, U., B. Thinkhamrop, and S. Kharmwan. 2005. Effectiveness of traditional Thai massage versus Swedish massage among patients with back pain associated with myofascial trigger points. *J Bodyw Mov Ther* 9(4): 298-309.

Chaitow, L. 2004. *Palpation and assessment skills.* 2nd ed. Edinburgh: Churchill Livingstone.

Chenot, J.F., A. Becker, C. Leonhardt, S. Keller, N. Donner-Banzhoff, E. Baum, M. Pfingsten, J. Hildebrandt, H.D. Basler, and M.M. Kochen. 2007. Use of complementary alternative medicine for low back pain consulting in general practice: A cohort study. *BMC Complement Altern Med* 7: 42.

Cherkin, D.C., D. Eisenberg, K.J. Sherman, W. Barlow, T.J. Kaptchuk, J. Street, and R.A. Deyo. 2001. Randomized trial comparing traditional Chinese medical acupuncture, therapeutic massage, and self-care education for chronic low back pain. *Arch Intern Med* 161(8): 1081-1088.

Cherkin, D.C., K.J. Sherman, J. Kahn, J.H. Erro, R.A. Deyo, S.J. Haneuse, and A.J. Cook. 2009. Effectiveness of focused structural massage and relaxation massage for chronic low back pain: Protocol for a randomized controlled trial. *Trials* 10(1): 96.

Cherkin, D.C., K.J. Sherman, J. Kahn, R. Wellman, A. Cook, E. Johnson, J. Erro, K. Delaney, and R.A. Deyo. 2011. A comparison of the effects of 2 types of massage and usual care on chronic low back pain. *Ann of Intern Med* 155: 1-9.

Chou, R., and L.H. Huffman. 2007. Nonpharmacologic therapies for acute and chronic low back pain: A review of the evidence for an American Pain Society/American College of Physicians clinical practice guideline. *Ann Intern Med* 147(7): 492-504.

Deyo, R., M. Battie, A. Beurskens, C. Bombardier, P. Croft, B. Koes, A. Malmivaara, M. Roland, M. Von Korff, and G. Waddell. 1998. Outcome measures for low back pain research: A proposal for standardized use. *Spine* 23(18): 2003-2013.

Eisenberg, D.M., R.B. Davis, S.L. Ettner, S. Appel, S. Wilkey, M.Van Rompay, and R.C. Kessler. 1998. Trends in alternative medicine use in the United States, 1990-1997: Results of a follow-up national survey. *JAMA* 280(18): 1569-1575.

Ernst, E. 1999. "Massage therapy for low back pain: a systematic review." *J Pain Symptom Manage* 17(1): 65-69.

Ernst, E. 2003. The safety of massage therapy. *Rheumatology* 42: 1101-1106.

Ezzo, J. 2007. What can be learned from Cochrane systematic reviews of massage that can guide future research? *J Altern Complem Med* 13(2): 291-296.

Farasyn, A., R. Meeusen, and J. Nijs. 2006. A pilot randomized placebo-controlled trial of roptrotherapy in patients with subacute non-specific low back pain. *J Back Musculoskelet* 19: 111-117.

Field, T., M. Hernandez-Reif, M. Diego, and M. Fraser. 2007. Lower back pain and sleep disturbance are reduced following massage therapy. *J Bodyw Mov Ther* 11:141-145.

Franke, A., S. Gebauer, K. Franke, and T. Brockow. 2000. Acupuncture massage vs. Swedish massage and individual exercise vs. group exercise in low back pain sufferers: A randomized controlled clinical trial in a 2-by-2 factorial design. *Forsch Komp Klass Nat* 7(6): 286-293.

Fregni, F., M. Imamura, H.F. Chien, H.L. Lew, P. Boggio, T.J. Kaptchuk, M. Riberto, W.T. Hsing, L.R. Battistella, and A. Furlan. 2010. International placebo symposium working group. Challenges and recommendations for placebo controls in randomized trials in physical and rehabilitation medicine: A report of the international placebo symposium working group. *Am J Phys Med Rehabil* 89(2): 160-172.

Furlan, A.D., M. Imamura, T. Dryden, and E. Irvin. 2008. Massage for low-back pain. *Cochrane Db Syst Rev* 8(4): CD001929.

Furlan, A.D., M. Imamura, T. Dryden, and E. Irvin. 2009. Massage for low back pain: An updated systematic review within the framework of the Cochrane Back Review Group. *Spine* 34(16): 1669-1684.

Geisser, M.E., E.A. Wiggert, A.J. Haig, and M.O. Colwell. 2005. A randomized, controlled trial of manual therapy and specific adjuvant exercise for chronic low back pain. *Clin J Pain* 21(6): 463-470.

Goats, G.C. 1994. Massage—The scientific basis of an ancient art: Part 2. Physiological and therapeutic effects. *Br J Sports Med* 28(3): 153-156.

Haraldsson, B., A. Gross, C.D. Myers, J. Ezzo, A. Morien, C.H. Goldsmith, P.M.J. Peloso, and G. Brønfort. 2006. Cervical overview group. Massage for mechanical neck disorders. *Cochrane Db Syst Rev* 3: CD004871.

Hernandez-Reif, M., T. Field, J. Krasnegor, and H. Theakston. 2001. Lower back pain is reduced and range of motion increased after massage therapy. *Int J Neurosci* 106(3-4): 131-145.

Hsieh, L.L., C.H. Kuo, M.F. Yen, and T.H. Chen. 2004. A randomized controlled clinical trial for low back pain treated by acupressure and physical therapy. *Prev Med* 39(1): 168-76.

Hsieh, L.L., C.H. Kuo, L.H. Lee, A.M. Yen, K.L. Chien, and T.H. Chen. 2006. Treatment of low back pain by acupressure and physical therapy: Randomised controlled trial. *BMJ* 332(7543): 696-700.

Kania, A., A. Porcino, and M. Verhoef. 2008. Value of qualitative research in the study of massage therapy. *Int J Ther Massage Bodywork* 1(2):6-11.

Lee, M.H.M., K. Itoh, and G.F.W. Yang. 1990. Physical therapy and rehabilitation medicine: Massage. In *The management of pain,* ed. J.J. Bonica, 1777-1778. Philadelphia: Lea and Febiger.

Little, P., G. Lewith, F. Webley, M. Evans, A. Beattie, K. Middleton, J. Barnett, K. Ballard, F. Oxford, P. Smith, L. Yardley, S. Hollinghurst, and D. Sharp. 2008. Randomised controlled trial of Alexander technique lessons, exercise, and massage (ATEAM) for chronic and recurrent back pain. *BMJ* 19(337): a884.

Liu, J., and S. Zhang. 2000. Treatment of protrusion of lumbar intervertebral disc by pulling and turning manipulations. *J Tradit Chin Med* 20: 195-197.

Mackawan, S., W. Eungpinichpong, R. Pantumethakul, U. Chatchawan, and T. Hunsawong. 2007. Effects of traditional Thai massage versus joint mobilization on substance P and pain perception in patients with non-specific low back pain. *J Bodyw Mov Ther* 11(1): 9-16.

Melzack, R., and P.D. Wall. 1996. *The challenge of pain.* 2nd ed. London: Penguin Books.

Moher, D., K.F. Schulz, and D.G. Altman. 2001. The CONSORT statement: Revised recommendations for improving the quality of reports of parallel-group randomized trials. *Ann Intern Med* 134(8): 657-662.

Morhenn, V.B., J.W. Park, E. Piper, and P.J. Zak. 2008. Monetary sacrifice among strangers is mediated by endogenous oxytocin release after physical contact. *Evol Hum Behav* 29: 375-383.

Moyer, C.A., J. Rounds, and J.W. Hannum. 2004. A meta-analysis of massage therapy research. *Psychol Bull* 130: 3-18.

Moyer, C.A., T. Dryden, and S. Shipwright. 2009. Directions and dilemmas in massage therapy research: A workshop report from the 2009 North American Research Conference on Complementary and Integrative Medicine. *Int J Ther Massage Bodywork* 2(2): 15-27.

Poole, H., S. Glenn, and P. Murphy. 2007. A randomised controlled study of reflexology for the management of chronic low back pain. *Eur J Pain* 11(8): 878-887.

Preyde, M. 2000. Effectiveness of massage therapy for subacute low-back pain: A randomized controlled trial. *CMAJ* 162(13): 1815-1820.

Quinn, F., C.M. Hughes, and G.D. Baxter. 2008. Reflexology in the management of low back pain: A pilot randomised controlled trial. *Complement Ther Med* 16(1): 3-8.

Rachlin, I. 2002. Physical therapy treatment approaches for myofascial pain syndromes and fibromyalgia; therapeutic massage in the treatment of myofascial pain syndromes and fibromyalgia. In *Myofascial pain and fibromyalgia. Trigger point management,* ed. E.S. Rachlin and I. Rachlin, 467-487. St. Louis: Mosby.

Roland, M., and J. Fairbank. 2000. The Roland-Morris Disability Questionnaire and the Oswestry Disability Questionnaire. *Spine* 25(24): 3115-3124.

Sagar, S., T. Dryden, and K. Wong. 2007. Massage therapy for cancer patients: A reciprocal relationship between body and mind. *Current Oncology* 14(2): 45-56.

Scott, J., and E.C. Huskisson. 1976. Graphic representation of pain. *Pain* 2: 175-184.

Sefton, J.M., C. Yarar, J.W. Berry, and D.D. Pascoe. 2010. Therapeutic massage of the neck and shoulders produces changes in peripheral blood flow when assessed with dynamic infrared thermography. *J Altern Complement Med* 16(7): 723-732.

Simons, D.G., J.G. Travell, and L.S. Simons. 1999. Apropos of all muscles: Trigger point release. In *Travell & Simons' myofascial pain and dysfunction: The trigger point manual. Upper half of body.* 2nd ed., ed. D.G. Simons, 94-177. Baltimore: Williams & Wilkins.

Vickers, A., and C. Zollman. 1999. ABC of complementary medicine. Massage therapies. *BMJ* 319(7219): 1254-1257.

Waddell, G. 1998. *The back pain revolution*. Edinburgh: Churchill Livingstone.

Yip, Y.B., and S.H. Tse. 2004. The effectiveness of relaxation acupoint stimulation and acupressure with aromatic lavender essential oil for non-specific low back pain in Hong Kong: A randomised controlled trial. *Complement Ther Med* 12(1): 28-37.

Zaproudina, N., T. Hietikko, O.O. Hänninen, and O. Airaksinen. 2009. Effectiveness of traditional bone setting in treating chronic low back pain: A randomised pilot trial. *Complement Ther Med* 17(1): 23-28.

Zhang, J.F., and W.H. Chen. 2004. Curative effect of nonoperative therapy for the lumbar disc herniation. *Chin J Clin Rehabil* 8: 2006-2007.

chapter 13

Anxiety and Depression

Christopher A. Moyer, PhD

Imagine someone dear to you is suffering. For weeks he has seemed tense, nervous, and sad, and he has abandoned the activities he used to enjoy. Though he looks tired, moves sluggishly, and reports having no energy, he is also unable to sleep. He confides to you that he is always worried, irritable, and unable to concentrate. Perhaps he even goes on to report feeling that things are hopeless and finding himself thinking about suicide.

Unfortunately, many readers will have little trouble imagining such a scenario because these are symptoms of anxiety and depressive disorders, which are surprisingly common. Anxiety disorders are the most common mental disorders in America; at least one in four Americans will have one during his or her lifetime. Depressive disorders are nearly as common; approximately one in five Americans will have one at some point (Kessler et al. 2005). Their prevalence appears to be increasing rapidly in many parts of the world (Cross-National Collaborative Group 1992).

Although these disorders are common, they are serious. They not only compromise quality of life, but also contribute to poor social functioning (Hecht, von Zerrsen, and Wittchen 1990; Koran, Thienemann, and Davenport 1996), decreased resistance to illness (Schleifer et al. 1996; Zorilla et al. 1996), unemployment (Dooley, Fielding, and Levi 1996), and even death (Fawcett et al. 1990; Unützer et al. 2002). In addition, their economic effect is staggering. Together, anxiety and depressive disorders cost the U.S. economy more than $120 billion annually (Greenberg et al. 1999), a recurring toll equivalent to the economic cost of Hurricane Katrina (Burton and Hicks 2005).

Fortunately, both psychotherapy (Wampold 2001) and medications (Mitte et al. 2005) can be effective for these disorders. However, each has significant limitations. Medications for anxiety and depression can interact with other medications (Spina and Scordo 2002), lead to undesirable side effects (Fava 2006), or simply fail to work for some patients (Rush et al. 2006). *Psychotherapy* can be expensive and time consuming (Seligman 1995). It does not work for all patients (Thase et al. 1997), and it is unavailable in some communities (U.S. Department of Health and Human Services 1997). Finally, the effectiveness of both is frequently limited by treatment noncompliance ("Dropping out of psychotherapy" 2005; Fava 2006). For these reasons, effective alternatives and complements to these conventional treatments would be of great value.

psychotherapy
▸ The therapeutic application of discussion and a range of behavioral interventions, within the context of an interpersonal relationship, to treat mental disorders or to assist a patient in coping with life problems.

ANXIETY AND DEPRESSION: OVERVIEW

Anxiety and depression are common conditions in modern life. Further, while they can be meaningfully distinguished from each other, it is also known that they are often present at the same time in a person. An overview of these conditions is presented here, with special attention devoted to details of particular relevance to massage therapy research and practice.

Anxiety

Barlow (2002) defines anxiety as a negative affect state that is accompanied by a self-focused shift in attention and a strong physiological response consistent with a state of readiness. Individual vulnerability to high anxiety is a function of biological, psychological, and social factors.

Though anxiety is typically unpleasant, we would not want to eliminate it from our lives. One of the oldest and most consistent psychological findings is that the right amount of anxious arousal, for a given situation, improves performance (Yerkes and Dodson 1908). Nevertheless, problems arise when anxiety is too high. Optimal concentration devolves into an obsessional focus that impedes clear, open thinking. Mild anticipation escalates into paralyzing worry. A feeling of readiness progresses unchecked to become tension, stiffness, headache, fatigue, and digestive troubles. Worst of all, severe anxiety can behave as if it has its own momentum, remaining detrimentally high even when the afflicted person knows there is no logical reason to be highly anxious. When anxiety is high, persistent, and unresponsive to a person's efforts to manage it, treatment is needed.

Assessing and Classifying Anxiety in MT Research

Three approaches to conceptualizing anxiety are most relevant for understanding MT research. Massage therapy research commonly distinguishes state anxiety from trait anxiety, utilizing treatment schedules and assessments that are specific to each. By contrast, MT research rarely uses diagnostic procedures that allow the identification of specific anxiety disorders, even though this approach is valuable, and is commonly used in other areas of clinical practice and research.

State Anxiety

State anxiety is a momentary emotional reaction to one's situation that can include apprehension, tension, worry, and heightened arousal of the autonomic nervous system. Logically, the intensity and duration of the emotional reaction is determined by the person's perception of a situation as threatening (Spielberger 1972).

In MT research, the concept of state anxiety is most useful when considering the effects of a particular session, or *single dose,* of MT. Because state anxiety is a momentary emotional reaction, it is reasonable to expect that a single dose of MT could have an immediate effect.

single dose

▸ In massage therapy research, this specifies the effect of one session of treatment, as opposed to the effect of a series of treatments.

Trait Anxiety

In contrast to the situational and transient nature of state anxiety, trait anxiety is a person's relatively stable proneness to experience anxiety. People with a high level of trait anxiety are more apt to perceive the world as dangerous and threatening, and are more likely to experience frequent and intense anxiety states, than persons with a low level of trait anxiety (Spielberger 1972).

In MT research, the concept of trait anxiety is most useful when considering the progressive effect of a series of MT treatments, or a *multiple-dose* effect. Because trait anxiety is known to be relatively stable within a person, and therefore resistant to change, we do not typically expect a single dose of MT to influence it greatly. Rather, assessment of trait anxiety is usually reserved for studies that include a series of MT treatments across a period of days, weeks, or months. Logically, it

multiple dose

▸ In massage therapy research, this specifies the effect of a series of treatments, as opposed to the effect of a single session of treatment.

could also be appropriate to examine whether MT's effect on trait anxiety continues after a course of treatment has ended.

Specific Anxiety Disorders

Almost all MT research concerned with anxiety has been limited to the assessment methods just discussed. However, anxiety is not itself a disorder. In clinical practice and in some clinical research, it is common to use a categorical approach in which a patient either does or does not meet the diagnostic criteria for one or more specific disorders that prominently feature anxiety. (This approach can be, and often is, used in combination with the approaches for assessing state and trait anxiety previously described.) In the United States and Canada, the predominant diagnostic system is the Diagnostic and Statistical Manual of Mental Disorders (DSM-IV-TR; American Psychiatric Association 2000), which includes 12 distinct anxiety disorders (box 13.1). Most other countries use a similar *nosology* contained in the International Statistical Classification of Diseases and Related Health Problems (ICD-10; World Health Organization 2007).

nosology

▸ A scientific system for the classification of diseases.

BOX 13.1

DSM-IV-TR Anxiety Disorders and Their Key Characteristics

- *Panic disorder without agoraphobia:* Presence of recurrent, unexpected panic attacks.
- *Panic disorder with agoraphobia:* Presence of recurrent, unexpected panic attacks, in combination with anxiety about places or situations in which escape might be difficult or embarrassing.
- *Agoraphobia without history of panic disorders:* Anxiety about places or situations in which escape might be difficult or embarrassing.
- *Specific phobia:* Intense and persistent fear that is excessive or unreasonable in response to specific objects or situations.
- *Social phobia:* Intense and persistent fear of social or performance situations in which one might be judged.
- *Obsessive-compulsive disorder:* Presence of recurrent, persistent thoughts, impulses, or images that cause anxiety or distress, or repetitive behaviors or mental acts the person feels driven to perform in response to an obsession.
- *Post-traumatic stress disorder:* The delayed onset of increased arousal, persistent avoidance, numbing of general responsiveness, or reexperiencing of a traumatic event in response to an event that involved the threat of death or serious injury to self or others.
- *Acute stress disorder:* The undelayed onset of increased arousal, persistent avoidance, numbing of general responsiveness, or reexperiencing of a traumatic event in response to an event that involved the threat of death or serious injury to self or others.
- *Generalized anxiety disorder:* Excessive anxiety and worry, over a period of 6 months or longer, that a person finds difficult to control.
- *Anxiety disorder due to a general medical condition:* Prominent anxiety, panic attacks, obsessions, or compulsions that are physiologically caused by a medical condition.
- *Substance-induced anxiety disorder:* Prominent anxiety, panic attacks, obsessions, or compulsions that are physiologically caused by a drug or medication.
- *Anxiety disorder not otherwise specified:* Presence of clinically relevant anxiety symptoms that do not correspond to one of the previously described anxiety disorders.

Diagnosis of these specific disorders is accomplished by means of a clinical interview, sometimes aided by use of an instrument such as the Structured Clinical Interview for DSM-IV Axis I Disorders (SCID I/P; First et al. 2002). Whether or not such an instrument is used, diagnosis is time intensive and requires considerable clinical expertise. Largely for these reasons, MT studies tend not to use diagnostic methods to identify or target specific anxiety disorders. However, a diagnostic approach will probably have to be adopted as the field progresses if we are to determine which specific anxiety disorders are responsive to MT.

Depression

The difficulty in defining depression becomes evident when we consider that it has been conceptualized in many different ways, including as a mood state, a symptom, a syndrome, a mood disorder, and a disease. For present purposes, it is important that we distinguish depression from ordinary unhappiness or a sad mood. However, when negative mood states are accompanied by mild to moderate deficits in motivation or cognition, vegetative signs, and disruptions in interpersonal relationships, a subclinical level of depression is indicated (Ingram and Siegle 2002). Because most MT studies have selected participants according to the presence of other conditions that may be associated with depression (e.g., fibromyalgia patients in Field et al. 2002; Alzheimer's patients in Scherder, Bouma, and Steen 1998), rather than selecting participants for whom depression is the primary complaint, it is likely that MT's effect on depression has been studied primarily with subclinical samples (Moyer, Rounds, and Hannum 2004; Coelho, Boddy, and Ernst 2008).

Assessing and Classifying Depression in MT Research

Anxiety and depression can be classified and assessed in a variety of ways, and this is evident in massage therapy research. The way or ways that are selected may depend on the specific population being researched, the time and resources available, researchers' preference for and familiarity with specific methods, and other factors. The various approaches to classification and assessment can influence the resultant research and its interpretation, such that a basic understanding of them is valuable.

Measuring Depression as a Continuous Variable

Several reliable and valid self-report instruments exist for the assessment of depression. These include the Center for Epidemiological Studies: Depression Scale (Radloff 1977) and the Beck Depression Inventory-II (Beck et al. 1988). Subscales of broader instruments, such as the Symptom Checklist-90-Revised (Derogatis 1983), can also be used. Such instruments are easy to administer, and yield a score that is easy to interpret, which makes them invaluable for research.

Specific Depressive Disorders and Diagnosis

Just as anxiety is not a specific disorder, neither is depression. Rather, it is a feature of several disorders that appear under the broad heading of mood disorders contained in DSM-IV-TR. As with anxiety disorders, MT research has not used the methods of clinical assessment necessary to identify specific depressive disorders.

comorbid

▸ Pertaining to a disorder or disease that occurs simultaneously with some other disorder or disease.

Comorbidity of Anxiety and Depression

Anxiety and depression are often *comorbid,* or present at the same time in a person. Anxiety may be present with or without depression, but recent evidence indicates that almost all patients with depression are also anxious (Barlow 2002; Brown et al. 2001). Further, though these conditions are manifestly different, they may originate from the same underlying genetic factors (Kendler et al. 1995). Refinements to current diagnostic procedures may see anxiety and depressive disorders contained together within a larger category. The comorbidity and conceptual overlap of anxiety and depression are relevant to MT research because MT may only need to have an effect on anxiety for it to also appear to be effective for depression.

EFFECTS OF MASSAGE THERAPY ON ANXIETY AND DEPRESSION

A clear picture of MT's effects comes from randomized controlled trials (RCTs), and there have been numerous RCTs that examine MT for anxiety. The picture is clearest when the results of the highest quality RCTs are combined in a meta-analysis, a summary of a research domain that quantifies the typical strength of an effect, its variability, and its statistical significance (Rosenthal 1995). This approach has been used to review the psychological effects of MT on adult (Moyer, Rounds, and Hannum 2004) and pediatric (Beider and Moyer 2007) recipients. The results of those reviews are summarized here, but readers requiring greater detail are advised to examine them directly.

Massage Therapy for Anxiety

The effect of massage therapy on anxiety has been researched more than any other outcome. Given the prevalence of anxiety and the role it may play in perpetuating other disorders and diseases, this focus is warranted. The promising effects of massage therapy on anxiety are reviewed here.

State Anxiety

MT reduces state anxiety in adults, though the effect is not as robust as is often reported. Across 21 MT RCTs that used 1,026 total research participants, the average recipient of single-dose MT had a posttreatment level of state anxiety that was lower than 64% of control group participants (Moyer, Rounds, and Hannum 2004), an effect considered "small to medium," according to statistical conventions in the behavioral sciences (Cohen 1988). A subsequent analysis to account for the possibility that this result could be influenced in a positive direction by publication bias indicated that the true effect may be even smaller and not statistically significant.

In pediatric recipients, MT's effect on state anxiety appears to be more consistent and stronger. However, this assertion should be evaluated cautiously, since the number of studies examining this effect is small. Across four MT RCTs that used 81 total research participants, the average child recipient of single-dose MT, at the beginning of a treatment series, had a posttreatment level of state anxiety that was lower than 72% of control group participants. In addition, Beider and Moyer (2007) separately examined the single-dose effects of the first and last treatments in a series to examine whether these differed (figure 13.1).

Effects of single-dose MT were significantly stronger when assessed at the end of a treatment series, such that the average child recipient of single-dose MT had a posttreatment level of state anxiety lower than 86% of control group participants. These effects are medium and large in magnitude, respectively, according to convention (Cohen 1988). The stronger single-dose effect observed at the final treatment in a series may be the result of children's increasing comfort with MT, or with their massage therapist, over the course of time.

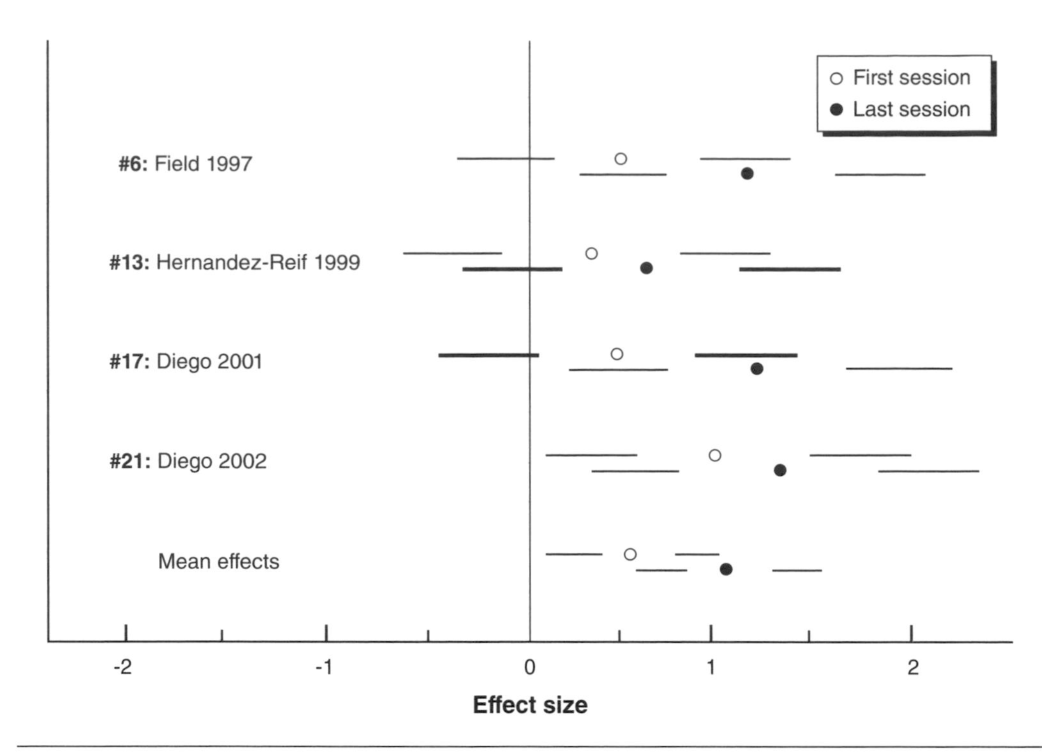

Figure 13.1 Single-dose mean effects and their 95% confidence intervals for MT to reduce state anxiety in pediatric recipients; note that effects are consistently stronger at last sessions than in first sessions.

Trait Anxiety

Results from seven MT RCTs, which used 194 total research participants, demonstrate that MT consistently lowers trait anxiety significantly more than controls do. (Among these studies, only one can be considered to have used a pediatric sample, and the results of that study are similar in magnitude to the six that used adult participants. Therefore, the results of all seven studies are considered together.) At the conclusion of a series of MT treatments, the average MT recipient had a level of trait anxiety that was lower than 77% of control group participants (Moyer, Rounds, and Hannum 2004), which is a medium to large effect (Cohen 1988).

MT for Depression

A series of MT treatments appears to consistently and substantially reduce depression in adult recipients. Across 10 MT RCTs, which used 249 total research participants, the average MT recipient had a lower posttreatment level of depression than 73% of control group participants (Moyer, Rounds, and Hannum 2004), which is a medium effect (Cohen 1988).

EXPLAINING MASSAGE THERAPY EFFECTS

On the whole, currently available evidence supports MT effects on anxiety and depression. How does MT accomplish these effects? Several theories are consistently asserted in research reports, but research designs that rigorously test these theories are rare. In addition, much MT research features analyses that lead researchers to overstate what is known about MT's actual causal mechanisms (Moyer 2009). Presently, the simplest and most accurate answer to the question "How does MT reduce anxiety and depression?" is "We don't know for certain."

Despite this, a review of these theories is still in order. Note that the following theories are not mutually exclusive. It is possible, perhaps likely, that more than one is responsible for MT effects on anxiety and depression.

Change in Balance of Autonomic Nervous System Activation

It is frequently asserted that MT shifts the balance of autonomic nervous system (ANS) activity, causing a reduction of activity in the sympathetic branch while promoting activation of the parasympathetic branch (Ferrell-Torry and Glick 1993; Hulme, Waterman, and Hillier 1999). This balance of ANS activity is associated with rest and recovery, including decreased cardiorespiratory activity and level of stress hormones, and feelings of calmness and well-being inconsistent with depression and anxiety.

Evidence in support of this theory is mixed. MT does consistently reduce blood pressure and heart rate, but its effect on the stress hormone cortisol is much too small to be a cause of the statistically robust effects that the treatment has on anxiety and depression (Moyer et al. 2011; Moyer, Rounds, and Hannum 2004; Beider and Moyer 2007).

Influence on Neurotransmitters

Field, Diego, and Hernandez-Reif (2007) contend that, by stimulating subcutaneous pressure receptors, MT increases levels of the neurotransmitters serotonin and dopamine, an effect that in turn leads to a decrease in depression. However, this conclusion is based on within-group effects, reviewed in Field and colleagues (2005), that disregard data from those studies' control groups. Further, the requisite pressure for MT to produce effects has only been examined in a single study that examined its importance in infant massage (Diego et al. 2004). The role of pressure in MT effects has not been established, in part because it is a difficult variable to study.

Muscle Tension

In a review of MT effects in pediatric samples, a desirable change in muscle tone was one of the largest effects. (The average MT recipient's posttreatment tonus was better than 82% of control group children.) Given that muscle tension is a key symptom of generalized anxiety disorder, one of the most common anxiety disorders, MT's potential to reduce that tension could largely explain its effect on anxiety. Because anxiety is so often comorbid with depression, this same mechanism might also explain MT's effect on that condition. Possibly, MT is only truly effective for anxiety, and its observed effect on depression is actually a second-order effect that is mediated by its effect on anxiety.

Interpersonal Attention and Parallels with Psychotherapy

It is notable that a series of MT treatments produces reductions of anxiety and depression that are similar in magnitude to those typically observed in psychotherapy research. In addition, MT parallels psychotherapy in structure; both therapies rely on repeated, private interpersonal contact between the practitioner and recipient, and similar session lengths and patterns are employed. MT intended to reduce anxiety and depression may be more similar to psychotherapy than has commonly been considered, which would have important ramifications for both education and research.

RECOMMENDATIONS FOR MASSAGE THERAPY PRACTICE

Though there is always more to be discovered, our current understanding of massage therapy, anxiety, and depression yields these recommendations for practice.

- Prevalence Demands Basic Knowledge. As previously noted, anxiety and depression are common. They are so common, in fact, that every massage therapist will eventually encounter these conditions in their practice. Therefore, to practice ethically and responsibly, all massage therapists, and not just those attempting to tailor their practice to serve these specific populations, need to have basic knowledge of these conditions.
- Benefits Can Be Asserted With Confidence. Massage therapists can be confident that MT has been scientifically demonstrated to reduce anxiety and depression, and that the benefits are substantial. Indeed, there are probably no other effects in MT research that have been as consistently demonstrated as these mental health benefits. Massage therapists can confidently and ethically assert these benefits when discussing MT with recipients, other health care professionals, and the public at large, though they should also take care to highlight important caveats. These include the following:
    - How MT produces these effects is not precisely known.
    - MT, like any treatment, works differently for different people, and will not work for everyone.
    - The magnitude of these effects likely depends on an optimal amount and pattern of treatments that are not yet known.
    - The best type of MT for reducing anxiety and depression has not yet been determined.
- Understand the Nature of Patient Self-Reports. Some MT patients who are anxious or depressed will know this about themselves and openly report it, but such patients are probably rare. Others will know that they have anxiety or depression, but unfortunately, will not report this out of embarrassment. Another subset of patients with anxiety or depression will not even know that they have such a condition. Instead, they are likely to believe that their symptoms indicate a physical, rather than psychological, problem. Persons with anxiety who are unaware of it as the cause of their symptoms may report digestive troubles, shortness of breath, sweating, difficulty sleeping, poor concentration, or general agitation. Persons unaware of depression as their underlying condition may report fatigue, sleep disturbances, difficulty performing everyday activities, loss of appetite, or listlessness (Taylor 2006). The key point is that some MT patients who are anxious or depressed will not state it plainly, so massage therapists need to be attentive to other indicators of these conditions. With depression especially, massage therapists should heed guidelines provided by the U.S. Preventive Services Task Force that advise clinicians to be alert to "depressive symptoms in adolescents and young adults, persons with a family or personal history of depression, those

with chronic illnesses, those who perceive or have experienced a recent loss, and those with sleep disorders, chronic pain, or multiple unexplained somatic complaints" (1996, 544-545).

• Assess Anxiety and Depression at Intake. Any professionally administered health intervention needs to begin with a procedure for collecting essential information about the patient's current health and motivations for seeking treatment. Though MT intake procedures undoubtedly vary widely according to therapists' training, practice settings, and individual levels of comfort and experience in performing the task (Walton 2005), every massage therapist should be asking about anxiety and depression at intake. In many settings, two simple questions (e.g., "Have you been anxious? Have you been depressed?"), given verbally or on an intake form, may be sufficient. Even these basic questions have the potential to provide important information and to open a channel for broader dialogue about the patient's health. Therapists who are apprehensive about asking these questions should note that affirmative answers need not require a series of invasive follow-up questions. Patients who admit to being anxious or depressed can be informed that MT may help, and provided with a referral to a mental health professional (see relevant following section). These steps, though basic and requiring little time, have great potential to benefit patients. Therefore, they should be a part of every massage therapist's intake procedures.

• Logically, massage therapists wishing to specialize in the treatment of anxiety and depression may find that more specialized assessment procedures are called for. As this specialty develops, administration and interpretation of well-validated standardized instruments, such as the Beck Depression Inventory (Beck et al. 1988) and the State-Trait Anxiety Inventory (Spielberger 1983), will be invaluable. Note, however, that the use of these instruments may require some training not currently within the scope of massage therapy, unless the practitioner is also credentialed in the practice of psychology. The eventual adoption of such instruments as part of an MT specialty would optimize assessment, facilitate communication with mental health professionals (e.g., when sharing information about specific cases), and help to legitimize MT as specialty for anxiety and depression.

• Network With Medical and Mental Health Professionals. A professional massage therapist should not see oneself only as a sole practitioner, but as one member of a larger health care community. This maximizes the likelihood of connecting one's patients with the health information and services that will most benefit them. In addition, opportunities for the massage therapist to learn and to increase one's patient base are also valuable. Professional connections with local medical and mental health professionals permit the massage therapist to offer referrals to anxious or depressed patients, and to receive referrals from those professionals.

• Recognize Limitations. Armed with the scientific findings that massage therapy reduces anxiety and depression, massage therapists should be enthusiastic about the treatment that they offer. But, it is essential to temper that enthusiasm with a respect for the limitations of this form of treatment. Massage therapists who intend to work with anxious and depressed patients must recognize that the evidence, while promising, is small and limited in scope compared to that which has been conducted on first-line treatments for these conditions. Further, because massage therapy for these conditions is a relatively recent phenomenon, the profession has not had the opportunity to incorporate specialized education and training pertaining to specific concerns that are raised by these conditions.

These concerns, which include advanced training in interpersonal communication, extensive knowledge of the factors that contribute to or cause anxiety and depression, clinical experience with other conditions that are a part of the picture in some cases of anxiety or depression, such as personality disorders or substance abuse, and the prevention of self-harm or suicide, are addressed in the training of medical and mental health professionals. They illustrate the tremendous importance of being networked with such professionals for the massage therapist who expects to treat anxious or depressed patients.

- Keep Up With the Latest Research. New MT research, much of it concerned with anxiety and depression, is being conducted all the time. Every practitioner should make the effort to keep up with the latest findings (see chapter 19).

Evidence-Based Treatment Guidelines

Because anxiety and depression are common and because they sometimes go unidentified, massage therapists should routinely ask patients if they are experiencing anxiety and depression as a part of intake procedures. They should also be networked with mental health professionals to facilitate patient referral and permit consultation as needed. Whether or not massage therapy is provided, patients with significant anxiety or depression should be referred to a mental health practitioner for assessment and treatment.

Based on the evidence, massage therapy is an effective treatment for patients suffering from anxiety and depression. A series of massage therapy treatments yields the best outcomes, though optimal dosing is not yet known. Massage therapist training, especially for therapists considering specializing in this area, should include development of interpersonal communication skills and basic understanding of the factors that contribute to anxiety, depression, and other mental health conditions. They should also provide related knowledge on substance abuse, prevention of self-harm or suicide, and the treatments commonly used for treatment of anxiety and depression. Providing patients with evidence-based information on methods of self-care for anxiety and depression, such as relaxation exercises, is also recommended.

DIRECTIONS FOR FUTURE RESEARCH

Moyer, Dryden, and Shipwright (2009) identified numerous directions for MT research, many of which apply to MT for anxiety and depression. Chief among these are the following:

1. Identification of the types of, and necessary pressure for, MT to optimally reduce anxiety and depression.
2. Neuroimaging studies that could document the effects of MT in the central nervous system.
3. Determination of optimal MT dosing.
4. Examination of MT used in combination with psychotherapy, medications, or both of these.
5. Examination of the therapeutic relationship that forms between massage therapist and recipient during treatment, and its importance in the delivery of antianxiety and antidepressant effects.
6. Cost-effectiveness studies that quantify the value of MT, in dollars and cents, for the treatment of anxiety and depression.
7. Longer-term longitudinal studies to determine the duration and maintenance of antianxiety and antidepressant effects, including those that may extend beyond the cessation of treatment.

Case Study

For six months, Sarah T., age 38, has found herself preoccupied with worries pertaining to her job, her marriage, and the health of her asthmatic son. She is almost always restless and fatigued, and has suffered from insomnia and frequent tension headaches. Within the last month, she has started to feel sad almost all the time, and sometimes feels an uncontrollable urge to cry. She has lost her normally healthy appetite, and has experienced difficulties concentrating and making decisions at work. At the urging of her husband and friends, who have noticed an increase in her symptoms, she reluctantly agreed to try weekly sessions of psychotherapy with Dr. Estella F., a clinical psychologist.

Using her clinical judgment in combination with results from the State-Trait Anxiety Inventory and the Beck Depression Inventory, Dr. F. diagnosed generalized anxiety disorder and major depressive disorder of mild severity. Treatment, however, proves more difficult. Sarah struggles with talk therapy, possibly due to her difficulty concentrating. She showed little improvement after four sessions. Dr. F. sensed that her patient was increasingly ambivalent about continuing psychotherapy, and worried that Sarah would prematurely terminate treatment. Further, even though Dr. F. told her that she might benefit from antianxiety or antidepressant medication, Sarah was opposed to this treatment option.

Dr. F. informed Sarah that she mlght benefit from massage therapy. Sarah was skeptical, but when Dr. F. points out that it is very safe and usually pleasant, and that research shows its effectiveness, she agreed that it was worth a try. Dr. F. secured Sarah's written consent to share aspects of her case with Helen S., a local massage therapist who is developing a specialty in MT for anxiety and depression.

Never having received a professional massage, Sarah was naturally apprehensive at her first appointment. She was reassured to learn that Helen welcomes feedback during the massage. She was pleasantly surprised at the overall feeling of wellness and relaxation she had when leaving her first appointment with Helen. She also appreciated the contrast between MT and psychotherapy. While she knows she needs to listen, talk, and concentrate in her psychotherapy sessions if they are going to be effective, she felt no such demands at her MT appointment. Sarah decided to continue with MT for at least a few more sessions.

As her comfort with MT increased, Sarah experienced its benefits more strongly and for a greater duration. The resulting symptom reduction changed her attitude in and commitment to psychotherapy. Dr. F. observed that Sarah had a newfound hope and that she was able to benefit more from the process of psychotherapy as her energy level gradually improved and her nervous tension gradually diminished.

After 12 weeks of psychotherapy and 8 weeks of MT, Sarah's level of depression, as indicated by the Beck Depression Inventory, was reduced to the nonclinical range. Her level of anxiety was also much reduced, but was still higher than the average. Sarah continued to struggle with worries, but had made considerable improvement. Psychotherapy was terminated with Dr. F.'s approval, albeit with the understanding that Sarah could return to treatment if her condition worsened. Sarah continues to receive MT twice a month, which she and Helen have agreed to try as a maintenance dose.

SUMMARY

Anxiety and depression are common and potentially serious conditions. Fortunately, a substantial amount of research has examined the effect of massage therapy on these conditions, and the results are consistent and promising. In light of these positive outcomes, massage therapists should familiarize themselves with and keep abreast of this research literature, work interprofessionally with medical and mental health experts, and prepare themselves to see these conditions in their practices. In addition, all massage therapists should ask about anxiety and depression as a part of intake procedures. Practitioners considering specializing in this area should also acquire training in effective interpersonal communication skills; a basic understanding of the factors that contribute to anxiety, depression, and other mental health conditions; and related knowledge on substance abuse, prevention of self-harm and suicide, and the treatments commonly used for treatment of anxiety and depression.

REFERENCES

Abrams, S.M. 1999. Attention-deficit/hyperactivity disordered children and adolescents benefit from massage therapy. *Dissertation Abstracts International* 60: 5218.

American Psychiatric Association. 2000. *Diagnostic and statistical manual of mental disorders: DSM-IV-TR*. Washington, DC: American Psychiatric Publishing.

Barlow, D.H. 2002. *Anxiety and its disorders: The nature and treatment of anxiety and panic.* 2nd ed. New York: Guilford Press.

Beck, A., N. Epstein, G. Brown, and R. Steer. 1988. An inventory for measuring clinical anxiety: Psychometric properties. *J Consult Clin Psych* 56(6): 893-897.

Beider, S., and C.A. Moyer. 2007. Randomized controlled trials of pediatric massage: A review. *Evid-Based Compl Alt* 4: 23-34.

Brown, T.A., L.A. Campbell, C.L. Lehman, J.R. Grisham and R.B. Mancill. 2001. Current and lifetime comorbidity of the DSM-IV anxiety and mood disorders in a large clinical sample. *J Abnorm Psychol* 110: 585-599.

Burton, M. L., and M. Hicks. 2005. Hurricane Katrina: Preliminary estimates of commercial and public sector damages. www.marshall.edu/cber/research/katrina/Katrina-Estimates.pdf.

Coelho, H.F., K. Boddy, and E. Ernst. 2008. Massage therapy for the treatment of depression: A systematic review. *Int J Clin Pract* 62(2): 325-333.

Cohen, J. 1988. *Statistical power analysis for the behavioral sciences.* 2nd ed. Hillsdale, NJ: Erlbaum.

Cross-National Collaborative Group. 1992. The changing rate of major depression: Cross-national comparisons. *JAMA* 268: 3098-3105.

Derogatis, L.R. 1983. *SCL-90-R administration, scoring and procedures manual.* Towson, MD: Clinical Psychometric Research.

Diego, M.A., T. Field, C. Sanders, and M. Hernandez-Reif. 2004. Massage therapy of moderate and light pressure and vibrator effects on EEG and heart rate. *Int J Neurosci* 114: 31-44.

Dooley, D., J. Fielding, and L. Levi. 1996. Health and unemployment. *Annu Rev Publ Health* 17: 449-465.

Dropping out of psychotherapy. 2005. *Harvard Mental Health Letter* 22: 3-4.

Ernst, E. 2003. The safety of massage therapy. *Rheumatology* 42: 1101-1106.

Fava, M. 2006. Prospective studies of adverse events related to antidepressant discontinuation. *J Clin Psychiat* 67: 14-21.

Fawcett, J., W.A. Scheftner, L. Fogg, D.C. Clark, M.A. Young, D. Hedeker, and R. Gibbons. 1990. Time-related predictors of suicide in major affective disorder. *Am J Psychiat* 146: 1189-1194.

Ferrell-Torry, A.T., and O.J. Glick. 1993. The use of therapeutic massage as a nursing intervention to modify anxiety and the perception of cancer pain. *Cancer Nurs* 16: 32-35.

Field, T., M. Hernandez-Reif, M. Diego, S. Schanberg, and C. Kuhn. 2005. "Cortisol decreases and serotonin and dopamine increase following massage therapy." *Int J Neurosci* 115(10): 1397-1413.

Field, T., M. Diego, C. Cullen, M. Hernandez-Reif, W. Sunshine, and S. Douglas. 2002. Fibromyalgia pain and substance p decrease and sleep improves after massage therapy. *J Clin Rheumatol* 8: 72-76.

Field, T., M. Diego, and M. Hernandez-Reif. 2007. Massage therapy research. *Dev Rev* 27: 75-89.

First, M.B., R.L. Spitzer, M. Gibbon, and J.B.W. Williams. 2002. *Structured clinical interview for DSM-IV-TR Axis I disorders, research version, patient edition with psychotic screen (SCID-I/P W/ PSY SCREEN).* New York: New York State Psychiatric Institute.

Greenberg, P.E., T. Sisitsky, R.C. Kessler, S.N. Finkelstein, E.R. Berndt, J.R. Davidson, J.C. Ballenger, and A.J. Fyer. 1999. The economic burden of anxiety disorders in the 1990s. *J Clin Psychiat* 60: 427-435.

Greenberg, P.E., R.C. Kessler, H.G. Birnbaum, S.A. Leong, S.W. Lowe, P.A. Berglund, and P.K. Corey-Lisle. 2003. The economic burden of depression in the United States: How did it change between 1990 and 2000? *J Clin Psychiat* 64: 1465-1475.

Hecht, H., D. von Zerssen and H.U. Wittchen. 1990. Anxiety and depression in a community sample: The influence of comorbidity on social functioning. *J Affect Disorders* 18: 137-144.

Hernandez-Reif, M., T. Field, J. Krasgenor, H. Theakston, Z. Hossain, and I. Burman. 2000. High blood pressure and associated symptoms were reduced by massage therapy. *J Bodyw Mov Ther* 4: 31-38.

Hernandez-Reif, M., T. Field, J. Krasgenor and H. Theakston. 2001. Lower back pain is reduced and range of motion increased after massage therapy. *Int J Neurosci* 106: 131-145.

Hulme, J., H. Waterman, and V.F. Hillier. 1999. The effects of foot massage on patients' perception of care following laparoscopic sterilization as day case patients. *J Adv Nurs* 30: 460-468.

Ingram, R.E. and G.J. Siegle. 2002. Contemporary methodological issues in the study of depression: Not your father's Oldsmobile. In *Handbook of depression,* eds. I.H. Gotlib and C.L. Hammen, 86-114. New York: Guilford Press.

Kendler, K.S., R.C. Kessler, E.E. Walters, C. MacLean, M.C. Neale, A.C. Heath and L.J. Eaves. 1995. Stressful life events, genetic liability, and onset of an episode of major depression in women. *Am J Psychiat* 152: 833-842.

Kessler, R.C., P. Berglund, O. Demler, R. Jin, K.R. Merikangas, and E.E. Walters. 2005. Lifetime prevalence and age-of-onset distributions of DSM-IV disorders in the national comorbidity survey replication. *Arch Gen Psychiat* 62: 593-602.

Koran, L.M., M.L. Thienemann, and R. Davenport. 1996. Quality of life for patients with obsessive-compulsive disorder. *Am J Psychiat* 153: 783-788.

Mitte, K., P. Noack, R. Steil and H. Hautzinger. 2005. "A meta-analytic review of the efficacy of drug treatment in generalized anxiety disorder. *J Clin Psychopharm* 24: 141-150.

Moyer, C.A. 2009. "Between-groups study designs demand between-groups analyses: A response to Hernandez-Reif, Shor-Posner, Baez, Soto, Mendoze, Castillo, Quintero, Perez, and Zhang." *Evid-Based Compl Alt* 6: 49-50.

Moyer, C.A., J. Rounds, and J.W. Hannum. 2004. A meta-analysis of massage therapy research. *Psych Bull* 130: 3-18.

Moyer, C.A., T. Dryden, and S. Shipwright. 2009. Directions and dilemmas in massage therapy research: A workshop report from the 2009 North American research conference on complementary and integrative medicine. *Int J Ther Massage Bodywork* 2: 15-27.

Moyer, C.A., L. Seefeldt, E.S. Mann, and L.M. Jackley. 2011. Does massage therapy reduce cortisol? A comprehensive quantitative review. *J Bodyw Mov Ther* 15: 3-14.

Radloff, L. 1977. The CES-D scale: A self-report depression scale for research in the general population. *Appl Psych Meas* 1: 385-401.

Rosenthal, R. 1995. Writing meta-analytic reviews. *Psych Bull* 118: 183-192.

Rush, A.J., H.T. Madhukar, S.R. Wisniewski, J.W. Stewart, A.A. Nierenberg, M.E. Thase, L. Ritz, M. M. Biggs, D. Warden, J. F. Luther, K. Shores-Wilson, G. Niederehe, and M. Fava. 2006. Bupropion-SR, sertraline, or venlafaxine-XR after failure of SSRIs for depression. *New Engl J Med* 354: 1231-1242.

Scherder, E., A. Bouma and L. Steen. 1998. Effects of peripheral tactile nerve stimulation on affective behavior of patients with probable Alzheimer's disease. *Am J Alzheimers Dis* 13: 61-69.

Schleifer, S.J., S.E. Keller, J.A. Bartlett, H.M. Eckholdt, and B.R. Delaney. 1996. Immunity in young adults with major depressive disorder. *Am J Psychiat* 153: 477-482.

Seligman, M.E.P. 1995. The effectiveness of psychotherapy. *Am Psychol* 50: 965-974.

Spielberger, C.D. 1972. Conceptual and methodological issues in anxiety research. In *Anxiety: Vol. 2. Current trends in theory and research,* ed. C.D. Spielberger, 481-493. New York: Academic Press.

———. 1983. *Manual for the state-trait anxiety inventory.* Palo Alto, CA: Consulting Psychologists Press.

Spina, E., and M.G. Scordo. 2002. Clinically significant drug interactions with antidepressants in the elderly. *Drugs Aging* 19: 299-320.

Taylor, S.E. 2006. *Health psychology.* 6th ed. New York: McGraw-Hill.

Thase, M.E., D.J. Buysse, E. Frank, C.R. Cherry, C.L. Cornes, A.G. Mallinger and D.J. Kupfer. 1997. Which depressed patients will respond to interpersonal psychotherapy? The role of abnormal EEG sleep profiles. *Am J Psychiat* 154: 502-509.

United States Department of Health and Human Services. 1997. Mental health providers in rural and isolated areas: Final report of the ad hoc rural mental health provider work group. www.mentalhealth.samhsa.gov/publications/allpubs/SMA98-3166/default.asp.

U.S. Preventive Services Task Force. 1996. *Guide to clinical preventive services.* 2nd ed. http://odphp.osophs.dhhs.gov/pubs/guidecps.

Unützer, J., D.L. Patrick, T. Marmon, G.E. Simon, and W.J. Katon. 2002. Depressive symptoms and mortality in a prospective study of 2,558 older adults. *Am J Geriat Psychiat* 10: 521-530.

Walton, T. 2005. Medical conditions in massage practice: Intake forms and questions, part I. www.massagetoday.com/mpacms/mt/article.php?id=13221.

Wampold, B.E. 2001. *The great psychotherapy debate.* Mahwah, NJ: Erlbaum.

World Health Organization. 2007. *International statistical classification of diseases and related health problems: ICD-10.* Geneva: WHO.

Yerkes, R.M., and J.D. Dodson. 1908. The relation of strength of stimulus to rapidity of habit-formation. *Journal of Comprehensive Neurologic and Psychology* 18: 459-482.

Zorilla, E.P., J.R. McKay, L. Luborsky, and K. Schmidt. 1996. Relation of stressors and depressive symptoms to clinical progression of viral illness. *Am J Psychiat* 153: 626-635.

chapter

14

Massage for Adults With a History of Sexual Trauma

Cynthia J. Price, PhD, LMT

Numerous studies have demonstrated the psychological and physical consequences of traumatic events, experiences that result in "intense fear, helplessness, or horror in response to an event" (American Psychiatric Association 2000). These can include exposure to sexual abuse or assault, rape, and domestic violence. The prevalence of sexually traumatic events is high. Childhood prevalence is estimated at 14% for males and 32% for females (Briere and Elliott 2003). Among adults, approximately 1 in every 10 women experiences sexual assault (Kessler et al. 1995). This rate is even higher, at 1 in every 4, among women in the military (Sadler et al. 2000).

To date, a number of studies, all with female participants, have investigated the benefit of massage therapy (MT) as a treatment for sexual trauma. This chapter provides an overview of the health issues associated with trauma, describes the results from the MT studies, discusses future directions for MT research specific to trauma treatment, and provides guidelines for practice. The chapter concludes with a case study, derived from one of the research studies, that illustrates some of the key issues in MT as treatment for sexual trauma.

OVERVIEW OF SEXUAL TRAUMA

The long-term effects of sexual trauma include dissociation, a disruption of the normally integrated experience of consciousness or psychological functioning, depression, *somatization,* anxiety, sleep problems, and difficulty trusting others (Briere and Runtz 1993). Studies of people seeking primary care (McCauley et al. 1997) and of veterans (Dobie et al. 2004) show significantly increased psychological and physical symptoms among those with a history of sexual trauma. Some people who live through traumatic experiences develop post-traumatic stress disorder (PTSD), depending on the type and severity of traumatic event, their history of previous trauma, and the perceived threat of violence (Breslau 2002).

somatization

▸ The expression of psychological stress as a physical symptom.

Post-traumatic stress disorder (PTSD) is an anxiety disorder that is characterized, in part, by difficulties in assessing the emotional environment and negotiating internal and external sensory and emotional cues (Thayer and Lane 2000). This disorder has an estimated lifetime prevalence of 8% in the general population. With the exception of exposure to military violence, women have twice the risk of men for developing PTSD (Kessler et al. 1995; Olff et al. 2007), which is likely due to their greater exposure to violent crimes associated with severe interpersonal distress (Seedat, Stein, and Carey 2005; Stein, Walker, and Forde 2000). Medical conditions, including poor cardiorespiratory and gastrointestinal health and diabetes, are all more common among people with PTSD (Kimerling 2004; Ciechanowski et al. 2004; Weisberg et al. 2002; Gill and Page 2006). The effect of trauma is societal as well as individual: The odds of teenage childbearing, marital instability, unemployment, and dropping out of high school or college are all significantly increased in persons with PTSD (Kessler 2000). The medical costs of treating PTSD are remarkably high. It is the most costly anxiety disorder to treat (Marciniak et al. 2005), reflecting, in part, the higher utilization of medical services by patients with PTSD (Tagay et al. 2005). These negative consequences associated with trauma and PTSD, for both individual patients and for society, highlight the need for effective care and treatment.

HEALING FROM TRAUMA AND ITS RELATIONSHIP TO THE BODY

Recovery from trauma involves reintegration of the self: a process of reestablishing trust and safety, regulation of emotions, and empowerment (Herman 1997). Sexual trauma is often accompanied by the discontinuity between self and body as a dissociative coping mechanism for the pain of the abuse (van der Kolk, van der Hart, and Marmar 1996; Timms and Connors 1992). Not surprisingly, the sense of separation from the self that characterizes dissociation can lead to client apprehension about getting MT, since it is common for sexual abuse survivors to fear the emotions associated with bodily sensation. The client may feel anxious about being touched or disconnected from the MT experience, and may aim to just get through it. She could also fear the emotions that could precipitate a dissociative response. Yet despite these potential obstacles to receiving and benefitting from MT, the desire to relieve their symptoms often motivates these adults to seek MT (Palinkas and Kabongo 2000; Price et al. 2007), as does the desire for increased *body awareness* and connection to sense of self (Price 2004; Price 2005). These issues, and how to address them therapeutically, are discussed in the MT clinical literature (Timms and Connors 1992; Benjamin 1996; Fitch and Dryden 2000).

body awareness

▸ The degree to which people attend to and have an accurate and healthy perception of their own body's appearance, condition, and functioning.

EFFECTS OF MASSAGE THERAPY FOR WOMEN WITH A HISTORY OF SEXUAL TRAUMA

The current amount of research on MT for adult women with a history of trauma is minimal, but the results are promising. Several studies (Field et al. 1997; Price 2005; Price 2006; Price 2007) show that MT is highly acceptable to women in recovery from sexual trauma. This is evidenced by high recruitment and retention rates and by data gathered in qualitative interviews in which participants report satisfaction with their MT experience. MT also reduces their levels of anxiety and depression, PTSD symptoms, dissociation, and the number and intensity of physical symptoms. In addition, body connection and body investment were increased with massage.

In one of my own studies (Price 2005), 7 out of the 12 women who received a standardized MT intervention met the diagnostic criteria for PTSD at baseline. At the 3-month follow-up, only 3 of the women met the criteria for current PTSD, which suggests that MT was a clinically effective adjunct to psychotherapy. A graphical account of their progress is displayed in figure 14.1.

Participants in that study also completed written questionnaires that asked about their experience receiving MT. Two primary themes emerged from their

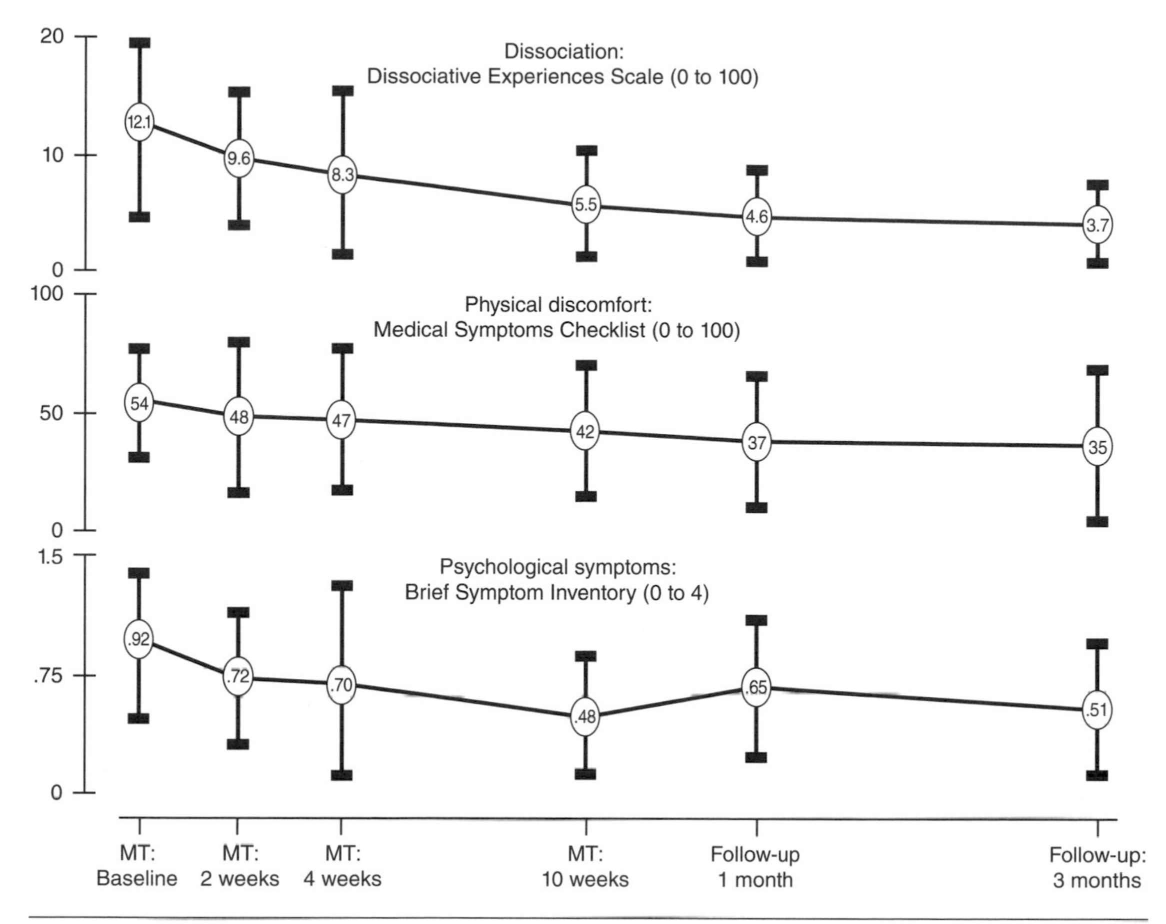

Figure 14.1 Mean values, +/- one standard deviation, for measures of dissociation, physical discomfort, and psychological symptoms across 10 weeks of massage therapy (MT) and 3 months of follow-up ($n = 11$). All three are significantly reduced across time (repeated measures ANOVAs, all $p < .01$).

qualitative responses, both of which indicate the high level of comfort and safety that participants experienced during MT. One of these themes was increased *self-awareness,* as evidenced by one participant's response that she is now "owning just how disconnected . . . [she is] at this point with [her] body." The other was increased *self-care,* exemplified by another response in which a participant said that she was "trying to learn to connect, accept, nurture, and take care of [her] body." In addition to these benefits, it is also important to point out that there were no adverse events observed in this study, nor in any of the other studies that have examined MT for trauma.

self-awareness

▸ The conscious consideration and knowledge of one's own feelings, desires, interests, and character.

self-care

▸ Any behavior or act that one can do for oneself in the pursuit of health or well-being.

EXPLAINING MASSAGE THERAPY EFFECTS

Given the small number of studies that have been conducted and the small samples in those studies, we cannot precisely estimate the magnitude of MT benefits for persons who have experienced trauma, nor do we know how MT produces the benefits that those studies suggest. However, one of these studies (Price 2007) found that a reduction of dissociation, facilitated by MT and leading to a more coherent sense of self, may be of particular importance. Dissociation was reduced steadily and consistently across the MT intervention period and at a 3-month follow-up. In addition, the reduction of dissociation in combination with improvement on all other mental and physical health outcomes that were assessed suggests a link between dissociation reduction and positive health outcomes.

This is consistent with the broader clinical (Timms and Connors 1992; Ford 1993; Fosha 2000; Kepner 2003) and research literatures (van der Kolk 2001; van der Kolk 2006), both of which emphasize the importance of connecting with and reclaiming the body in trauma recovery. Massage therapy research of participants' perception that MT improved their self-efficacy, or their belief in their ability to accomplish goals or address challenges, may also play a role in positive massage outcomes (Price 2005). These research findings support the theory that embodiment is a key factor in the recovery process and that MT may play a unique role in the path toward embodiment for trauma survivors.

RECOMMENDATIONS FOR MASSAGE THERAPY PRACTICE

Providing therapy to clients with trauma and PTSD can be challenging due to the emotional and psychological issues that can arise and the risk of vicarious traumatization, in which the therapist experiences some trauma by internalizing the client's stories of abuse or assault (Pearlman and Saakvitne 2005). While MT does not focus on verbal exploration of traumatic experience as does psychotherapy, it is not uncommon for clients to share their memories once a trust relationship is established (Timms and Connors 1992; Fitch and Dryden 2000). Thus, it is important that massage therapists have adequate skills for working with emotional and psychological issues, should they arise, and adequate supervision to provide professional support and guidance when working with clients who are in trauma recovery, such as from a psychotherapist with trauma expertise. Identification of psychotherapists with this specialty can be accomplished through interprofessional networking. The American Psychological Association's online psychologist locator (http://locator.apa.org) can also be useful for this purpose.

Evidence-Based Treatment Guidelines

The most important issue in the delivery of MT to trauma survivors involves maintaining client safety and comfort, particularly in response to client dissociation. MT research supports trauma-specific treatment guidelines, described in the clinical literature, that outline the need for sensitivity when working with trauma survivors who may request that certain areas of the body not be touched, or who may feel a lack of safety or comfort at times in an MT session (Benjamin 1996; Fitch and Dryden 2000). Protocols used in three of the MT for trauma studies included frequent and consistent verbal check-ins to assess participants' comfort and customization to maximize delivery of sensitive care and feelings of comfort and safety.

Comfort and safety ensure that the client can relax to the fullest degree possible. This promotes trust between the therapist and client, facilitates self-connection and awareness, and reduces protective response patterns. It is important that the massage therapist discuss the importance of comfort and safety with the client. The client should agree on strategies for maximizing these elements during a session. An emphasis on learning to receive soothing touch by staying present and connected with their bodily sensations will help facilitate clients' ability to negotiate emotional responses in massage therapy. It is imperative that the massage therapist verbally check in with the client throughout the session and stay attentive to any indication of client discomfort or feelings of insecurity, while also being prepared to respond with flexibility and creativity to the client's needs.

DIRECTIONS FOR FUTURE RESEARCH

The small amount of MT research on trauma recovery means that there is plenty yet to be examined. First and foremost, more research, including larger studies, is needed. Additional research with women, as well as new research with men, would be beneficial. In addition, we should learn if subsets of the population exist for whom MT is especially useful, such as people with complex trauma resulting from multiple and varied incidents, clients with single assault experiences, and military veterans. The clinical effectiveness of MT, whether as a stand-alone or adjunctive treatment, is important for us to understand so that we learn whether it reduces psychological and physical distress, facilitates long-term functioning, and helps to reduce health care costs associated with childhood sexual abuse and PTSD.

It is also important for new research to examine how MT results in the reduction of symptoms for those suffering from the consequences of trauma. What are the underlying psychological and physiological changes that actually cause the benefits of MT in this population? Research designed to address these gaps in our

Case Study

Carol J. is a Caucasian female in her mid-40s who was physically abused by both parents throughout childhood and who was sexually assaulted on more than one occasion around 6 years of age. She also reports having been raped more than once as a young adult. Presently, she works at a demanding full-time job and lives with her two children. She is divorced. For 3 years, she has had regular sessions with her psychotherapist Dr. Sara S., who has recently referred her for MT with Rebecca G., a massage therapist that she knows and trusts.

At the first MT appointment, Rebecca asked Carol to sign an agreement that permits her to exchange information pertinent to Carol's case with Dr. S. Rebecca also encouraged Carol to discuss her MT experiences with Dr. S. if any psychological issues come up during or between MT sessions. Rebecca also administered some questionnaires pertaining to Carol's symptoms of psychological distress, physical distress, and trauma, which will enable progress to be tracked.

Carol informed Rebecca that she has had fewer than 10 massages in her life. She later revealed that she experienced some physical tension and discomfort at times during the session, including a feeling of constriction in her throat, neck pain, and coldness in her hands and feet. She said that while she is aware of her physical tension, she often does not feel as if she is in her body. In other words, she does not have a strong sense of physical connection to herself. Carol expressed a desire to increase her awareness and sense of connectedness with her body.

Carol attended eight weekly MT sessions and quickly developed a strong and trusting relationship with Rebecca. Although she had to work hard to stay present and to attend to her sensory experiences while receiving MT, she felt rewarded with increased positive sensations and emotional awareness. Previously, Carol tended to avoid her bodily sensations, since they were often associated with painful memories, anxiety, and fear. As she became more comfortable during MT sessions, Carol increasingly experienced her body as a source of joy and peace. This was new and exciting, and she felt that this profoundly helped her to heal.

(continued)

Case Study *(continued)*

At the completion of eight weeks of MT, Rebecca readministered the set of symptom questionnaires, as well as a written questionnaire focused on Carol's overall MT experience. Carol's responses indicated that her symptoms had remarkably improved. There was an overall reduction in her symptoms of psychological distress, particularly symptoms of anxiety and interpersonal sensitivity. Her trauma symptoms also improved to a remarkable degree, and with the exception of fatigue, every physical symptom she had also showed improvement. Carol also indicated that through MT, she had experienced a "safe inner place" inside herself. She went on to state that "relaxation does not merely move me to a pleasant, neutral place; it is deeply satisfying and pleasurable. This is very significant in connection with my sense of overall safety in the world. To find this inner safe place is a great gift."

Carol elected to continue MT on a weekly basis because she found it helpful in her trauma treatment. Dr. S. and Rebecca conferred occasionally during Carol's treatment, particularly in times of heightened emotional content in the sessions or in times of heightened stressful life events for Carol that might affect her MT session experience. Carol noted that attending concurrent massage and psychotherapy was very helpful for her. In particular, she was aware that she gained increased capacity to connect and explore emotions in psychotherapy as a result of increased relaxation and sense of safety that had emerged in massage.

knowledge will help us to develop evidence-based guidelines and treatment programs that are targeted to certain subgroups and are capable of being integrated into mainstream care.

SUMMARY

The effects of trauma range widely, and can include various forms of somatization, symptoms of anxiety or depression, and sleep difficulties. In some cases, as in post-traumatic stress disorder, the deleterious effects do not appear until considerable time has passed since the trauma occurred. Although it is based on a limited number of studies, evidence exists that massage therapy can be beneficial for trauma survivors. Massage may promote healthy body awareness, reduce dissociation, and encourage self-care and feelings of self-efficacy. Logically, massage therapy with a trauma survivor, and especially with a survivor of sexual trauma, demands a careful and cautious approach. Massage therapists working with this population should be prepared to check on the recipient's level of comfort frequently. They must take extra care to stay present during the session. They must also be prepared to work interprofessionally with mental health care professionals with expertise in this area. All aspects of trauma and its treatment are potential areas for future massage therapy research. As larger studies are completed, we can expect our understanding of massage therapy for trauma to be rapidly improved.

REFERENCES

American Psychiatric Association (APA). 2000. *Diagnostic and statistical manual of mental disorders*. Revised 4th ed. Washington: American Psychiatric Association.

Benjamin, B. 1996. Massage and bodywork with survivors of abuse (Part V). *Massage Therapy Journal* 35(3).

Blackburn, J., and C. Price. 2007. Implications of presence in manual therapy. *J Bodyw Mov Ther* 11: 68-77.

Briere, J., and M. Runtz. 1993. Childhood sexual abuse: Long-term sequelae and implications for psychological assessment. *J Interpers Violence* 8(3): 312-330.

Briere, J., and D. Elliott. 2003. "Prevalence and psychological sequelae of self-reported childhood physical and sexual abuse in a general population sample of men and women." *Child Abuse Neglect* 27(10): 1205-1222.

Breslau, N. 2002. Gender differences in trauma and posttraumatic stress disorder. *J Gend Specif Med* 5(1): 34-40.

Ciechanowski, P.S., E.A. Walker, J.E. Russo, E. Newman, and W.J. Katon. 2004. Adult health status of women HMO members with posttraumatic stress disorder symptoms. *Gen Hosp Psychiatry* 26(4): 261-268.

Dobie, D.J., D. R. Kivlahan, C. Maynard, K. R. Bush, T. M. Davis, and K. A. Bradley. 2004. "Post-traumatic Stress Disorder in female VA patients: Association with self-reported health problems and functional impairment." *Archives of Internal Medicine* 164(4): 394-400.

Field, T., M. Hernandez-Reif, S. Hart, O. Ouintin, L. Drose, T. Field, C. Kuhn, and S. Schanberg. 1997. Effects of sexual abuse are lessened by massage therapy. *J Bodyw Mov Ther* 1(2): 65-69.

Fitch, D., and T. Dryden. 2000. Recovering body and soul from post-traumatic stress disorder. *Massage Therapy Journal* 39(1): 41-62.

Ford, C. 1993. *Compassionate touch.* New York: Simon and Schuster.

Fosha, D. 2000. *The transforming power of affect: A model for accelerated change.* New York: Basic Books.

Gill, J.M., and G.G. Page. 2006. Psychiatric and physical health ramifications of traumatic events in women. *Issues Ment Health Nurs* 27(7): 711-734.

Herman, J. 1997. *Trauma and recovery: The aftermath of violence—From domestic abuse to political terror.* New York: Harper Collins.

Kepner, J. 2003. *Psychotherapy with adult survivors of childhood abuse.* London: Routledge.

Kessler, R.C. 2000. Posttraumatic stress disorder: The burden to the individual and to society. *J Clin Psychiatry* 61(5): S4-S14.

Kessler, R.C., A. Sonnega, E. Bromet, M. Hughes, and C.B. Nelson. 1995. Posttraumatic stress disorder in the National Comorbidity Survey. *Arch Gen Psychiatry* 52(12): 1048-1060.

Kimerling, R. 2004. An investigation of sex differences in nonpsychiatric morbidity associated with posttraumatic stress disorder. *J Am Med Womens Assoc* 59(1): 43-47.

Marciniak, M., M. Lage, E. Dunayevich, J. Russell, L. Bowman, R. Landboom, and L. Levine. 2005. "The Cost of Treating Anxiety: The Medical and Demographic Correlates that Impact Total Medical Costs." *Depression and Anxiety* 21: 178-184.

McCauley, J., D. E. Kern, K. Kolodner, L. Dill, A. F. Schroeder, H. K. DeChant, J. Ryden, L. R. Derogatis, and E. B. Bass. 1997. "Clinical characteristics of women with a history of childhood abuse: unhealed wounds." *JAMA* 277 (17):1362-8.

Olff, M., W. Langeland, N. Draijer, and B.P. Gersons. 2007. Gender differences in posttraumatic stress disorder. *Psychol Bull* 133(2): 183-204.

Palinkas, L.A., and M.L. Kabongo. 2000. The use of complementary and alternative medicine by primary care patients. A SURF*NET study. *J Fam Pract* 49(12): 1121-1130.

Pearlman, L., and K. Saakvitne. 2005. *Trauma and the therapist: Countertransference and vicarious traumatization in psychotherapy with incest survivors*. New York: Norton.

Price, C.J. 2002. Body-oriented therapy as an adjunct to psychotherapy in recovery from childhood abuse: A case study. *J Bodyw Mov Thers* 6(4): 228-236.

———. 2004. Characteristics of women seeking body-oriented therapy as an adjunct to psychotherapy during recovery from childhood sexual abuse. *J Bodyw Mov Ther* 8: 35-42.

———. 2005. Body-oriented therapy in recovery from child sexual abuse: An efficacy study. *Altern Ther Health Med* 11(5): 46-57.

———. 2006. Body-oriented therapy in sexual abuse recovery: A pilot-test comparison. *J Bodyw Mov Ther* 10: 58-64.

———. 2007. Dissociation reduction in body therapy during sexual abuse recovery. *Complement Ther Clin Pract* 13(2): 116-128.

Price, C.J., B. McBride, L. Hyerle, and D.R. Kivlahan. 2007. Mindful awareness in body-oriented therapy for female veterans with post-traumatic stress disorder taking prescription analgesics for chronic pain: A feasibility study. *Altern Ther Health Med* 13(6): 32-40.

Sadler, A. G., B. M. Booth, D. Nielson, and B. N. Doebbeling. 2000. “Health-related consequences of physical and sexual violence: Women in the military.” *Obstetrics & Gynecology* 96(3): 473-480.

Seedat, S., D.J. Stein, and P.D. Carey. 2005. Post-traumatic stress disorder in women: Epidemiological and treatment issues. *CNS Drugs* 19(5): 411-427.

Stein, M.B., J.R. Walker, and D.R. Forde. 2000. Gender differences in susceptibility to posttraumatic stress disorder. *Behav Res Ther* 38(6): 619-628.

Tagay, S., S. Herpertz, M. Langkafel, and W. Senf. 2005. Posttraumatic stress disorder in a psychosomatic outpatient clinic. Gender effects, psychosocial functioning, sense of coherence, and service utilization. *J Psychosom Res* 58(5): 439-446.

Thayer, J.F., and R.D. Lane. 2000. A model of neurovisceral integration in emotion regulation and dysregulation. *J Affect Disord* 61(3): 201-216.

Timms, R.J., and P. Connors. 1992. *Embodying healing: Integrating bodywork and psychotherapy in recovery from childhood sexual abuse*. Orwell: Safer Society Press.

van der Kolk, B.A. 2001. The assessment and treatment of complex PTSD. In *Traumatic Stress,* ed. R. Yehuda, American Psychiatric Press.

———. 2006. Clinical implications of neuroscience research in PTSD. *Ann N Y Acad Sci.* 1071: 277-293.

van der Kolk, B.A., O. van der Hart, and C. Marmar. 1996. Dissociation and information processing in posttraumatic stress disorder. In *Traumatic stress: The effects of overwhelming experience on mind, body and society,* ed. B. van der Kolk, C. McFarlane, and L. Weisaeth. New York: Guilford Press.

Weisberg, R.B., S.E. Bruce, J.T. Machan, R.C. Kessler, L. Culpepper, and M.B. Keller. 2002. Nonpsychiatric illness among primary care patients with trauma histories and posttraumatic stress disorder. *Psychiatr Serv* 53(7): 848-854.

chapter

15

Scars

Ania Kania, BSc, RMT

Scarring, the biological process by which normal skin is replaced after injury or disease, can negatively affect a client's physical abilities and psychological health. Nerve impairment, compromised joint function, or damage to underlying soft tissue can be a source of significant discomfort, pain, and pruritus (itching), a common symptom associated with the formation of scar tissue. Discomfort with scarring can range from mild to severe. Scarring can also cause sleep disturbance and can restrict daily activities (Bell and Gabriel 2009). Scars that cause disfigurement can also be a source of psychological distress (Edwards 2003). As such, a holistic treatment approach that addresses these various areas and prevents the development of abnormal scars or pathologies, such as contractures, is crucial for optimal outcomes.

Massage therapy (MT) can play an important role in the treatment of clients, both adults and children, with scars. Scar tissue can be treated with techniques such as lymphatic drainage, Swedish techniques, *fascial techniques,* and *transverse frictions.* Restrictions of surrounding soft tissues can also be treated with a variety of massage techniques. Psychological symptoms or conditions can be treated through a relaxation-based approach. However, in order to provide safe and effective MT, it is necessary to have a thorough understanding of the condition and treatment options that is based on research and practice-based experience. This chapter provides an overview of how scars are formed and the different types of scars. It also reviews research literature published to date on massage in the treatment of scars, outlines treatment recommendations based on research and practice experience, and proposes directions for future research directions.

fascial techniques

▸ A broad category of massage techniques intended to affect connective tissue.

transverse frictions

▸ A nongliding, repetitive fascial technique intended to produce movement between fibers of dense connective tissue.

OVERVIEW OF THE CONDITION: SCAR TISSUE

A scar is the end product of a series of physiological processes that repair tissue damaged by mechanical forces, surgical incisions, thermal agents (such as hot liquid or fire), chemicals, or electricity. Scars have a unique structure distinct from the tissue they replace. Generally, larger and deeper scars are more problematic, requiring more time for full recovery due to the extensive tissue damage

---

The practice experience of Nancy Keeney Smith and her willingness to share her experience and approach in the treatment of children with scars informed the development of the treatment recommendations presented in this chapter.

sustained, the greater potential for complications, and the negative effect on the client's quality of life and psychological state (Aarabi, Longaker, and Gurtner 2007; Edgar and Brereton 2004).

Phases of Normal Wound Healing and Scar Formation

Scars result when a wound is deeper than the epidermis. Wound healing moves through three distinct and overlapping phases: inflammation, proliferation, and remodeling. The specific steps that take place in each of these phases are summarized in table 15.1.

The wound healing process is initiated at the time of injury and can last as long as 2 years. The duration of each phase and the resulting quality of the scar depend on factors such as the depth and area of damage, the extent of tissue loss (particularly the epithelial layer), the prior health of the client, and genetic factors (Aarabi, Longaker, and Gurtner 2007; Romo et al. 2008).

Table 15.1 Three Phases of Wound Healing

Wound healing phase	Description
Phase 1: inflammatory process	The inflammatory response consists of vascular and cellular responses initiated at the time of injury in response to damage. • The clotting cascade is initiated and includes the release of platelet-derived growth factors (PDGF) and transforming growth factors beta (TGF-β), which attract neutrophils and macrophages to the injured site. This results in the creation of a protective layer and swelling. (Aarabi et al. 2007; Romo et al. 2008)
Phase 2: proliferative phase	As inflammation subsides, new tissue production begins. This process can take 3 to 5 weeks. • New blood vessels are formed, ensuring a rich nutrient supply to support new tissue. • If the basal membrane of the epidermis is intact, new epithelial cells begin to replace the damaged epithelial layer. • Granulation tissue is formed, which provides the materials required for collagen to be produced and deposited. • This newest collagen (type I) forms thick bundles that are the key structural material of the scar. • The wound edges begin to move closer together to facilitate wound closure. (Romo et al. 2008)
Phase 3: remodeling (maturation) phase	The synthesis and breakdown of collagen reach equilibrium. This phase can last 6 months to 2 years, depending on the size and depth of the wound. • The collagen formed in the proliferative phase is remodeled; the type III collagen is replaced by type I collagen. • Water is reabsorbed from the scar tissue. • Collagen fibers reorganize along lines of tension, resulting in increased tensile strength and decreased thickness. • The vascular networks created in the proliferative phase are broken down, reducing the scar's redness. (Romo et al 2008)

Types of Scars

A good quality scar is characterized as soft, pliable, and flat. It should have a color similar to that of the surrounding skin. However, a number of factors may negatively influence the wound healing process, resulting in the formation of an abnormal scar. Two types of abnormal scars have been distinguished: hypertrophic and keloid.

hypertrophic scar

▸ A type of scar that is red, raised, and rigid, and which stays within the boundaries of the original injury.

Hypertrophic scars (see figure 15.1) are characterized by redness, rigidity, and elevation greater than surrounding tissue due to a buildup of excess collagen fibers; however, they stay within the confines of the original lesion. They most frequently occur from surgical incisions or second- or third-degree burns (Atiyeh 2007; Edgar and Brereton 2004), and they generally begin to form 3 to 5 weeks after wound closure. Though the development of hypertrophic scars is not well understood, factors thought to contribute include prolonged or recurring inflammation, delayed epithelialization during wound healing, and high mechanical tension on the healing tissue (Aarabi, Longaker, and Gurtner 2007). Sometimes, hypertrophic scars soften and flatten spontaneously over time. However, to ensure that the scar does not develop into a thick, restricted mass, treatment that includes the use of pressure garments is necessary (Mustoe et al. 2002; Sheridan 2007).

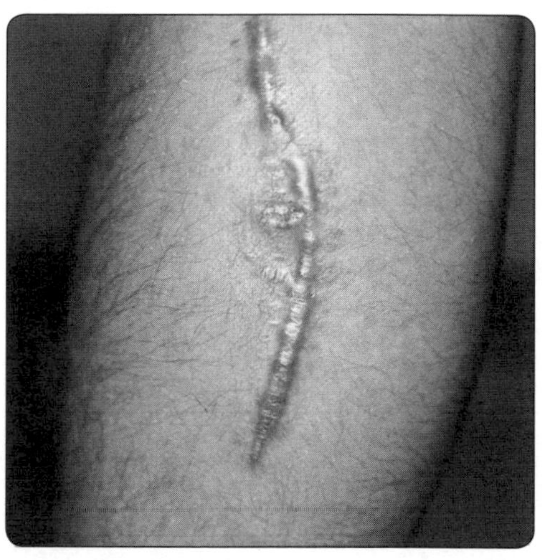

Figure 15.1 Hypertrophic Scar

Image reprinted with permission from eMedicine.com, 2010.

Keloid scars (see figure 15.2) are benign growths that do not regress with time (Edwards 2003). They are characterized by a mass of elevated scar tissue that spreads beyond the margins of the original wound (Atiyeh 2007; Edwards 2003). They most commonly develop on the shoulders, neck, chest, upper arms, and face. Though the likelihood of an abnormal scar developing is increased by poor or compromised conditions in the initial stages of wound healing, keloids can also occur even if initial wound healing and closure occurs quickly and without complications. The causes of keloid formation are not fully understood, but persons who are between 10 and 30 years of age and of African-American, Hispanic, or Asian descent, or who come from a family with a history of keloid scarring are at higher risk. Recent studies suggest that they may be caused by a disruption of the maturation phase of wound healing, since keloids contain higher levels of immature collagen (Aarabi, Longaker, and Gurtner 2007; Kokoska and Prendiville 2007; Wihelmi 2008).

keloid scar

▸ A type of scar that produces an abundance of elevated scar tissue that spreads beyond the boundaries of the original injury.

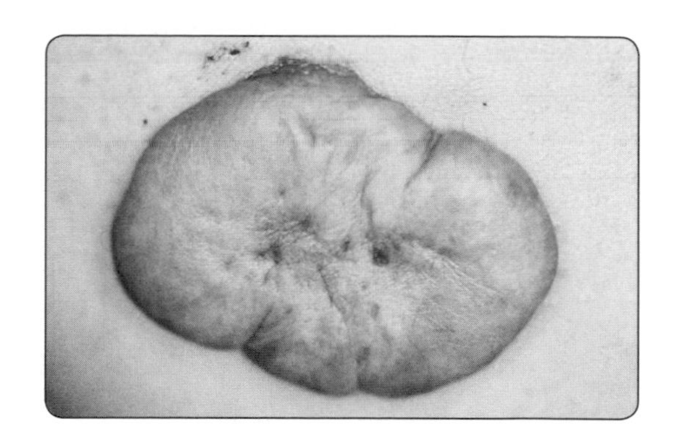

Figure 15.2 Keloid scar

Image reprinted with permission from eMedicine.com, 2010.

EFFECTS OF MASSAGE THERAPY IN THE TREATMENT OF SCAR TISSUE

A literature search identifies seven studies on massage therapy for scar treatment; these are summarized in table 15.2.

Note that all seven studies are concerned with scars resulting from burns and that all of the studies are small (the largest of the set has 30 subjects). The massage intervention was predominantly studied as a complementary treatment rather than as a main treatment. Application of treatments varies across the studies from nearly immediately after injury to as long as 2 years later. Five of the studies investigated the application of MT directly to the scar tissue.

Table 15.2 Summary of Research Studies on Massage Therapy in the Treatment of Individuals With Scars

Study	Research design	Subjects	Treatment details	Findings
Boersen (2001)	Case report	Individual with burn scar on dorsal region of foot 7 months postinjury	Subject received daily 30-minute sessions of Swedish techniques for 1 week.	Pain and pruritis were eliminated by end of treatment period, and subject's tolerance for standing increased from 17 minutes to over 90 minutes.
Field et al. (1998)	Randomized controlled trial	28 adults undergoing burn treatment	All subjects received standard care; in addition, subjects randomized to massage received daily back massage 20 minutes in duration and using Swedish techniques for 1 week.	Massage subjects had significant within-group reductions of anxiety, cortisol, depression, anger, and pain; between-groups effects are not presented.
Hernandez-Reif et al. (2001)	Randomized controlled trial	24 children undergoing burn treatment	All subjects received standard care; in addition, subjects randomized to massage received 15-minute sessions applied to nonburned body regions before dressing changes.	Children who received massage exhibited fewer distress behaviors during the dressing change, as rated by their nurses.
Morien et al. (2008)	Clinical pseudo-experiment	8 children who had received skin grafts, 2 or more years prior, for treatment of 3rd-degree burns	All subjects received a 20- to 25-minute massage including effleurage, petrissage, and friction techniques, applied to scar tissue, daily for 5 days. A correspondingly scarred region on the other side of each subject's body, which was not massaged, served as a control.	Massaged tissue showed a significant improvement in range of motion, while control tissue was not significantly improved. Subjects' mood was not significantly changed during treatment period.
Patino et al. (1999)	Randomized controlled trial	30 children with hypertrophic scarring	All subjects were treated with pressure garments; in addition, subjects received 10-minute friction massage daily for 3 months.	Massage had no significant effects on vascularity, pliability, or height of hypertrophic scars; some massage subjects reported decrease in pruritis.

Study	Research design	Subjects	Treatment details	Findings
Silverberg et al. (1996)	Randomized controlled trial	10 adults with burn scars	All subjects received standard care; in addition, subjects randomized to massage received 10 to 15 minutes of soft tissue mobilization.	No difference between groups in range of motion, scar pliability, or vascularity.
Tsamis (2005)	Case report	Individual with a 2nd-degree burn scar 4 months postinjury	Fascial, lymphatic, passive stretching, and Swedish techniques were administered at 4 treatments in a 1-month period.	Pain, pruritis, and scar sensitivity decreased and range of motion and scar appearance were improved during treatment period.

Two studies did not focus on massage as a strategy to reduce the pain and anxiety resulting from burn treatment, which is frequently arduous.

A range of massage approaches and protocols were used in these studies, but in most cases, individual sessions were short. In some cases, they were only 10 minutes in duration, which may not provide a valid test of clinical utility. Nevertheless, reductions of anxiety, distress, pain, and pruritus, and improvements of scar quality observed in some of these studies are promising. These results begin to reinforce subjective clinical evidence that massage is of value in scar treatment. At the same time, it is clear that more research is needed.

EXPLAINING MASSAGE THERAPY EFFECTS

Several mechanisms of action of massage have been proposed to explain the effects massage therapy may have on scar tissue. Scar pliability may increase as massage realigns collagen fibers during scar formation and remodeling (Edgar and Brereton 2004; Edwards 2003; LaFrano 2001; Morien, Garrison, and Smith 2008). It is also postulated that the direct mechanical effect of massage may break down adhesions of the scar to underlying tissue, allowing for increased movement of the scar tissue and underlying soft tissues and increased range of motion in affected joint structures (Silverberg, Johnson, and Moffat 1996). The mechanical effects may also displace fluid in maturing scar tissue, flattening the scar (Wieting and Cugalj 2008). While these are plausible theories, it must be noted that they still require scientific examination.

RECOMMENDATIONS FOR MASSAGE THERAPY PRACTICE

Given the relatively small amount of research studies that have been conducted on scar massage, current treatment recommendations must be based on the existing research combined with a considerable portion of practice-based experience.

At each stage of the healing process, MT should be framed within a holistic approach, such that the massage therapist treats the client and not just the scar. Based on need, such an approach requires consideration of the scar tissue, underlying tissues, compromised compensatory structures, and psychological symptoms that may arise due to discomfort associated with the scarring, scar treatments, or the physical appearance of the scars (Edgar and Brereton 2004). Further, when developing a treatment plan, it is important to identify which massage technique or combination of techniques will be administered, along with the direction, depth, and pressure with which they are applied. These decisions should be informed by the current scar condition, the level of inflammation, the patient's tolerance for treatment, and the goals of the treatment. Regular reassessment, using subjective reports, observation, and standardized outcome measures, such as the McGill Pain Questionnaire (Melzack 1975) and the Vancouver Burn Scar Scale (Baryza and Baryza 1995), is required to track progress and to adapt the treatment plan as the case evolves. The following sidebar provides a summary of factors to consider when planning treatment.

Evidence-Based Treatment Guidelines

Factors to consider when developing a treatment plan for clients presenting with scars include the following:

- Stage of healing.
- Healing progress.
- Age of the scar.
- Health state of the client.
- In the early stages of wound healing, the wound and newly forming scar should be monitored for indicators of abnormal scar tissue formation, increased swelling, or slow scab formation.
- Scar is considered immature if it is red, raised, or rigid.
- Scar is considered mature if it is avascular (pale), flat, pliable, and soft.
- Scar maturation may take anywhere from 6 months to 5 years; during this time, the scar will continue to change.
- Changes in the scar tissue and wound healing process will require modifications and alterations of the massage treatment plan. Consider the goals and concerns of the client.

Acknowledgemnts: The work with burn survivors done by the massage therapy team, specifically Kimberly Boersen-Gladman and Zoran Jelicic, at St. John's Rehab Hospital in Toronto, ON provides a significant contribution to understanding approaches to MT treatment planning and provision to clients with scar tissue.

Inflammatory Phase

During the inflammatory phase, the primary focus is on the prevention of problematic or abnormal scars and the reduction of potentially negative effects on underlying and surrounding tissue (Atiyeh 2007; Edwards 2003; Mustoe et al. 2002). Massage should emphasize an optimal healing environment within which the wound can heal and a functional, good quality scar can develop. In addition, treatment goals during this phase are likely to include the reduction or management of swelling, reduction or management of pain, treatment of compensatory structures affected by the injury, and provision of psychological support. Areas that can be treated during this phase include soft tissue proximal to the wound, compensatory structures, and noninjured tissues. Massage techniques may be applied in the area of the scar, but it is important that newly forming scar tissue is not distorted or stretched. Lymphatic drainage techniques should be applied proximal to the wound site with light pressure that is directed away from the scar. Treatment of compensatory structures is based on needs specific to each case. Treatment to uninjured areas to provide psychological support may be initiated in the context of a relaxation focus. Logically, session length and the number of sessions will be based on the goals of the treatment, tissue response, and the client's tolerance to massage.

Proliferative Phase

As the scar forms, the new tissue is fragile and may be susceptible to breakdown in response to treatments that are too aggressive. It is highly recommended that communication (and patient consent for communication) with the health care team be obtained prior to MT treatment. Collaborative, interprofessional care is essential in scar treatment. Collaborative practice happens when multiple health workers from different professional backgrounds work together with patients, families, caregivers, and communities to deliver the highest quality of care (World Health Organization 2010). For further discussion on the importance of collaborative interprofessional education for massage therapists, please see chapter 18.

Goals of a massage treatment during the proliferative phase may include reduction or management of swelling; reduction or management of pain due to numerous causes, including physical activity, dressing changes, the healing process, and physical therapy; reduction or management of pruritus; promotion of scar pliability; reduction of adhesions and restrictions in the tissue; maintenance of, or increase in, range of motion in joints that may be affected by adjacent injury or scarring; prevention of contracture formation; treatment of compensatory structures; and provision of psychological support. Lymphatic drainage, Swedish, and gentle passive stretching techniques may be applied to tissues around the new scar during the proliferative phase, with movement carefully applied toward tissue resistance. Toward the end of this stage, massage may be applied along the scar's margin and slowly into the scar, but treatment of the scar region should not exceed 20 minutes. The scar should not be stretched.

At this stage, the amount of manipulation that the scar can be subjected to depends on the health of the tissue and the patient's tolerance. Working within that tolerance, the amount of manipulation and pressure applied to scar tissue should be gradually increased across treatments. Aggressive or vigorous massage techniques that may exacerbate inflammation or compromise the healthy formation of new tissue should be avoided. Continual assessment of the healing process and of the patient's ongoing response to treatment is crucial during this stage.

Remodeling Phase

At this stage, the scar has tensile strength. Massage may be applied directly to the scar tissue. Massage may also be used as a complement in managing symptoms such as tightness or pain related to the scar tissue.

Treatment goals during this phase may include reduction or management of swelling, reduction or management of pain, reduction or management of pruritus, promotion of scar pliability, reduction of adhesions and restrictions in the tissue, maintenance of (or increase in) range of motion in joints that may be affected by adjacent injury or scarring, treatment of compensatory structures, and provision of psychological support. In this phase, Swedish, fascial, transverse friction, and passive stretching techniques may be applied to the scar tissue. Swedish and fascial techniques can be applied in all directions. They should begin to challenge restrictions within the scar tissue, so long as the degree of challenge is built up gradually across treatments and is always kept within the patient's level of tolerance. Further, duration of treatment applied directly to the scar should not exceed 30 minutes.

In this phase, the scar's permanent or semipermanent appearance, which can have an effect on psychological health, is likely to become evident. From a holistic perspective, MT during this phase can promote relaxation and can reduce anxiety and depression (see chapter 13). It may even help patients to accept changes to their appearance by facilitating optimal body–mind integration (see chapter 14 on massage for adults with a history of sexual trauma).

Mature Scar Tissue

Currently, there is no research on the effectiveness of massage therapy in producing changes to mature scar tissue. However, clinical experience suggests that scar massage may reduce the sensation of tightness and improve the softness and color of the scar. Research is needed to confirm or refute these possible benefits and to develop effective treatment recommendations. Until then, the treatment of mature scars should be based on the remodeling phase of tissue healing.

Abnormal Scars

Research on massage therapy for hypertrophic scars is largely absent. Given the ongoing inflammation present in hypertrophic scar tissue, Swedish and fascial techniques and transverse frictions should be applied with caution, since they may exacerbate inflammation. Application of lymphatic drainage may be most appropriate in the reduction or management of associated edema.

No highly effective treatment for keloid scars has yet been identified and no research on massage therapy for keloids has been conducted. This makes their treatment problematic. Conservative treatment includes application of pressure, pharmacotherapy, laser therapy, and radiotherapy. If the keloid scar is unresponsive, surgical excision can be conducted when growth has ceased (Romo et al. 2008).

Contraindications to Treatment

To provide optimally effective care, treatment must avoid inappropriate therapies and techniques. Massage of scar tissue is contraindicated whenever there is an open wound, evidence of tissue fragility, a breakdown of scar tissue, or cutaneous or systemic infection (Atiyeh 2007; Ludwig 2000). In addition, even in cases where MT may be a useful component of treatment, it may be inappropriate for it to be the single or dominant form of treatment. Treatment of scars, particularly those resulting from major trauma, such as second- or third-degree burns, often requires a multidisciplinary team that can provide coordinated and comprehensive treatment to achieve optimal outcomes. Massage therapists can be an important part of such a team by contributing their expertise in understanding and treating soft tissue in support of optimal scar development, by maximizing the health and functionality of the underlying and surrounding tissues, and by ameliorating psychological symptoms associated with scarring. Whether the massage therapist is an official member of the rehabilitation team or not, regular communication with the patient's other health care providers is essential for optimal and ethical care.

DIRECTIONS FOR FUTURE RESEARCH

Given the relative paucity of MT research on massage therapy for scar treatment, prevention, and management, combined with its increased application in these areas, there is significant need for investigation in this area. Research is needed to more precisely determine when MT should be introduced to the scar formation process, if massage is effective in treating abnormal and mature scars, and which techniques and protocols are most effective in treating scar tissue. Similarly, research should examine the optimal ways to integrate massage therapy into a multidisciplinary or interprofessional team-based approach to scar rehabilitation. Also needed are investigations of the potentially adverse effects of scar massage. This is of particular importance in the treatment of hypertrophic scars. Finally, scar massage research has focused primarily on burns. Research is also needed on the treatment of surgical scars, such as those resulting from mastectomy, organ transplants, and heart surgery, which often result in functional limitations that may be effectively addressed with massage therapy.

Massage therapy is considered a standard therapy in the treatment of scar tissue (Demling and DeSanti 2001; Edwards 2003; Mustoe et al. 2002; Sheridan 2007). In rehabilitation centers specializing in the treatment of scars and burns, it is routinely used in the management of scar tissue, occupying a place in 52% of treatment protocols (Atiyeh 2007). The experience of massage therapists working in these settings is an invaluable source of information that could contribute to our knowledge of specific treatment approaches and techniques. A survey of best practices, drawn from the practitioners of scar massage, could substantially inform the safe and effective provision of this treatment, while simultaneously revealing the limits of current knowledge to guide the development of research reflective of and relevant to current practices.

Finally, within the current climate of financial restraint and conservative resource allocation in health care, there is an increased demand for evidence of treatment's cost-effectiveness. Anecdotal evidence suggests that massage therapy may reduce symptoms and speed recovery in instances where scarring plays a primary or major role. Cost-effectiveness studies, capable of demonstrating the value of massage therapy in dollars and cents, should be conducted. These may be the key to an increased acceptance and integration of massage therapy in scar treatment.

Case Study

Teresa M. is a 40-year-old woman who sustained second-degree burns from cooking oil that splashed onto the dorsal surface of her right hand. She received immediate emergency care at the time of injury 2 months prior. She was later referred to massage therapy by her physician due to limited scar-tissue mobility, tightness, and pruritus. At an assessment to determine the suitability of scar massage, massage therapist Karen J. observed the scar to be intact, closed, and red, with thickened, darker edges. Residual swelling extended to the surrounding area and into four digits. In addition to massage therapy, Teresa was also receiving physical therapy twice weekly to increase the range of motion of her wrist and digits.

(continued)

Case Study *(continued)*

Assessment

Teresa reported a sensation of constant tightness in the scar tissue. This feeling was severe in the morning, but decreased to a moderate level as the day progressed. Teresa also reported moderate levels of pruritus, which worsened at night and frequently awakened her. She rated the severity of her pruritus as 6 out of a possible 10, where 10 represented the worst possible case. Physical examination by Karen revealed that the scar tissue was fully adhered to the underlying structures and that full wrist extension was limited by discomfort at the scar site. Flexion of the digits was also limited, which impaired Teresa's ability to hold objects such as a pen or brush.

Treatment

Teresa received a 1-hour massage twice weekly for 4 weeks. During each treatment, lymphatic techniques were applied to the right arm and hand. Gradually, fascial techniques (c-bowing and s-bowing) of moderate pressure and Swedish techniques (fingertip kneading, thumb kneading) with water-based lotion were administered to the scar tissue. Pressure ranged from mild to moderate, based on the progress of the scar and Teresa's comfort. Muscles of the right forearm were also treated for soft-tissue restrictions and trigger points. Treatment concluded with Swedish massage of the left arm, shoulders, and neck. Teresa was also taught to self-massage her scar and was instructed to do so daily.

Reassessment

Teresa reported a decrease in the pruritus, rating it as 3 by the end of the first week and then 1 by the end of the second week, by which time it no longer awakened her. Swelling was visibly reduced. Mobility also showed signs of improvement, indicated by the scar's ability to glide over underlying structures. By the end of the third week, Teresa reported only mild pruritus that could be managed with self-massage. She was also able to fully flex her fingers and grasp objects with minimal difficulty. Wrist extension was no longer limited by the discomfort in the scar tissue, and scar mobility had improved such that the scar glided easily and skin rolling was possible. In light of this progress, Karen modified the treatment plan to one massage session weekly for 2 weeks, followed by treatment only as needed.

SUMMARY

Massage therapy (MT) can play an important role in the treatment of clients with scars. Scar tissue can be treated with MT techniques, such as lymphatic drainage, Swedish techniques, and fascial techniques, including transverse frictions. The correct approach depends on an understanding and ability to identify the three general stages of wound healing—the inflammatory phase, the proliferative phase, and the remodelling/maturation phase—since each of these requires a different approach to facilitate optimal healing and to reduce risk of harm to fragile tissues.

Presently, research on scar massage is limited. Treatment guidelines come primarily from practice-based evidence. These include a holistic approach to care and inclusion of therapeutic support for the client as a person in addition to MT treatment of the scar. Further research is necessary to more fully understand to what extent MT reduces symptoms and speeds recovery, especially in instances where scarring plays a primary or major role in healing. Cost-effectiveness studies should also be included in future research, the results of which may be the key to an increased acceptance and integration of massage therapy in scar treatment.

REFERENCES

Aarabi, S., M. Longaker, and G. Gurtner. 2007. Hypertrophic scar formation following burns and trauma: New approaches to treatment. *PLoS Med* 4 (9). www.plosmedicine.org/article/info:doi%2F10.1371%2Fjournal.pmed.0040234.

Atiyeh, B. 2007. Nonsurgical management of hypertrophic scars: Evidence-based therapies, standard practices and emerging methods. *Aesthet Plast Surg* 31: 468-492.

Baryza M.J., and G.A. Baryza. 1995. The Vancouver scar scale: An administrative tool and its interrater reliability. *J Burn Care Rehabil* 16: 535-538.

Bell, P., and V. Gabriel. 2009. Evidence-based review for treatment of post-burn pruritus. *J Burn Care Res* 30: 55-61.

Boersen, K. 2001. Treating post-burn pain and injury: Massage therapy in rehabilitation. Case report. *Rehab and Community Care Medicine* Fall: 56-57.

Chapman, T. 2007. Burn scar and contracture management. *J Traum* 62(6): S8.

Demling, R., and L. DeSanti. 2001. Scar management strategies in wound care. *Rehab Management.* www.rehabpub.com/features/892001/3.asp.

Edgar, D., and M. Brereton. 2004. ABC of burns—Rehabilitation after burn injury. *Brit Med J* 329: 343-345.

Edwards, J. 2003. Scar management. *Nursing Standard* 17(52): 39-42.

Field, T., M. Peck, S. Krugman, T. Tuchel, S. Schanberg, C. Kuhn, and I. Burman. 1998. Burn injuries benefit from massage therapy. *J Burn Care Rehab* 19: 241-244.

Goutos, I., P. Dziewulski, and P. Richardson. 2009. Pruritus in burns: Review article. *J Burn Care Res* 30(2): 221-228.

Hernandez-Reif, M., T. Field, S. Largie, S. Hart, M. Redzepi, B. Nierenberg, and M. Peck. 2001. Children's distress during burn treatment is reduced by massage therapy. *J Burn Care Rehab* 22:191-195.

Kokoska, M.S., and S. Prendiville. 2007. Hypertrophic scarring and keloids. http://emedicine.medscape.com/article/876214-overview.

LaFrano, C. 2001. Scar tissue massage. *Massage Magazine*, May/June 91:151.

Ludwig, L. 2000. Wounds and burns: Injuries that break the skin. In *Clinical massage therapy: Understanding, assessing and treating over 70 conditions,* eds. F. Rattray and L. Ludwig, 249-263. Toronto, ON: Talus.

Melzack R. 1975. The McGill pain questionnaire: Major properties and scoring methods. *Pain* 1: 277-299.

Morien, A., D. Garrison, and N. Smith. 2008. Range of motion improves after massage in children with burns: A pilot study. *J Bodyw Mov Ther* 12: 67-71.

Mustoe, T., R. Cotter, M. Gold, F. Hobbs, A. Ramelet, P. Shakespeare, M. Stella, L. Teot, F. Wood, and U. Ziegler. 2002. International clinical recommendations on scar management. *Plast Reconstr Surg* 110: 560-571.

Patino, C., C. Novick, A. Merlo, F. Benaim. 1999. Massage in hypertrophic scars. *J Burn Care Rehab* 10: 268-271.

Romo, T., J. Pearson, H. Yalamanchili, and R. Zoumalan. 2008. Wound healing, skin. http://emedicine.medscape.com/article/884594-overview.

Sheridan, R. 2007. Burn rehabilitation. http://emedicine.medscape.com/article/318436-overview.

Silverberg, R., J. Johnson, and M. Moffat. 1996. The effects of soft tissue mobilization on the immature burn scar: Results of a pilot study. *J Burn Care Rehab* 17(3): 252-259.

Tsamis, R. 2005. Massage treatment of a 4 month old, second degree burn. *Journal of Soft Tissue and Manipulation* 12(4): 12-13.

Wihelmi, B. 2008. Wound healing, widened and hypertrophic scars. http://emedicine.medscape.com/article/1298541-overview.

Wieting, M., and A. Cugalj. 2008. Massage, traction and manipulation. http://emedicine.medscape.com/article/324694-overview.

World Health Organization. 2010. Framework for action on interprofessional education and collaborative practice. http://whqlibdoc.who.int/hq/2010/WHO_HRH_HPN_10.3_eng.pdf.

chapter

16

Fibromyalgia

Douglas Nelson, LMT, NMT

Fibromyalgia syndrome (FMS) is characterized by widespread muscle aches and pain lasting longer than 3 months. Other symptoms common to FMS include fatigue, nonrestorative sleep, inability to tolerate exercise, and difficulty in cognitive function. Depression, irritable bowel syndrome, systemic lupus erythematosus, headaches, and anxiety disorders are all more likely to be present in persons with FMS. The condition is more common in women than in men (Neumann and Buskila 2003). In addition, evidence exists of familial and genetic factors in FMS, particularly in female first-degree relatives (Bradley 2008). The exact number of FMS sufferers is difficult to determine with precision, and estimates range from 0.5% to 5% of the population. Diagnoses of FMS in the United States now exceed six million cases, and FMS accounts for up to 30% of patients in a typical rheumatology practice (Bennett 2005).

Classification of FMS as a disorder by the American College of Rheumatology did not take place until 1990, and the World Health Organization did not officially recognize FMS until 1993. Fibromyalgia is classified as a syndrome, rather than as a disease, because it is diagnosed by the presenting symptoms without a known cause. People with FMS have symptoms for an average of 6 years prior to diagnosis (Barker 2005), during which time their symptoms and complaints may not be taken seriously by family, friends, and health care providers. This environment of skepticism can add emotional stress and conflict to the physical symptoms of FMS. Similarly, the historical absence of a clear diagnostic standard has served to frustrate both health care providers and FMS sufferers. Currently, the American College of Rheumatology's diagnostic criteria for FMS is centered on tissue sensitivity in 18 specific anatomical locations (figure 16.1). A diagnosis of FMS is given if 11 or more of these points are tender in response to 4 kg of pressure, and if the pain is widespread and has lasted for more than 3 months.

These areas of tissue sensitivity are called *tender points,* and it is important for diagnosis and treatment to differentiate them from *trigger points.* Trigger points have three characteristics: a taut band of tissue, a local twitch response when stimulated, and the referral of sensation to a distant area. Tender points do not refer to other areas and do not have a taut band of tissue, but they are sensitive to palpation. Deactivation of an offending trigger point will reduce or eliminate pain and discomfort. By contrast, in FMS, elimination of a tender point has little or no effect on the person's overall pain, since the tender point is a symptom of the condition, but not its cause.

tender points

▸ Anatomical sites that are sensitive to palpation, but which do not have the taut tissue, twitch response, or sensation referral associated with trigger points.

trigger points

▸ Hyperirritable sites in skeletal muscle associated with a taut band of tissue, a local twitch response when stimulated, or the referral of sensation to a distant anatomical site.

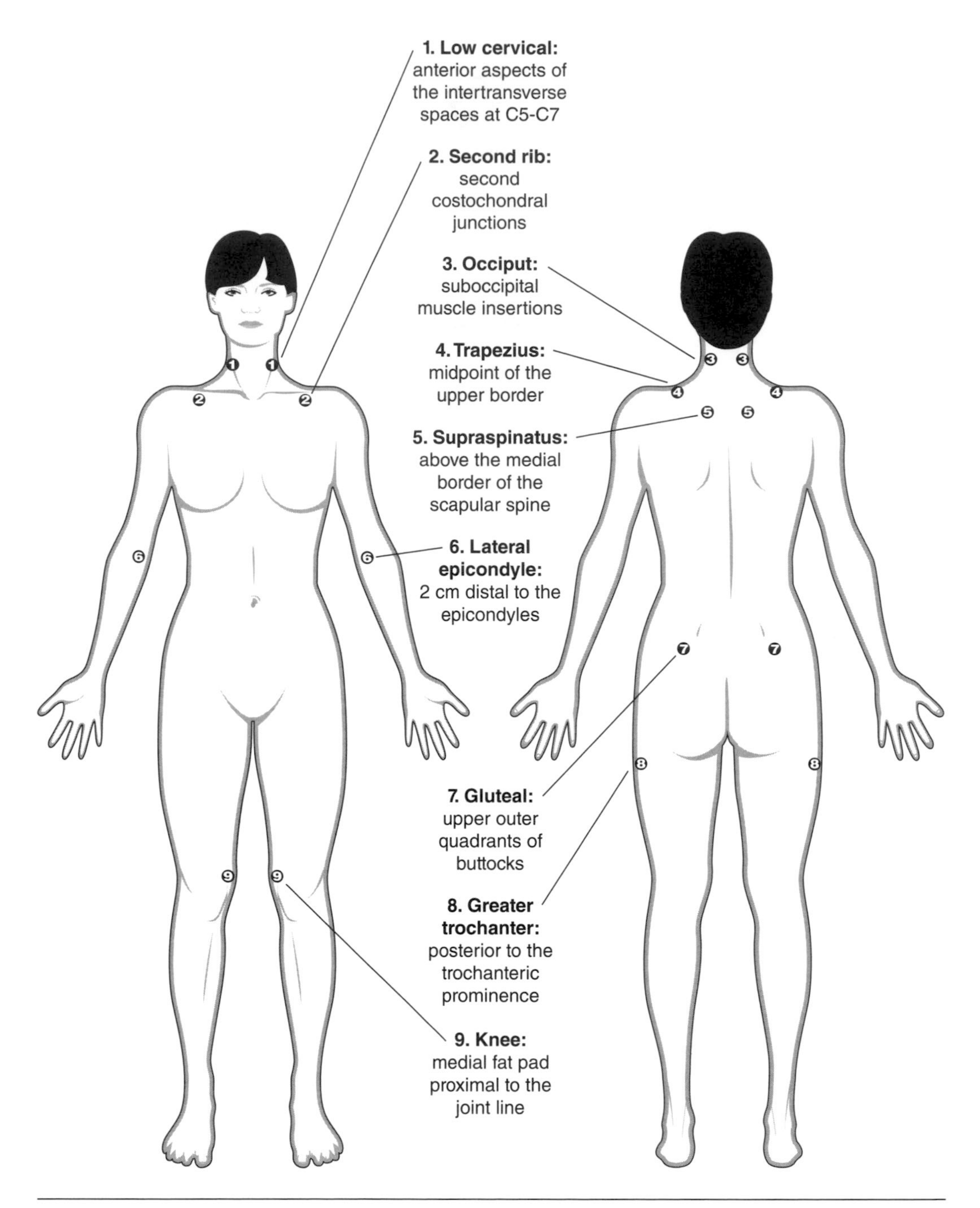

Figure 16.1 Fibromyalgia Tender Points

Reprinted, by permission, from J. Dedhia and M. Bone, 2009, "Pain and fibromyalgia," *Continuing Education in Anesthesia Critical Care and Pain* 9(5):162-166.

substance P

▸ A neurotransmitter involved in the transmission of pain and inflammatory processes.

Recent breakthroughs in medical imaging are providing important new clues as to how people with FMS process pain. Neuroscience imaging techniques have uncovered differences in specific brain regions in patients with FMS as compared with healthy controls (Harris et al. 2007; Guedj 2008). In addition, levels of nerve growth factor and the quantity of *substance P* nociceptors are elevated in FMS sufferers (Giovengo, Russell, and Larson 1999). Some evidence shows that levels of serotonin, a neurotransmitter that plays a role in pain and sleep disturbances, may also be elevated (Russell 2001). While these findings could eventually lead to increasingly objective diagnostic tests, presently they bolster the theory that FMS is caused or maintained by an alteration in the afflicted person's ability to process pain.

THEORIZED CAUSES OF FMS

Though the cause of fibromyalgia is not known, there are several plausible theories. These include the influences of central sensitization, reduced microcirculation, peripheral input, anxiety and depression, and sleep disturbance.

Central Sensitization

Central sensitization occurs when there is hyperactivity and amplification of sensory processing in the brain, which increases peripheral tissue responsiveness to sensory input, such as touch (Desmeules et al. 2003; Staud et al. 2003). In FMS, a widely distributed pattern of hypersensitivity to touch, or *allodynia,* may be caused by central sensitization. This contrasts with myofascial pain syndrome, in which the injury and subsequent touch sensitivity originate and remain in the peripheral branch of the nervous system. Because the hypersensitivity in FMS may originate in the central nervous system, it can affect the whole body relatively equally, rather than in a lateralized regional presentation, as seen in myofascial pain syndrome. Recent evidence suggests that allodynia in FMS is present not only in the 18 tender points presently used for diagnosis, but throughout the entire body (Staud 2008). This may explain the lack of consensus of exact tender point locations among early FMS researchers. An additional central sensitization symptom in some FMS sufferers is auditory hypersensitivity (Geisser et al. 2008).

allodynia

▸ When pain is generated by stimuli, such as ordinary touch, that would not ordinarily cause pain.

Central sensitization may be a cause of FMS, but what causes or triggers central sensitization? Possibilities include trauma and certain types of injury. Ledingham and colleagues (1993) found that 15% of FMS sufferers linked their development of the syndrome with a traumatic event. Persons with traumatic neck injuries were 13 times more likely to develop FMS than persons with traumatic injuries to the lower extremities (Buskila et al. 2005).

Reduced Microcirculation

Strobel and colleagues (1997) found that microcirculation in muscle, assessed in the trapezius, was reduced in FMS. Muscular contraction associated with exercise normally creates its own temporary decrease in vascular circulation. Since microcirculation in FMS may already be reduced, it is hypothesized that the additional reduction of microcirculation caused by exercise creates hypoxia, leading to increased pain.

Although exercise is ordinarily one of the most efficient ways to promote overall circulation, it may present a problem in FMS. It is not uncommon for people with FMS to experience pain after exercise, particularly aerobic exercise (Busch et al. 2008). Since higher levels of aerobic activity may increase symptoms in this population, some researchers have explored increasing activities of daily living (ADL) as a substitute for exercise. In one study, the cumulative effect of a moderate increase in ADL was a decrease in FMS symptoms without negative aftereffects (Fontaine and Haaz 2007). Possibly, massage therapy might provide FMS sufferers with the same type of benefit as moderately increased ADL, but this has yet to be tested.

Increased pain from exercise in FMS may also be due to descending inhibition. During activation of muscular activity, the sensory experience of pain is generally dampened by this mechanism, in which pain decreases during activity that originates, or descends from, the central nervous system. Because the central nervous system may be altered in FMS sufferers, the mechanism of descending inhibition may be impaired (Kosek, Eckholm, and Hannson 1996). In addition, the mechanism of descending inhibition is thought to be less efficient in women (Wickelgren 2009), which could account for their increased incidence of FMS.

Peripheral Input

Studies show that a high percentage of people with FMS have trigger points in addition to FMS tender points (Baldry, Yunus, and Inanici 2001). These peripherally generated stimuli may exacerbate central sensitization by increasing the volume of sensory signals flowing toward the brain. Logically, decreasing the amount of peripheral input should serve to decrease central sensitization, such that reduction or elimination of trigger points in an FMS sufferer has the potential to reduce syndrome severity.

Comorbidity of Anxiety and Depression

Clinical levels of anxiety and depression are often present in combination with FMS. One study found that anxiety is present in 32% of FMS sufferers, and depression may be present in as many as 70% of cases (Thieme, Turk, and Flor 2004). Reducing anxiety and depression with MT is important in the treatment of FMS (see chapter 13).

Sleep Disturbances

Persons with FMS often have disturbed sleep patterns (Moldofsky 2008). Depriving healthy people of slow-wave sleep actually produces symptoms very similar to FMS, which leads researchers to hypothesize that disturbed sleep could be a cause of FMS. Since improved sleep reduces FMS symptoms, FMS patients are often prescribed sleep medications. Sleep improvement should be one of the primary goals in the treatment of FMS. This goal may be facilitated by MT, which has been shown in some studies to increase sleep quality (Soden et al. 2004).

EFFECTS OF MASSAGE THERAPY FOR FIBROMYALGIA

Several primary studies have examined the effects of massage therapy on persons with fibromyalgia, with varying results. Some did not show significant improvement. University of Miami's Touch Research Institute has conducted two randomized controlled trials of massage therapy for fibromyalgia (Sunshine et al. 1996; Field et al 2002). However, each of these omits the between-groups test results and related statistical details necessary to determine if massage therapy outperformed control groups, a common shortcoming in massage therapy research (Moyer 2007). Alnigenis and colleagues (2001) completed a pilot study that compared 10 sessions of Swedish massage over 24 weeks to standard physician care for fibromyalgia. Group differences were not statistically significant, though the statistical power of this pilot study may have been too low to definitively uncover treatment effects.

Other studies showed positive results of MT. Brattberg (1999) compared 15 sessions of connective tissue massage to a control condition over a period of 10 weeks. At the end of treatment, massage recipients with fibromyalgia reported significantly less pain, fewer negative effects on their lives as a result of fibromyalgia, and better quality of life. Lemstra and Olszynski (2005) randomly assigned 79 persons with fibromyalgia to either receive standard care or a combination treatment consisting of exercise, informational lectures, and two sessions of massage therapy. At the end of the 6-week intervention period, the combination treatment group had significantly better self-perceived health status and lower levels of depressed mood and pain than the standard care group. Further, most of these benefits were still evident at a 15-month follow-up assessment. Ekici and colleagues (2009) conducted a randomized controlled trial that compared two types of massage. Women with fibromyalgia received either manual lymph drainage or connective tissue massage five times per week for 3 weeks. Both groups showed improvement from baseline and had similar outcomes for pain reduction, but scores on the Fibromyalgia impact questionnaire significantly favored manual lymph drainage as the more effective treatment. The authors concluded that "both methods . . . seemed to be useful" (Burckhardt, Clark, and Bennett 1991, 132).

Two reviews of fibromyalgia treatments have also examined massage therapy. Sim and Adams (2002), in a review of nonpharmacological treatments for fibromyalgia, found no strong evidence for any single intervention, though they did conclude there was preliminary support for aerobic exercise as an intervention. Because the types of massage examined in individual studies varied, they found that it was difficult to impossible to draw definitive conclusions about the effectiveness of massage for fibromyalgia. Similarly, Goldenberg, Burckhardt, and Crofford (2004) concluded that there was only weak evidence for the efficacy of massage therapy in the treatment of fibromyalgia, as compared with modest to strong evidence in support of various medications, consistent aerobic exercise, cognitive–behavioral therapy, strength training, acupuncture, biofeedback, hypnotherapy, and balneotherapy. Their final clinical recommendation was that education, medication, exercise, cognitive–behavioral therapy, or some combination of these four treatments should be preferred, based on current evidence.

EXPLAINING MASSAGE THERAPY EFFECTS

While the evidence in support of massage therapy for fibromyalgia is mixed, this is clearly an area where further research is needed. Some studies do show positive effects, and the studies that do not exhibit such effects may fail to do so not because the treatment is ineffective, but because the studies may have been underpowered or have suffered from other methodological shortcomings.

Given this state of evidence, we can only speculate about the ways in which massage therapy positively affects fibromyalgia. One possibility is that massage therapy reduces fibromyalgia symptoms enough to permit greater movement and activity. This would be consistent with the finding that exercise is one of the most effective interventions for fibromyalgia. Other possibilities are that massage therapy promotes microcirculation in a way that undermines the condition (Mori et al. 2004; Hinds et al. 2004), promotes better sleep (Field et al. 2002), somehow improves or recalibrates a faulty mechanism of pain processing in the nervous system, or reduces the comorbid anxiety and depression that, left untreated, perpetuate the condition.

RECOMMENDATIONS FOR MASSAGE THERAPY PRACTICE

A wide variance of MT approaches exists for treatment of FMS. Based on best available evidence and clinical experience, the following clinical guidelines are suggested.

Evidence-Based Treatment Guidelines

- Take a thorough health history, especially in regard to medications.
- Maintain good client communication. Preferences and response to pressure vary widely among clients. Attempt to quiet the central nervous system with soothing MT techniques (Matarán-Peñarrocha et al. 2009).
- Encourage slow breathing (Zautra et al. 2010).
- Reduce peripheral input by treating trigger points. Be cautious about overtreating and overstimulating the nervous system.
- Promote local microcirculation or improve quality of sleep.
- Be mindful that treatment of FMS takes patience and time (Brattberg 1999).
- Encourage exercise, at a level and intensity tolerable to the patient, between massage therapy sessions (Sim and Adams 2002; Goldenberg, Burckhardt, and Crofford 2004).
- Encourage patients to explore other professionally administered treatments, such as medication or cognitive–behavioral therapy, for which consistent evidence of effectiveness already exists (Goldenberg, Burckhardt, and Crofford 2004).

DIRECTIONS FOR FUTURE RESEARCH

More research needs to be done in all phases of the MT treatment of FMS. A comparative study with different types of MT to determine which are most effective would certainly be valuable. Many other questions also need to be addressed. Are direct manipulations, such as deep-tissue techniques, more helpful than indirect approaches, such as *craniosacral therapy?* What dosage pattern produces the best results? What session length is optimal? How can MT be administered to best improve sleep quality? Does MT treat FMS by increasing microcirculation or by reducing central sensitization? What are the best ways to test these theories?

craniosacral therapy

▸ A bodywork modality that attempts to manipulate the cranial and sacral bones in conjunction with the therapist's perception of the pulsating rhythm of the recipient's cerebrospinal fluid.

Case Study

Bea L. struggled with undiagnosed muscular pain and discomfort for many years. After recently meeting with a physiatrist, she was diagnosed with FMS. Although various medications have provided some relief, Bea continues to experience frequent pain of unknown origin, especially in her shoulders and neck. The pain is worse after a workday, during which Bea sorts mail. Positional stress caused by her workplace environment and activities are likely a factor. Most of her pain is distributed equally over her shoulders, extending to the middle of her thorax. Bea's physiatrist refers her to massage therapist Cal J.

After taking a thorough health history, conducting a physical assessment, and explaining the current evidence for MT in the treatment of FMS, Cal proposes a conservative approach with regard to length of sessions, frequency of treatments, and depth of pressure, since Bea has never received MT before. Early treatment goals are reduction of pain and improved sleep. As treatment progresses, Bea adapts to MT. She can tolerate deeper pressure and longer sessions, which permits Cal to focus on trigger-point reduction. In addition, based on his knowledge of the research literature, he encourages her to gradually increase daily living activities. Cal also helps Bea to reduce her workplace-related physical stressors by suggesting the need for frequent short breaks and specific stretches and deep-breathing exercises that reduce muscular tension in her mid- to upper back and shoulders.

Eventually Cal varies the frequency of Bea's treatments and takes care to track the results in his treatment notes. He also encourages Bea to keep an FMS journal. Eventually, through some trial and error, they are able to lengthen the time between MT sessions and arrive at an optimal maintenance schedule, supplemented by mild exercise. Bea still has occasional episodes of pain, but the duration of these episodes is shorter and her quality of life is improved. Bea continues to see Cal for MT once a month on average, with additional sessions added in response to acute flare-ups of FMS symptoms.

SUMMARY

Fibromyalgia is a condition that either is now occurring with greater frequency or is just now beginning to be recognized by professionals. Both may also be true. Though its causes are not understood, it is known to be highly comorbid with anxiety, depression, and sleep disturbance. It may result from an alteration of the nervous system's ability to process pain effectively. Scientific evidence in support of massage therapy as a treatment for fibromyalgia is mixed, though this state of the evidence is likely a function of the small number of studies that have been conducted and their variable methodological quality. Based on current evidence, massage therapy may be especially useful in combination with exercise, medications, or cognitive–behavioral therapy, which are currently recognized as the most effective interventions for fibromyalgia. Massage therapy may also be of particular value to patients who are not responsive to these interventions or who cannot pursue them. Further research is needed to refine our understanding of massage as a treatment for fibromyalgia and to uncover its specific mechanisms of action for this condition.

REFERENCES

Alnigenis, M.N.Y., J.D. Bradley, J. Wallick, and C.L. Emsley. 2001. Massage therapy in the management of fibromyalgia: A pilot study. *J Musculoskelet Pain* 9(2): 55-67.

Baldry, P., M.B. Yunus, and F. Inanici. 2001. *Myofascial pain and fibromyalgia syndromes*. Edinburgh: Churchill Livingstone.

Barker, K. 2005. *The fibromyalgia story*. Philadelphia: Temple University Press.

Bennett, R. 2005. Fibromyalgia: Present to future. *Current Rheumatology Reports* 7(5): 371-376.

Bradley, L. 2008. Family and genetic influences on fibromyalgia syndrome. *J Musculoskelet Pain* 16(1-2): 49-57.

Brattberg, G. 1999. Connective tissue massage in the treatment of fibromyalgia. *Eur J Pain* 3(3): 235-244.

Burckhardt, C.S., S.R. Clark, and R.M. Bennett. 1991. The fibromyalgia impact questionnaire: Development and validation. *J Rheumatol* 18(5): 728-733.

Busch, A. J., P. Thille, K. Barber, C. L. Schachter, J. Bidonde, and B. K. Collacott. 2008. "Best-practice: E-model – prescribing physical activity and exercise for individuals with fibromyalgia." *PTP* 24(3): 151-166.

Buskila, D., L. Neumann, G. Vaisberg, D. Alkalay, and F. Wolfe. 2005. Increased rates of fibromyalgia following cervical spine injury: A controlled study of 161 cases of traumatic injury. *J Arthritis Rheum*40(3): 446-452.

Desmeules, J.A., C. Cedraschi, E. Rapiti, E. Baumgartner, A. Finckh, P. Cohen, P. Dayer, and T.L. Vischer. 2003. Neurophysiologic evidence for a central sensitization in patients with fibromyalgia. *Arthritis Rheum* 48: 1420-1429.

Ekici, G., Y. Bakar, T. Akbayrak, and I. Yuksel. 2009. Comparison of manual lymph drainage and connective tissue massage in women with fibromyalgia: A randomized controlled trial. *J Manipulative Physiol Ther* 32(2): 127-133.

Field, T., M. Diego, C. Cullen, M. Hernandez-Reif, W. Sunshine, and S. Douglas. 2002. Fibromyalgia pain and substance p decrease and sleep improves after massage therapy. *J Clin Rheumatol* 8(2): 72-76.

Fontaine, K.R. and S. Haaz. 2007. "Effects of lifestyle physical activity on health status, pain and function, in adults with fibromyalgia syndrome." *J Musculoskeletal Pain* 15(1):3-9.

Geisser, M.E., J.M. Glass, L.D. Rajcevska, D.J. Clauw, D.A. Williams, P.R. Kileny, and R.H. Gracely. 2008. A psychophysiological study of auditory and pressure sensitivity in patients with fibromyalgia and healthy controls. *J Pain* 9(5): 417-422.

Giovengo, S.L., J. Russell, and A.A. Larson. 1999. Increased concentration of nerve growth factor in cerebrospinal fluid of patients with fibromyalgia syndrome. *J Rheumatol* 26: 1564-1569.

Goldenberg, D.L., C. Burckhardt, and L. Crofford. 2004. Management of fibromyalgia syndrome. *JAMA* 292(19): 2388-2395.

Guedj, E. 2008. Clinical correlate of brain SPECT perfusion abnormalities in fibromyalgia. *J Nucl Med* 49(11): 1798-1803.

Harris, R.E., D.J. Clauw, D.J. Scott, S.A. McLean, R.H. Gracely, and J. Zubieta. 2007. Decreased central μ-opioid receptor availability in fibromyalgia. *J Neurosci* 27(37): 10000-10006.

Hinds, T., I. McEwan, J. Perkes, E. Dawson, D. Ball, and K. George. 2004. Effects of massage on limb and skin blood flow after quadriceps exercise. *Med Sci Sports Exerc* 36(8): 1308-1313.

Kosek, E., J. Eckholm, and P. Hannson. 1996. Modulation of pressure pain thresholds during and following isometric contraction in patients with fibromyalgia and in healthy normal controls. *Pain* 64: 415-423.

Ledingham, J., S. Doherty, and M. Doherty. 1993. Primary fibromyalgia syndrome: An outcome study. *Br Soc Rheumatology* 32(2): 139-142.

Lemstra, M., and W.P. Olszynski. 2005. The effectiveness of multidisciplinary rehabilitation in the treatment of fibromyalgia: A randomized controlled trial. *Clin J Pain* 21(2): 166-174.

Matarán-Peñarrocha, G., A.M. Castro-Sánchez, G.C. García, C. Moreno-Lorenzo, T.P. Carreño, and M. Zafra. 2009. Influence of craniosacral therapy on anxiety, depression and quality of life in patients with fibromyalgia. http://ecam.oxfordjournals.org/cgi/reprint/nep125v1.

Moldofsky, H. 2008. The assessment and significance of the sleep/waking brain in patients with chronic widespread musculoskeletal pain and fatigue syndromes. *J Musculoskeletal Pain* 16(1-2): 37-48.

Mori, H., H. Ohsawa, T. Tanaka, E. Taniwaki, G. Leisman, and K. Nishijo. 2004. Effect of massage on blood flow and muscle fatigue following isometric lumbar exercise. *Med Sci Monit* 10(5): 173-178.

Moyer, C.A. 2007. Between-groups study designs demand between-groups analyses: A response to Hernandez-Reif, Shor-Posner, Baez, Soto, Mendoze, Castillo, Quintero, Perez, and Zhang. *Evid Based Complement Alternat Med* 6(1): 49-50.

Neumann, L., and D. Buskila. 2003. Epidemiology of fibromyalgia. *Curr Pain Headache Rep* 7: 362-368.

Russell, J. 2001. Fibromyalgia syndrome. In *Bonica's Management of Pain, 3rd ed.,* ed. J.D. Loeser, S.H. Butler, C.R. Chapman, and D.C. Turk. Philadelphia: Lippincott Williams and Wilkins.

Sim, J., and N. Adams. 2002. Systematic review of randomized controlled trials of nonpharmacological interventions for fibromyalgia. *Clin J Pain* 18(5): 324-326.

Soden, K., K. Vincent, S. Craske, C. Lucas, and S. Ashley. 2004. A randomized controlled trial of aromatherapy massage in a hospice setting. *Palliat Med* 18(2): 87-92.

Staud, R. 2008. The role of peripheral input for chronic pain syndromes like fibromyalgia syndrome. *J Musculoskeletal Pain* 16(1-2): 67-74.

Staud, R., R. Cannon, A. Mauderli, M.E. Robinson, D.D. Price, and C.J. Vierck Jr. 2003. Temporal summation of pain from mechanical stimulation of muscle tissue in normal controls and subjects with fibromyalgia syndrome. *Pain* 102: 87-95.

Strobel, E.S., M. Krapf, M. Suckfull, W. Bruckle, W. Fleckenstein, and W. Muller. 1997. Tissue oxygen measurement and 31P magnetic resonance spectroscopy in patients with muscle tension and fibromyalgia. *Rheumatol Int* 16: 175-180.

Sunshine, W., T.M. Field, O. Quintino, K. Fierro, C. Kuhn, I. Burman, and S. Schanberg. 1996. Fibromyalgia benefits from massage therapy and transcutaneous electrical stimulation. *J Clin Rheumatol* 2(1): 18-22.

Thieme, K., D. Turk, and H. Flor. 2004. Comorbid depression and anxiety in fibromyalgia syndrome: Relationship to somatic and psychosocial variables. *Psychosom Med* 66: 837-844.

Wickelgren, I. 2009. "I do not feel your pain." *Scientific American Mind* 20(5): 50-57.

Zautra, A., R. Fasman, M. Davis, and A. Craig. 2010. The effects of slow breathing on affective responses to pain stimuli: An experimental study. *Pain* 149(1): 12-18.

chapter 17

Cancer

Janice E. Post-White, PhD, RN, FAAN

Patients with cancer seek massage to help manage symptoms and side effects of cancer-related treatment and to help them cope with the anxiety, stress, and tension associated with this life-altering diagnosis. As more evidence proves it to be safe, massage is increasingly offered as an adjunctive therapy for cancer. This chapter reviews the evidence for safety, efficacy, and indications for massage for adults and children with cancer.

The diagnosis of cancer and its treatment creates uncertainty and anxiety, and disrupts family and work activities. Although many cancers are now curable, patients and families fear death, disability, and distressing symptoms. Multiple symptoms of pain, fatigue, sleep disruption, nausea or vomiting, anxiety, depression, and changes in body image and self-esteem all increase distress. Cancer survivors often face ongoing health issues secondary to treatment. And when treatment fails, end-of-life care focuses on managing symptoms, improving quality of life, and supporting the family. Evidence-based interventions are needed for managing symptoms and promoting wellness.

Massage therapy (MT) is one of the integrative therapies most often used for adults and children with cancer (Boon, Olatunde, and Zick 2007; Myers, Walton, and Small 2008; Post-White, Fitzgerald, Hageness, et al. 2009; Van Cleve et al. 2004). As part of treatment, touch can be comforting, healing, and nurturing, and can counter the invasiveness of some necessary procedures. Massage therapies studied in patients with cancer include Swedish massage, *aromatherapy massage, reflexology, acupressure,* and manual lymphatic drainage.

aromatherapy massage

▸ A modality that combines massage with application of essential oils to promote health and wellness.

reflexology

▸ A massage modality based on the theory that reflex points in the feet, hands, and head correspond to vital organs, and that those organs can be influenced by stimulation of the reflex points.

acupressure

▸ A massage-like modality treatment derived from acupuncture in which manual pressure, rather than needles, is applied to acupuncture points.

EFFECTS AND SAFETY OF MASSAGE THERAPY IN CANCER CARE

This section reviews research evidence on the safety, feasibility, and effectiveness of MT across the cancer care spectrum in both children and adults and examines the effectiveness and limitations of MT to reduce both cancer- and treatment-related symptoms, such as pain, depression, anxiety, nausea, and fatigue. It also presents the limited evidence on improved biological and immune-response outcomes. It considers the adaptation of treatment sometimes necessary for this population and notes special precautions, such as avoiding radiation sites. In addition, it debunks the myth that MT must be avoided by persons with cancer.

Safety

adverse event

▸ Any unfavorable symptom or unintended harm associated with the use of a treatment or intervention intended to be therapeutic.

Serious *adverse events* are rare and massage is generally safe when given by credentialed and experienced practitioners (Corbin 2009; Deng et al. 2009). More than 60 trials provide evidence for the feasibility and safety of massage for children and adults at every phase of the cancer experience. In a systematic review of 10 studies involving 386 patients with cancer, one case report of a skin rash was the only adverse event reported (Wilkinson, Barnes, and Storey 2008). Other anecdotal reports in patients with cancer include headache, lightheadedness, muscle tenderness, or general feeling of unwellness for a day or two following deep tissue massage. Adverse effects can often be prevented with awareness, modification of touch and pressure, and changes to positioning. The Society for Integrative Oncology recommends the use of massage for cancer pain and anxiety, but cautions against the use of deep or intense pressure near cancer lesions or enlarged lymph nodes, radiation field sites, intravenous catheters and medical devices, and anatomic distortions, or in patients with a bleeding tendency (Deng et al. 2009).

metastasis

▸ The spread of a disease, such as cancer, from one site of the body to another, nonadjacent site.

It is a myth that massage spreads cancer (Corbin 2005; Ernst 2003). *Metastasis* of cancer cells is a complex interaction of structural, biochemical, hormonal, immunological, and genetic factors that control cell growth, adhesion, angiogenesis, cell signaling, and mobility. However, inflammation, pain, or sensitivity to pressure are other reasons practitioners should use a gentle touch and avoid direct or deep massage over a surgical or tumor site, or in a limb distal to lymph node removal. Other problems requiring modification of the depth or location of touch include infection, skin irritation, platelet or clotting disorders, bone metastasis, and nausea. Deep massage should be avoided in fields of radiation, since the skin may be fragile and the underlying tissue may be fibrotic or edematous. No oils or lotions should be used on the field of treatment during the course of radiation. Rocking motions should be avoided with patients who are experiencing nausea (Gecsedi 2002). Practicing diligent hand washing and using clean equipment and linens will reduce the risk of infection.

Caution should be used for patients with cancer-related pain. Massage will not resolve pain resulting from pressure of the tumor on surrounding sites, nerve impingement (radiating pain), or bone pain from metastases. Light-touch massage can reduce anxiety or distress, whereas deep massage can worsen the pain by increasing inflammation or causing fragile bones to break.

It is important to assess and adapt touch for each client. In one study, children declined therapeutic massage if they were feeling nauseated, in pain, or ill, but responded positively to light and comforting caress of their arms or legs from their parents (Post-White, Fitzgerald, Savik, et al. 2009). Long, slow, light touch triggers a parasympathetic (relaxing) response, whereas deep massage stimulates the sympathetic nervous system, which increases heart rate and blood pressure and may lead to distress. To provide safe and effective massage, MacDonald (2007) recommends reducing the pressure, slowing the strokes, shortening the session length, and working gently.

Cancer treatment can leave patients feeling lonely and vulnerable. Children may be particularly sensitive to experiencing changes in body image and being unclothed. Asking permission and proceeding gently when touching an amputated limb stump, a bald head, or a scar, even if it is well healed, conveys compassion and respect. Massage to the abdomen can trigger emotional responses. Calm, confident, and loving touch can be restorative and healing as the patient adjusts to a new body image and sense of self. (See chapter 14.)

Efficacy and Effectiveness

Efficacy is the assessment of whether treatment works under controlled conditions in a clinical trial. Controls within the study design reduce bias and eliminate alternate explanations for observed effects, resulting in a cause-and-effect prediction of a given probability. A treatment is efficacious when it proves to be superior to placebo or control conditions. By contrast, *effectiveness* is the assessment of whether treatment works in a typical clinical setting and is clinically relevant. Both are important to assessing the value of massage to the care of persons with cancer.

efficacy

▸ The ability of a treatment or intervention to work under controlled conditions, such as in a laboratory.

effectiveness

▸ The ability of a treatment or intervention to work under uncontrolled, real-world conditions, such as in a hospital or treatment center.

Several excellent summaries and systematic reviews evaluate the efficacy of massage research for children and adults with cancer. They include detailed tables of study samples, design, massage techniques, and findings (Ernst 2009; Fellowes, Barnes, and Wilkinson 2008; Hughes et al. 2008; Jane et al. 2008; Myers, Walton, and Small 2008; Russell et al. 2008; Wilkinson, Barnes, and Storey 2008; Beider and Moyer 2007). This chapter summarizes the findings and includes additional research published subsequent to the reviews.

Studies in Adults With Cancer

The most consistent and strongest effect of massage, aromatherapy massage, and foot reflexology in adults with cancer is reduced anxiety (table 17.1). Although most studies measure short-term effects, Wilkinson and colleagues (2007) found patients experienced less anxiety 2 weeks after 4 weekly aromatherapy massage sessions. Future research should determine the length of effects experienced following massage and the clinical relevance is for short-term reduction of anxiety.

Massage reduced depressive symptoms or depressed mood in some patients (table 17.1). Treatment with a single massage therapist over time was more effective than having different therapists in reducing depression in breast cancer survivors (Listing et al. 2009).

In most studies, massage relieved pain immediately after the session (table 17.1). However, some studies found no effect or only selective effects (Weinrich and Weinrich 1990). In *longitudinal studies,* Listing and colleagues (2009) found pain was reduced after 5 weeks of twice-weekly massage, while Kutner and others (2008) found similar pain-reduction effects for both massage and simple touch. In two other studies, patients used fewer analgesics after receiving massage (Post-White et al. 2003; Wilkie et al. 2000). Massage appears to be most effective for short-term relief of pain (Liu and Fawcett 2008). However, many of the studies assessing pain are limited by small sample sizes, inclusion of different stages of cancer and sources of pain, or a lack of control conditions (Cassileth and Vickers 2004; Currin and Meister 2008; Ferrell-Torry and Glick 1993; Sturgeon et al. 2009). More research is needed to determine the long-term effects and the clinical relevance of massage as an adjunct for pain control.

longitudinal study

▸ A type of research that examines change in one or more groups over a period of time.

The effect of massage on nausea is inconclusive, with some studies showing effectiveness and other studies showing no effect (table 17.1). Specific stimulation of the P6 acupressure point was more effective for nausea than body massage (Dibble et al. 2000; Dibble et al. 2007; Shin et al. 2004).

Although massage is standard care for *lymphedema* (Williams et al. 2002), other symptoms have not been studied sufficiently to draw conclusions. Patients report improved energy following massage, but few studies demonstrate effects on fatigue (table 17.1). In longitudinal studies, fatigue remained lower 6 weeks after 10 sessions of biweekly massage (Listing et al. 2009), but massage was not quite

lymphedema

▸ A condition, caused by a compromised lymphatic system, in which tissues swell due to retention of fluid.

significantly better ($p = 0.057$) than control groups in reducing fatigue after four weekly massage sessions (Post-White et al. 2003).

Anecdotal and research evidence exist to support the use of massage for comfort, pleasure, and respite from the stress of cancer. Massage is generally accepted to promote relaxation, relieve muscle tension (Pruthi et al. 2009), and improve quality of life for patients receiving cancer treatment (Sturgeon et al. 2009) or at the end of life (Kutner et al. 2008; Smith et al. 2009). Patients, caregivers, and family members benefit from both giving and receiving massage (Field et al. 2001; Goodfellow 2003).

Early massage studies are limited by small sample sizes, high dropout rates, and lack of comparison groups or analysis between groups. Almost half of the early studies either lack a control group or fail to use randomization to groups. More recent studies in adults use randomized controlled trials (RCT) with larger sample sizes of 100 to 300 subjects (Campeau et al. 2007; Kutner et al. 2008; Mehling et al. 2007; Post-White et al. 2003). Considerable variation remains in the depth of touch and the types and dose of massage administered in individual studies, which makes comparisons among studies difficult and limits the translation of findings to practice.

Studies in Children With Cancer

Although massage is used clinically for children with cancer, only five studies have tested its effectiveness. Consistent with adult studies, decreased anxiety was the most commonly observed effect in children receiving massage for a variety of conditions (Beider, Mahrer, and Gold 2007) and for cancer (table 17.1). Other findings included improved mood (Field et al. 2001; Haun, Graham-Pole, and Shortley 2009), reduced discomfort (Haun, Graham-Pole, and Shortley 2009; Phipps et al. 2005), and decreased heart rate (Post-White, Fitzgerald, Savik, et al. 2009) and respiratory rate (Haun, Graham-Pole, and Shortley 2009). In these small studies, massage did not lower blood pressure (Haun, Graham-Pole, and Shortley 2009; Post-White, Fitzgerald, Savik, et al. 2009), lessen symptoms of pain, nausea, and fatigue, or reduce cortisol levels (Post-White, Fitzgerald, Savik, et al. 2009). Phipps and colleagues (2004) found that massage reduced the time to engraftment after bone marrow transplant, but had no effects on mood or symptoms. Importantly, these studies support the feasibility and safety of both massage for children with cancer provided by both therapists (Haun, Graham-Pole, and Shortley 2009; Phipps et al. 2004; Phipps et al. 2005; Post-White, Fitzgerald, Savik, et al. 2009) and parents (Field et al. 2001; Phipps et al. 2004; Phipps et al. 2005). In two studies on the effects of massage for parents of children with cancer, parents reported less anxiety (Post-White, Fitzgerald, Savik et al. 2009), less fatigue, and greater vigor (Iwasaki 2005).

Conducting massage research in children with cancer presents unique challenges. Small sample sizes and low statistical power are common problems (Beider and Moyer 2007; Phipps et al. 2004; Phipps et al. 2005), as are lack of standardization in dose, frequency, and style of massage (Underdown et al. 2006). Few self-reporting instruments are validated for children, and parent proxy reports are often an inaccurate reflection of the child's perspective. Multisite studies make larger sample sizes possible, but they usually also require standardization of massage across settings, which may limit the effectiveness of treatment and the generalizability of study results. This is important because children often have unique needs and very specific tolerances and preferences that make standardization problematic. When children are undergoing treatment for cancer, massage therapists need to consider their health status and energy level, as well as their families' overwhelming schedules. More than one massage session may be needed to help the child feel comfortable with therapist-provided massage.

Table 17.1 Studies Testing Effectiveness of Massage in Reducing Symptoms in Patients With Cancer

	ADULTS WITH CANCER		CHILDREN WITH CANCER	
Symptom	Positive effects of massage	No effect of massage	Positive effects of massage	No effect of massage
Anxiety	Ahles et al. 1999; Campeau et al. 2007; Corner, Cawley, and Hildebrand 1995; Hernandez-Reif et al. 2004; Hernandez-Reif et al. 2005; Jane et al. 2009; Post-White et al. 2003; Quattrin et al. 2006; Stephenson et al. 2007; Tsay et al. 2008; Wilkie et al. 2000; Wilkinson et al. 2007	Billhult, Bergbom, and Stener-Victorin 2007; Billhult et al. 2008; Listing et al. 2009	Field et al. 2001; Haun, Graham-Pole, and Shortley 2009; Phipps et al. 2005; Post-White, Fitzgerald, Savik et al. 2009	
Depression/ depressed mood	Listing et al. 2009; Hernandez-Reif et al. 2004; Hernandez-Reif et al. 2005; Mehling et al. 2007; Post-White et al. 2003; Soden et al. 2004		Field et al. 2001; Haun, Graham-Pole, and Shortley 2009	Phipps et al. 2004; Phipps et al. 2005
Pain	Cassileth and Vickers 2004; Corner, Cawley, and Hildebrand 1995; Currin and Meister 2008; Grealish, Lomansey, and Whiteman 2000; Hernandez-Reif et al. 2004; Jane et al. 2009; Kutner et al. 2008; Listing et al. 2009; Mehling et al. 2007; Post-White et al. 2003; Smith et al. 2002; Stephenson et al. 2007; Tsay et al. 2008; Weinrich and Weinrich 1990; Wilkie et al. 2000	Soden et al. 2004; Sturgeon et al. 2009		Post-White , Fitzgerald, Savik et al. 2009
Nausea	Ahles et al. 1999; Billhult, Bergbom, and Stener-Victorin 2007; Grealish, Lomansey, and Whiteman 2000	Mehling et al. 2007; Post-White et al. 2003		Post-White, Fitzgerald, Savik et al. 2009; Phipps et al. 2005
Fatigue	Ahles et al. 1999; Cassileth and Vickers 2004; Hernandez Reif et al. 2005; Listing et al. 2009	Post-White et al. 2003		Post-White, Fitzgerald, Savik et al. 2009

Biological and Immunological Effects of Massage in Children and Adults With Cancer

The weakest evidence for massage effects is in biological and immunological outcomes. Some responses of the autonomic nervous system (heart rate, blood pressure) consistently decrease immediately following massage (Ahles et al. 1999; Billhult et al. 2009; Grealish, Lomasney, and Whiteman 2000; Post-White et al. 2003;

Post-White, Fitzgerald, Savik, et al. 2009; Wilkie et al. 2000). However, effects on salivary cortisol and immunological measures of stress are often insignificant. Only Stringer, Swindell, and Dennis (2008) found decreased serum cortisol and prolactin 30 minutes after massage compared to a control group. No differences were captured beyond 30 minutes, suggesting a short-term response of this circulating stress-related hormone. Similarly, only one study by Billhult and colleagues (2009) showed a stabilizing effect of a massage on cytotoxicity of natural killer (NK) cells, with no change in numbers of NK cells.

Hernandez-Reif and colleagues (2004; 2005) provide the strongest evidence to date for biological and immunological effects in response to massage. Although sample sizes in one study were too small to compare immune effects by group (2005), increases in number of NK cells and positive psychological outcomes were associated with increases in dopamine and serotonin immediately after massage and again 5 weeks later. By contrast, Billhult and colleagues (2008) found no changes in oxytocin in patients with cancer, even though oxytocin has been shown to increase after repeated massage in other populations and in highly controlled studies using rat models (Lund et al. 2002; Wikstrom, Gunnarsson, and Nordin 2003).

Lack of evidence is not synonymous with lack of effect. Because of individual variability in immune responses and differential effects of acute and chronic stress, immunological effects are difficult to capture and to compare to normative values or standards. Detecting changes in response to massage requires large sample sizes, large effects, or both. Effects may also be missed because of an emphasis on single cross-sectional assessments or a measurement schedule that does not capture circulating responses to massage. Alternately, statistically significant effects can be found and erroneously attributed to massage if distributions are skewed or if other important variables (e.g., sleep, infection, medications) are uncontrolled. Statistical significance does not imply clinical significance; short-term immune changes captured on isolated posttest assessments may not have clinical relevance. Longitudinal studies will provide findings of greater clinical relevance.

EXPLAINING MASSAGE THERAPY EFFECTS

A stress-reducing mechanism is most often used to explain how massage affects symptoms and, possibly, immune response. Although *psychoneuroimmunology* (PNI) theory is not specific to cancer alone, the cascade of stressful events preceding or resulting from cancer triggers the release of corticotrophin-releasing hormone from the pituitary gland, cortisol from the adrenal cortex, and epinephrine and noradrenaline from the adrenal medulla. This results in the suppression of NK cells and T lymphocytes, critical immune cells that control and kill cancer cells.

psychoneuroimmunology theory

▸ A framework for understanding health and the delivery of health care that accounts for the interactions between patients' perceptions and behaviors, their brain function, and the performance of their immune system.

It is theorized that massage downregulates this sympathetic stress response through stimulation of tissue receptors, which leads to reduced cortisol and increased blood and lymph flow to provide oxygen and nutrients to cells and tissues, as well as positive emotional responses that release tension and promote relaxation. The resultant positive mood states and beliefs, which are perceived and processed through the amygdala in the hypothalamus, release dopamine, endogenous opiates, and oxytocin. These activate the vagus nerve and the parasympathetic nervous system (Kolcaba et al. 2004; Lund et al. 2002), and decrease salivary and urinary cortisol (Field et al. 2005; Diego et al. 2004).

However, despite enthusiasm for this theory, massage therapy research fails to detect consistent reductions of stress hormones (Moyer 2008; Moyer et al. 2011). Neurohormone and cytokine responses are often fleeting, and they have intricate feedback systems. NK cells and oxytocin are also known to be both downregulated and upregulated in response to stress, making these effects difficult to capture and interpret. Massage effects are likely complex, and they are mediated by diverse central, peripheral, and local tissue responses (Sagar, Dryden, and Myers 2007).

RECOMMENDATIONS FOR MASSAGE THERAPY PRACTICE

Massage can be safely and feasibly adapted for patients with cancer at any stage of disease. Oncology massage therapists require specific training about what to expect when the patient has cancer. They should weigh the potential risks with the expected benefits (Grant et al. 2008) and modify treatment approaches for patients at the end of life (Smith et al. 2009). Massage should be avoided near or above tumor sites, surgical areas, radiation fields, or intravenous lines. Only light touch is appropriate for patients with bleeding tendencies, those in postoperative recovery, or those who are nauseated or cachectic. Therapists providing massage to children with cancer should have experience with pediatric massage. Consideration should be given for changes in body image and for childrens' preferences in terms of clothing worn or the presence of a parent in the room. Some younger children respond favorably if a parent receives massage first or if their parents are trained to provide the massage. Parents and caregivers benefit from both giving and receiving massage.

Although evidence to explain how massage works is inconclusive, RCTs consistently show that massage reduces pain and anxiety related to cancer. Although the effects are less consistent, massage may also help reduce depression, nausea, and fatigue. Insufficient evidence exists that massage improves immune responses. At this time, there are few recommendations for dose and frequency of massage for specific outcomes. Most studies measure only immediate effects, and little is known about the long-term effects or clinical relevance of ongoing massage. The best guidance is to individualize massage sessions to client preferences and needs and to carefully assess and document responses to massage. More than one session may be needed to observe benefits, with most studies showing the strongest effects when a series of massages is given.

Some believe that if patients want massage, and if it does no harm and provides emotional or physical benefit, then RCTs are not needed to demonstrate a higher level of efficacy. While this approach has appeal in an environment of limited resources, lack of evidence makes it hard to justify services and obtain reimbursement for massage in hospital or outpatient settings. Evidence is needed to demonstrate that massage is a healing intervention that can reduce emotional consequences or symptom distress and improve quality of life in patients undergoing cancer treatment.

Evidence-Based Treatment Guidelines

- Massage is recommended as part of multimodality treatment for cancer patients experiencing anxiety or pain (Deng et al. 2009).
- Massage therapists treating patients with cancer should be trained in how and when to modify techniques.
- Avoid deep or intense pressure near cancer lesions or enlarged lymph nodes, radiation field sites, medical devices (such as indwelling intravenous catheters), and anatomic distortions (such as postoperative changes), or in patients with a bleeding tendency (Deng et al. 2009).

- Adapt the massage technique, length, and depth according to the patient's age, symptoms, tolerance, and experience with previous massage. When in doubt, always choose a light touch.
- Assess and document effectiveness, outcomes, and any adverse reactions or responses.
- Offer massage or teach willing family members to give massage to spouses, children, siblings, and other family members.

DIRECTIONS FOR FUTURE RESEARCH

Future research is needed to address the methodological weaknesses of small sample sizes, lack of control groups, diversity of outcome measures, lack of standardization, and inconsistent blinding of researchers. RCTs with adequately powered sample sizes to detect effects are needed to validate massage for management of cancer-related symptoms across all phases of cancer care. Replication of study findings is essential to establish efficacy for symptom management and quality-of-life outcomes. Studies are specifically needed that test the effects of massage on fatigue, dyspnea, sleep quality, nausea, wound healing, and immune responses in patients, as well as the management of long-term effects and promotion of well-being in survivors. Also needed are studies that determine the best timing for massage interventions.

The clinical relevance of massage will depend on determining the effects that last beyond the time immediately following massage sessions and those that affect overall function or quality of life. Understanding the underlying mechanisms of how massage reduces symptoms or improves physiological outcomes will help to determine who is most likely to benefit and how the effects can be sustained. Efficacy studies also are needed to determine the value of massage for siblings, parents, spouses, and caregivers. Massage can be safe and effective, but clearly, more studies are needed to validate the efficacy of massage in cancer care.

Case Study

Sahara S. is an 8-year-old girl receiving chemotherapy for cancer. Massage therapist Candace B. first saw her when she was intubated in the pediatric intensive care unit. The chemotherapy affected her neurological function, and she was unable to speak or move her extremities. Although the oncologist referred Sahara to Candace, it was Sahara's grandfather who specifically knew that she had always liked touch and that she had relaxed during massage in previous hospitalizations. Her mom wanted Sahara to relax and to have something to look forward to at the hospital.

Simple massage techniques were chosen to counter the invasiveness of procedures that are a usual part of hospitalization. Candace started with light stroking of Sahara's arms and hands with lotion, and then did light effleurage on her back while Sahara lay on her side. Because Sahara seemed comfortable, Candace avoided repositioning her. Instead, she massaged Sahara's torso and limbs, which were easily accessible, while taking care to avoid the tubes and lines. As she massaged, Candace attended to how Sahara received the massage by watching her carefully and with intention to best assess how she responded to the touch. Candace modified her technique in response to Sahara's feedback, providing facilitated stretches to the extremities to relax tight muscles. Because Sahara couldn't speak, Candace looked for facial expressions of pain or pleasure, and felt how muscles softened or tightened in response to gentle touch. She was pleased to notice, from a look at the vital signs monitor, that the child's oxygen saturation increased and her heart rate decreased, which are indicative of increasing relaxation. She also caught a glimpse of a slight smile from Sahara.

Candace continued to treat Sahara when she received chemotherapy treatments. During one session, it was clear from Sahara's facial expressions that she felt too tired and nauseated to receive massage that day, so Candace simply sat with Sahara. She gently touched her but did not move her for the remainder of the session. Sahara drifted to sleep.

Because Sahara experienced symptom relief from the massages, Candace taught Sahara's parents a basic 5-minute massage that they could do at home between hospital visits. Candace showed them how to avoid Sahara's medical devices and answered their questions about safety. She also explained when to avoid massage, such as when Sahara had a fever or infection. After a week, Candace phoned Sahara's parents to see how everyone was doing with the massages. They reported that they found the massage easy to do, and that they had no questions or concerns. They said that they felt good about giving their daughter brief massages at bedtime, usually two or three times per week. They also reported that Sahara seemed to sleep better (more deeply and longer) on the nights she received massage and that they also benefited from the time they spent with her using the new skill they had learned. Candace suggested that they might also benefit from receiving massage to reduce the stress and fatigue associated with their daughter's treatment for cancer. She provided them with contact information for one of her colleagues who worked in their hometown.

Sahara continued to respond well to her cancer treatments. Her voice recovered, and after several months, her cancer was diagnosed as being in remission. At her 1-year checkup, Sahara's parents told Candace how beneficial the massages, both in hospital and at home, had been for Sahara. They also reported how much they had also benefited from both giving and receiving massages during that stressful time. Sahara was returning to all the activities she loved before she got sick, but she still occasionally asked her parents for a bedtime massage. These massages continued to be a special, shared time.

SUMMARY

Persons with cancer can use massage to manage symptoms and side effects of cancer-related treatment and to help them cope with the anxiety, depression, fatigue, insomnia, pain, and stress associated with this life-altering diagnosis. Evidence increasingly supports the safety of massage provided by trained therapists who adapt their treatment to the individual needs of the patient.

Although the effects of massage on the immune system are disputed and little is known about its exact mechanisms of action, sufficient evidence of its benefits support massage as an adjunctive therapy for a variety of cancers. Massage therapists working with patients with cancer should use an evidence-based approach to minimize risk and maximize benefits. They should also account for the patient's social context, which may include providing emotional support and massage to members of the patient's family and social support group. Across all stages of cancer, and for children, adults, and those at the end of life, well-trained massage therapists have the potential to reduce suffering, provide comfort, and help the patient to cope with the difficult challenges that this condition presents.

REFERENCES

Ahles, T.A., D.M. Tope, B. Pinkson, S. Walch, D. Hann, M. Whedon, B. Dain, J.E. Weiss, L. Mills, and P.M. Silberfarb. 1999. Massage therapy for patients undergoing autologous bone marrow transplantation. *J Pain Symptom Manag* 19(3): 157-163.

Beider, S., and C.A. Moyer. 2007. Randomized controlled trials of pediatric massage: A review. *Evid-Based Compl Alt* 4(1): 23-34.

Beider, S., N.E. Mahrer, and J.I. Gold. 2007. Pediatric massage therapy: An overview for clinicians. *Pediatr Clin N Am* 54(6): 1025-1041.

Billhult, A., I. Bergbom, and E. Stener-Victorin. 2007. Massage relieves nausea in women with breast cancer who are undergoing chemotherapy. *J Altern Complem Med* 13(1): 53-57.

Billhult, A., C. Lindholm, R. Gunnarsson, and E. Stener-Victorin. 2008. The effect of massage on cellular immunity, endocrine and psychological factors in women with breast cancer—A randomized controlled clinical trial. *Auton Neurosci-Basic* 140: 88-95.

Billhult, A., C. Lindholm, R. Gunnarsson, and E. Stener-Victorin. 2009. The effect of massage on immune function and stress in women with breast cancer—A randomized controlled trial. *Auton Neurosci-Basic* 150(1-2): 111-115.

Boon, H.S., F. Olatunde, and S.M. Zick. 2007. Trends in complementary/alternative medicine use by breast cancer survivors: Comparing survey data from 1998 and 2005. *BMC Women's Health* 7(4). www.biomedcentral.com/1472-6874/7/4.

Campeau M.P., R. Gaboriault , M. Drapeau, T. Nguyen, I. Roy, B. Fortin, M. Marois, and P.F. Nguyen-Tan. 2007. Impact of massage therapy on anxiety levels in patients undergoing radiation therapy: Randomized controlled trial. *J Soc Integr Oncol* 5(4): 133-138.

Cassileth B.J., and A.J. Vickers. 2004. Massage therapy for symptom control: Outcome study at a major cancer center. *J Pain Symptom Manag* 28(3): 244-249.

Corbin, L.W. 2005. Safety and efficacy of massage therapy for patients with cancer. *Cancer Control* 12: 158-164.

———. 2009. Massage therapy. In *Integrative Oncology,* ed. Donald I. Abrams and Andrew T. Weil, 232-243. New York: Oxford University Press.

Corner, J., N. Cawley, and S. Hildebrand. 1995. An evaluation of the use of massage and essential oils on the well being of cancer patients. *Int J Palliat Nurs* 1(2): 67-73.

Currin, J., and E.A. Meister. 2008. A hospital-based intervention using massage to reduce distress among oncology patients. *Cancer Nursing* 31(3): 214-221.

Deng, G.E., M. Frenkel, L. Cohen, B.R. Cassileth, D.I. Abrams, J.L. Capodice, K.S. Courneya, T. Dryden, S. Hanser, N. Kumar, D. Labriola, D. W. Wardell, and S. Sagar. 2009. Evidence-based clinical practice guidelines for integrative oncology: Complementary therapies and botanicals. *J Soc Integr Oncol* 7(3): 85-120.

Dibble, S.L., J. Chapman, K.A. Mack, and A.S. Shih. 2000. Acupressure for nausea: Results of a pilot study. *Oncol Nurs Forum* 27(1): 41-47.

Dibble, S.L., J. Luce, B.A. Cooper, J. Israel, M. Cohen, B. Nussey, and H. Rugo. 2007. Acupressure for chemotherapy-induced nausea and vomiting: A randomized clinical trial. *Oncol Nurs Forum* 34(4): 813-820.

Diego, M., T. Field, C. Sanders, and M. Hernandez-Reif. 2004. Massage therapy of moderate and light pressure and vibrator effects on EEG and heart rate. *Int J Neurosci* 114(1): 31-44.

Ernst, E. 2003. The safety of massage therapy. *Rheumatology* 42(9): 1101-1106.

———. 2009. Massage therapy for cancer palliation and supportive care: A systematic review of randomised clinical trials. *Support Care Cancer* 17(4): 333 -337.

Fellowes, D., K. Barnes, and S. Wilkinson. 2008. Aromatherapy and massage for symptom relief in patients with cancer. *Cochrane Db Syst Rev* Issue 4. CD002287. pub3.

Ferrell-Torry, A.T., and O.J. Glick. 1993. The use of therapeutic massage as a nursing intervention to modify anxiety and the perception of cancer pain. *Cancer Nursing* 16(2): 93-101.

Field, T., C. Cullen, M. Diego, M. Hernandez-Reif, P. Sprinz, K. Beebe, B. Kissell, and V. Bango-Sanchez. 2001. Leukemia immune changes following massage therapy. *J Bodyw Mov Ther* 5: 271-274.

Field, T., M. Hernandez-Reif, M. Diego, S. Schanberg, and C. Kuhn. 2005. Cortisol decreases and serotonin and dopamine increase following massage therapy. *Int J Neurosci* 115(10): 1397-1413.

Gecsedi, R.A. 2002. Massage therapy for patients with cancer. *Clin J Oncol Nurs* 6(1): 52-54.

Goodfellow, L.M. 2003. The effects of therapeutic back massage on psychophysiologic variables and immune function in spouses of patients with cancer. *Nurs Res* 52(5): 318-328.

Grant, K.E., J. Balletoo, D. Gowan-Moody, D. Healey, D. Kincaid, W. Lowe, and R.S. Travillian. 2008. Steps toward massage therapy guidelines: A first report to the profession. *Int J Ther Massage Bodywork* 1(1): 19-36.

Grealish, L.O., A. Lomansey, and B. Whiteman. 2000. Foot massage: A nursing intervention. *Cancer Nursing* 23: 237-243.

Haun, J.N., J. Graham-Pole, and B. Shortley. 2009. Children with cancer and blood diseases experience positive physical and psychological effects from massage therapy. *Int J Ther Massage Bodywork* 2(2): 7-14.

Hernandez -Reif, M., G. Ironson, T. Field, J. Hurley, G. Katz, M. Diego, S. Weiss, M.A. Fletcher, S. Schanberg, C. Kuhn, and I. Burman. 2004. Breast cancer patients have improved immune and neuroendocrine functions following massage therapy. *J Psychosom Res* 57(1): 45-52.

Hernandez-Reif, M., T. Field, G. Ironson, J. Beutler, Y. Vera, J. Hurley, M.A. Fletcher, S. Schanberg, C. Kuhn, and M. Fraser. 2005. Natural killer cells and lymphocytes increase in women with breast cancer following massage therapy. *Int J Neurosci* 115(4): 495-510.

Hughes, D., E. Ladas, D. Rooney, and K. Kelly. 2008. Massage therapy as a supportive care intervention for children with cancer. *Oncol Nurs Forum* 35(3): 431-442.

Iwasaki, M. 2005. Interventional study on fatigue relief in mothers caring for hospitalized children—Effect of massage-incorporating techniques from oriental medicine. *Kurume Med J* 52: 19-27.

Jane, S., D.J. Wilkie, B.B. Gallucci, and R.D. Beaton. 2008. Systematic review of massage intervention for adult patients with cancer: A methodological perspective. *Cancer Nursing* 31(6): E24-E35.

Jane, S., D.J. Wilkie, B.B. Gallucci, R.D. Beaton, and H. Huang. 2009. Effects of a full-body massage on pain intensity, anxiety, and physiological relaxation in Taiwanese patients with metastatic bone pain: A pilot study. *J Pain Sympt Manag* 37(4): 754-763.

Kolcaba, K., T. Dowd, R. Steiner, and A. Mitzel. 2004. Efficacy of hand massage for enhancing the comfort of hospice patients. *Journal of Hospice and Palliative Nursing* 6(2): 91-102.

Kutner, J.S., M.C. Smith, L. Corbin, L. Hemphill, K. Benton, B.K. Mellis, B. Beaty, S. Felton, T.E. Yamashita, L.L. Bryant, and D.L. Fairclough. 2008. Massage therapy versus simple touch to improve pain and mood in patients with advanced cancer. *Ann Intern Med* 149: 369-379.

Listing, M., A. Reißhauer, M. Krohn, B. Voigt, G. Tjahono, J. Becker, B.F. Klapp, and M. Rauchfuß. 2009. Massage therapy reduces physical discomfort and improves mood disturbances in women with breast cancer. *Psychooncology* 18(12): 1290-1299.

Liu, Y., and T.N. Fawcett. 2008. The role of massage therapy in the relief of cancer pain. *Nursing Standard* 22(21): 35-40.

Lund, I., Y. Ge, L. Yu, K. Uvnas-Moberg, J. Wang, C. Yu, M. Kurosawa, G. Agren, A. Rosen, M. Lekman, and T. Lundeberg. 2002. Repeated massage-like stimulation induces long-term effects on nociception: Contribution of oxytocinergic mechanisms. *Eur J Neurosci* 16(2): 330-338.

MacDonald, G. 2007. *Medicine hands: Massage therapy for people with cancer.* Forres, UK: Findhorn Press.

Mehling, W.E., B. Jacobs, M. Acree, L. Wilson, A. Bostrom, J. West, J. Acquah, B. Burns, J. Chapman, and F.M. Hecht. 2007. Symptom management with massage and acupuncture in postoperative cancer patients: A randomized controlled trial. *J Pain Sympt Manag* 33(3): 258-266.

Moyer, C.A. 2008. Affective massage therapy. *Int J Ther Massage Bodywork* 1(2): 3-5.

Moyer, C.A., L. Seefeldt, E.S. Mannand, and L.M. Jackley. 2011. Does massage therapy reduce cortisol? A comprehensive quantitative review. *J Bodyw Mov Ther* 15: 3-14.

Myers, C.D., T. Walton, and B.J. Small. 2008. The value of massage therapy in cancer care. *Hematol Oncol Clin N* 22: 649-660.

Phipps, S., M. Dunavant, S. Rai, X. Deng, and S. Lensing. 2004. The effects of massage in children undergoing bone marrow transplant. *Massage Ther J* 43(3): 62-71.

Phipps, S., M. Dunavant, E. Gray, and S. Rai. 2005. Massage therapy in children undergoing hematopoetic stem cell transplantation: Results of a pilot trial. *J Cancer Integr Med* 3(2): 62-70.

Post-White, J., M.E. Kinney, K.S. Savik, J.B. Gau, C. Wilcox, and I. Lerner. 2003. Therapeutic massage and healing touch improve symptoms in cancer. *Integr Cancer Ther* 2(4): 332-344.

Post-White, J., M. Fitzgerald, S. Hageness, and S.F. Sencer. 2009. Complementary and alternative medicine use in children with cancer and general and specialty pediatrics. *J Pediatr Oncol Nurs* 26(1): 7-15.

Post-White, J., M. Fitzgerald, K.S. Savik, M.C. Hooke, A.B. Hannahan, and S.F. Sencer. 2009. Massage therapy for children with cancer. *J Pediatr Oncol Nurs* 26: 16-28.

Pruthi, S., A.C. Degnim, B.A. Bauer, R.W. DePompolo, and V. Nayar. 2009. Value of massage therapy for patients in a breast clinic. *Clin J Oncol Nurs* 13(4): 422-425.

Quattrin, R., A. Zanini, S. Buchini, D. Turello, M.A. Annunziata, C. Vidotti, A. Colombatti, and S. Brusaferro. 2006. Use of reflexology foot massage to reduce anxiety in hospitalized cancer patients in chemotherapy treatment: Methodology and outcomes. *J Nurs Manag* 14(2): 96-105.

Russell, N.C., S. Sumler, C.M. Beinhorn, and M.A Frenkel. 2008. Role of massage therapy in cancer care. *J Altern Complem Med* 14(2): 209-214.

Sagar, S.M., T. Dryden, and C. Myers. 2007. Research on therapeutic massage for cancer patients: Potential biologic mechanisms. *J Soc Integr Oncol* 5(4): 155-162.

Shin, Y.H., T.I. Kim, M.S. Shin, and H. Juon. 2004. Effect of acupressure on nausea and vomiting during chemotherapy cycle for Korean postoperative stomach cancer patients. *Cancer Nursing* 27(4): 267-274.

Smith, M.C., J. Kemp, L. Hemphill, and C.P. Vojir. 2002. Outcomes of therapeutic massage for hospitalized cancer patients. *J Nurs Scholarship* 34: 257-262.

Smith, M.C., T.E. Yamashita, L.L. Bryant, L. Hemphill, and J.S. Kutner. 2009. Providing massage therapy for people with advanced cancer: What to expect. *J Altern Complem Med* 15(4): 367-371.

Soden, K., K. Vincent, S. Craske, C. Lucas, and S. Ashley. 2004. A randomized controlled trial of aromatherapy massage in a hospice setting. *Palliat Med* 18(2): 87-92.

Stephenson, N.L., M. Swanson, J. Dalton, F.J. Keefe, and M. Engelke. 2007. Partner-delivered reflexology: Effects on cancer pain and anxiety. *Oncol Nurs Forum* 34(1): 127-132.

Stringer, J., R. Swindell, and M. Dennis. 2008. Massage in patients undergoing intensive chemotherapy reduces serum cortisol and prolactin. *Psych Oncol* 17: 1024-1031.

Sturgeon, M., R. Wetta-Hall, T. Hart, M. Good, and S. Dakhil. 2009. Effects of therapeutic massage on the quality of life among patients with breast cancer during treatment. *J Altern Complem Med* 15(4): 373-380.

Tsay, S., H. Chen, S. Chen, H. Lin, and K. Lin. 2008. Effects of reflexotherapy on acute postoperative pain and anxiety among patients with digestive cancer. *Cancer Nursing* 31(2): 109-115.

Underdown, A., J. Barlow, V. Chung, and S. Stewart-Brown. 2006. Massage intervention for promoting mental and physical health in infants aged under six months. *Cochrane Lib* 4: CD005038.

Van Cleve, L., E. Bossert, P. Beecroft, K. Adlard, O. Alvarez, and M.C. Savedra. 2004. The pain experience of children with leukemia during the first year after diagnosis. *Nurs Res* 53(1): 1-10.

Weinrich, S., and M. Weinrich. 1990. The effect of massage on pain in cancer patients. *Appl Nurs Res* 3: 140-145.

Wilkie, D.J., J. Kampbell, S. Cutdshall, H. Halabisky, H. Harmon, L.P. Johnson, L. Weinacht, and M. Rake-Marona. 2000. Effects of massage on pain intensity, analgesics, and quality of life in patients with cancer pain. *Hospice J* 15: 31-53.

Wikstrom, S., T. Gunnarsson, and C. Nordin. 2003. Tactile stimulus and neurohormonal response: A pilot study. *Int J Neurosci* 113: 787-793.

Wilkinson, S.M., S.B. Love, A.M. Westcombe, M.A. Gambles, C.C. Burgess, A. Cargill, T. Young, E.J. Maher, and A.J. Ramirez. 2007. Effectiveness of aromatherapy massage in the management of anxiety and depression in patients with cancer: A multicenter randomized controlled trial. *J Clin Oncol* 25(5): 532-539.

Wilkinson, S. M., K. Barnes, and L. Storey. 2008. Massage for symptom relief in patients with cancer: Systematic review. *J Adv Nurs* 63(5): 430-439.

Williams, A.F., A. Vadgama, P. Franks, and P.S. Mortimer. 2002. A randomized controlled crossover study of manual lymphatic drainage therapy in women with breast cancer-related lymphoedema. *Eur J Cancer Care* 11(4): 254-261.

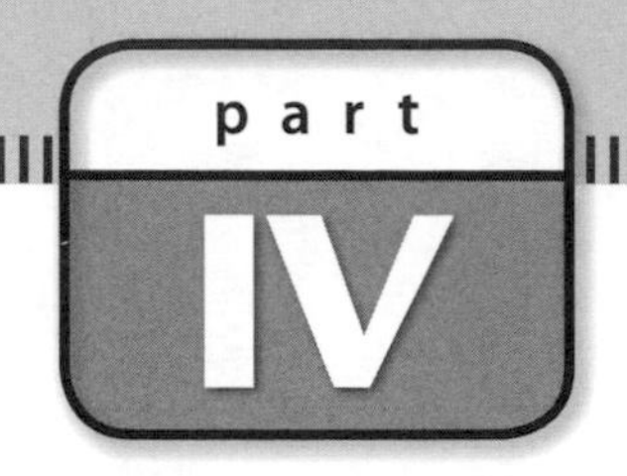

CONNECTING RESEARCH AND PRACTICE

How will research advance the profession of massage therapy? While chapters in the preceding section specifically illustrated how research and practice can be integrated in the treatment room, the chapters presented here show how the integration of research into the broader profession will lead to better, safer, and more effective practice.

chapter

18

Integrating Massage Therapy Research and Education

Trish Dryden, MEd, RMT

"In evidence informed care, research literacy is arguably as important as any other means of gathering patient related information, including, for example, case history taking and interpretation of physical examination findings. If this is indeed so, professional programs and schools should ensure that their curricula devote adequate attention to preparation of students with respect to research methods, the evaluation of evidence, and its application in the clinical setting. Ideally, this learning should not be compartmentalized. It should permeate the education of students in both didactic and clinical settings, and there are a number of approaches to curriculum design that emphasize the development of both an evidence informed orientation and skills related to research literacy."

(Finch 2007, 79)

With increasing numbers of people utilizing massage therapy (MT) for a variety of health issues, the profession must take increased responsibility to ensure public safety and improve health outcomes (Barnes, Bloom, and Nahin 2009; Esmail 2007). Preparing competent, ethical therapists, both before graduation and throughout their careers, is an inherent component of professional responsibility in the field of massage (NCCAM 2010; CMTO 2010). MT educators need to embrace this increased responsibility through research literacy and research capacity-building curricula, teacher education, and instructional delivery models that enhance evidence-informed skills for clinical decision making, and collaborative, client-centered practice. This chapter explores educational strategies that support increased safety and efficacy for clients, and encourages collaboration within and across disciplines. It concludes with a discussion of future directions in integrating MT research and education.

ENSURING SAFETY, BUILDING CAPACITY

As MT becomes more widely accepted, consumers, health care practitioners, government agencies, professional associations, and researchers are asking important questions about the safety and effectiveness of massage as a health care intervention. Furthermore, increased health insurance reimbursement for MT brings an increased requirement for accountability (Barnes, Bloom, and Nahin 2009; Esmail 2007; Millbank Memorial Fund 1998). Public and private stakeholders need to know which massage practices work best for clients in various circumstances. Clear and accurate information on the safety and effectiveness of MT must be generated through research and translated to practice in a variety of ways, including the development of guidelines for best practice (Grant et al. 2008). Underlying the concept of professional responsibility are assumptions about clinicians' educational preparation and capacity to assess and apply evidence to practice from a variety of sources, including research, clinical experience, and client preferences (Sackett et al. 1996).

Other health care providers also need clear and accurate information on the safety and effectiveness of massage therapy. Cohen and Kemper (2005) created a framework of questions for guiding pediatricians in making responsible, ethical, and legally defensible clinical decisions regarding the use of complementary and alternative medicine (CAM) for children. Their framework can be adapted and applied to diverse health care professionals to guide the use of MT for clients of all ages:

1. Will use of MT otherwise divert the client from necessary medical treatment?
2. Is the MT treatment selected known to be unsafe or ineffective?
3. Have the proper parties consented to the use of MT?
4. Is the risk–benefit ratio of the proposed MT treatment acceptable to a reasonable, similarly situated clinician? Does the MT treatment have at least minority acceptance or support in the medical literature?

Implicit in Cohen and Kemper's framework are key assumptions about the educational preparation of health professionals in ethical and legal professional responsibilities; research literacy, which is the ability to find, understand, critically assess and apply research evidence to practice, including the capacity to assess the relative risks and benefits of treatment from a biomedical perspective; and attitudes toward evidence-based practice (EBP), an approach to decision making in which the clinician uses the best evidence available, in consultation with the patient, to decide which course of action suits the patient best. While it can be argued that medical and nursing programs teach evidence-based practice (Straus et al. 2005) and increasingly offer varying levels of curricula in CAM (Verhoef and Brundin-Mather 2007; Lee et al. 2007), it is not known what specifically is taught about the safety and effectiveness of MT. However, equally little is known of what is taught in MT training programs about conventional health care, evidence-based practice, and MT research.

As several chapters in this book discuss, there is increasing evidence that MT is a safe and effective treatment for a variety of conditions and that it is an increasingly popular choice of treatment for many consumers. Many conventional health care practitioners have started referring patients to massage even if they know little about MT educational preparation, regulation, or research (Sherman et al. 2005; Verhoef and Page 1998). MT is also included as one of the modalities, along with chiropractic, naturopathic, and traditional Chinese medicine, that now constitute in aggregate form what is increasingly referred to as *integrative health care* (IHC), rather than complementary or alternative medicine (CAM) (Porcino and McDougall 2009; IRCIMH 2011). This interesting philosophical shift toward identifying MT as a component of an integrative health care system is ripe with both opportunity and challenge for the MT profession. What is not known is whether MT professionals are ready to embrace an integrated health care system that appears increasingly willing to include them as members.

Implications for the high levels of educational preparation and professional responsibility consistent with increased integration with conventional systems of health care are not universally embraced by the massage profession (Kelly et al. 2005). Diversity in values, regulation, and educational preparation in MT make it difficult to assess to what extent current educational practices in MT address research literacy, research capacity, and evidence-based practice curricula. Given the diversity of educational preparation of massage therapists, which vary widely in terms of time—U.S. programs range from 100 to 1,000 hours (averaging approximately 600 hours), Canadian programs are between 2,200 and 3,300 hours, and programs in some parts of Eastern Europe and China require a 4-year baccalaureate degree (American Massage Therapy Association 2010; Gowan-Moody and Baskwill 2005; NCCAM 2010)—it is hard to understand what the average massage therapist knows. To what extent do massage therapists have the skills needed to apply evidence to practice, communicate evidence-informed treatment plans with other health care professionals, or participate in integrated health care or research teams? If we accept the argument that research literacy and interprofessional communication represent a core of minimal entrance-to-practice requirements for an integrated health care system, are massage therapists ready and willing to participate? What steps are being taken, and which should be taken, to ensure and accelerate professional responsibility and readiness?

A national study on research literacy and capacity in Canadian CAM programs (Dryden et al. 2004) found that two-thirds of participants identified that their school offered research curricula within the academic program, although no common definition emerged for research course, *research literacy,* or *research capacity*. In addition, diverse teacher experience and training in both curriculum development and in research skills influenced a school's ability to address issues of research literacy and evidence-informed practice education. The concept of readiness across three domains—institutional, societal, and professional—emerged as means of predicting the existence of a research curriculum or a research program within a school, and, in some cases, across a discipline. It also provides a useful framework (table 18.1).

research literacy

▸ The combination of skills necessary to locate, read, understand, critically evaluate, and apply research evidence.

research capacity

▸ The combination of advanced skills, in addition to research literacy, necessary to actually conduct research.

Table 18.1 Readiness for Delivering and Developing Research Literacy Curricula in CAM Schools

Domain	Research curricula
Institutional readiness	• Perceived differences in fiscal resources for public vs. private educational institutions • Evaluation and research values embedded in the culture of the school • Financial stability • Salaried teachers and the provision of teacher training • Research literacy/capacity resources (libraries, designated librarians, computers, publication subscriptions, Internet and database access)
Societal readiness	• Legislative certification, regulation, or recognition • Accreditation of schools and availability of student bursaries • Primacy of the Western, evidence-based approach to health practice • Market driven trends: graduate employment rates, profitability, and competitiveness among schools • Student preferences: shorter, more affordable programs that are closer to home
Professional readiness	• Codes of ethics, standards of practice • Competency-based guidelines • Prerequisite educational level for entry to programs • Diversity of instructional design and delivery • Evidence of innovative learning models

Reprinted, by permission, from T. Dryden et al., 2004, *Research requirement: Literacy amongst complementary and alternative health care practitioners – phase I & phase II* (Ottawa, ON: Natural Health Products Directorate, Health Canada).

By using the framework to assess the institutional, societal, and professional readiness of a program or discipline to offer research education, many common gaps and needs were identified. Over the past decade, in recognition of the need for increased research literacy, research capacity, and interprofessional skills in the MT profession, leaders within the profession in both Canada and the United States have systematically promoted activities that accelerate the adoption of evidence-informed practice, including the following: development of research-literacy curricula (Dryden and Achilles 2003; Hymel 2003), increased numbers of research texts (Menard 2009; Andrade and Clifford 2008; Hymel 2006; Field 2006; Rich 2002), invitational research think tanks, research conferences, increased funding for research, annual competitions for student and practitioner case reports (Massage Therapy Foundation 2010a - 2010f), an open-access, peer-reviewed MT research journal (IJTMB 2010), online research networks (e.g., NZTMRC; IN-CAM; PedCAM; ISCMR; Massage Therapy Foundation), and increased support of sophisticated policy and advocacy work (IHPC; CAHCIM) for practice standards and regulation at local, national, and international levels (see chapter 1 for a historical overview). A further step planned for the field is the creation of evidence-informed, best-practice guidelines by an international and interdisciplinary committee (Grant et al. 2008).

BOX 18.1
Expected Outcomes of Best-Practice Guidelines

- Increased understanding by other stakeholders of massage and the profession of massage therapy.
- MTs will experience greater confidence and will take pride in their education, ethical practice, and professional quality of care.
- Heightened awareness of the complementary nature and integrative capacity of massage therapy for health care and wellness.
- Strengthened motivation and basis for referrals and payments to MTs as a result of clearer and more precisely defined measures of care.
- Recognition for a diversity of massage therapy approaches to client care within the global perspective of health care and wellness.
- Continued awareness of massage practitioners for providing safe and responsible care to their clients and patients.

Given the level of strategic activity, at least in North America, for promoting research, evidence-informed practice, and interprofessional communication, are MT programs keeping pace? Assessing the overall state of MT curricula is beyond the scope of this chapter. However, a review of best practices in teaching research literacy and EBP may help MT students, practitioners, and teachers assess their own experience and skills. It will also point to future directions.

TEACHING RESEARCH LITERACY AND EVIDENCE-BASED PRACTICE (EBP)

The skills needed for research literacy and EBP have been traditionally taught in medical education as stand-alone courses or workshops. However, knowledge was better retained or translated to practice when the learning was integrated into clinical settings rather than taught in traditional settings (Coomarasamy and Kahn 2004).

Early educational programs in MT research literacy also focused on stand-alone classes and workshops, principally on critical appraisal techniques, with no direct requirement to apply these skills directly in the clinical setting. In one of the first online research-literacy courses for massage therapists, learners showed significant gains in their knowledge of research-literacy skills and improved attitudes towards evidence-informed practice (Achilles and Dryden 2002). Little is known, however, concerning learners' long-term retention of that knowledge, application of the skills to practice, or increased use of EBP.

Among medical professions, studies on teaching that integrated EBP into clinical settings in real time, which includes asking answerable clinical questions or going online to find the evidence and applying it to immediate practice or treatment planning, support the usefulness of these kinds of interventions for improvements in skills, attitudes, and behavior. Stand-alone courses are equally effective for improving knowledge, but not skills, attitudes, and behavior (Coomarasamy and Kahn 2004). Clearly, it is important to integrate EBP teaching and research-literacy skills into clinical practice.

Consistent with best practices in adult learning, integrating EBP and research literacy into all aspects of MT programs increases the opportunity for real-world, real-time learning and the likelihood of behavioral change in practitioners. In addition, adult learning is best accomplished when it is facilitated through coaching and mentoring (Das, Malick, and Khan 2008). Since MT programs vary widely in terms of requirements for teacher training and supervised clinical work with clients, opportunities for MT students and practitioners to observe exemplary role models using EBP in the clinical setting and to practice the skills for themselves may be rare in many jurisdictions and schools.

In addition, skills acquisition in taking health histories, performing clinical assessments, planning treatments, keeping records, learning about pathophysiology, and assessing treatment outcomes all vary widely in MT programs. Without strong assessment skills and a working knowledge of pathophysiology, integrating EBP into training and practice is a challenge. In order to successfully incorporate real-time EBP activities into their lesson plans, teachers of science and clinical courses will need time and training, as well as access to online journals and databases, professional librarians, and computers in their classrooms, clinics, and labs. However, the ubiquity of smart phones and other personal data devices, along with wireless Internet access and growing numbers of digitally literate students (and one hopes, teachers), are likely to facilitate the incorporation of real-time EBP more easily and economically into diverse MT learning environments than in the past (Higher Ed Café 2010). In one innovative program, research-literacy skills are taught online through the use

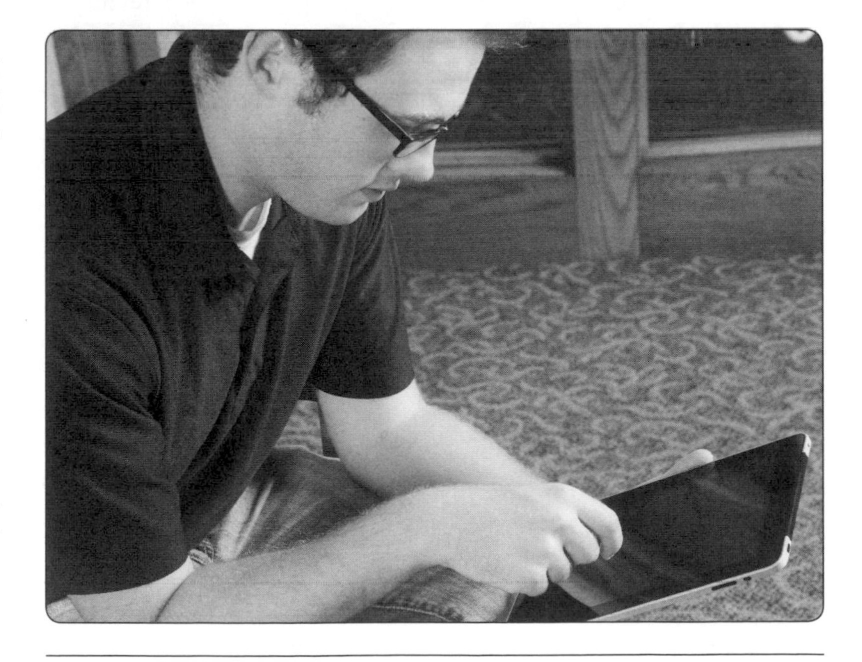

Smart phones and other personal data devices, like the iPad, are likely to facilitate the incorporation of real-time EBP more easily and economically into diverse MT learning environments.

of a graphic novel. Learners engage in didactic activities that are integrated components of a compelling and futuristic storyline (Atack et al. 2010). Gaming and online case simulation as instructional delivery methods for teaching research literacy and EBP need to be further developed in MT education and evaluated for effectiveness and learner satisfaction.

just in time

▸ Used to describe systems and procedures that deliver materials immediately as required.

Access to *just-in-time* online EBP modules for busy MT professionals will help accelerate the uptake of best evidence to practice (see chapter 20 for information on clinical case reports). The creation of easy-to-access pathways between MT programs and degree-granting postsecondary institutions will enable the cross-training of massage therapists in disciplines such as adult education, research methods, health administration, and specializations in diverse subject areas within the sciences and humanities. As noted earlier, it is anticipated that recent innovations will drive changes in the incorporation of EBP and research literacy at all levels. Utilization of electronic health records systems in MT, including the necessary creation of a coordinated system for reporting adverse events, would rapidly accelerate the kinds of information needed to develop best-practice guidelines and to answer key questions about client safety. To ensure their use by MT students and massage therapists in the field, both at the entry level and throughout their practices, educators, professional associations, and regulatory bodies need to mandate and evaluate competencies in research literacy and EBP through career-long learning and quality-assurance requirements.

More studies are needed to evaluate the effectiveness of EBP education in MT. Kirkpatrick's hierarchy is a useful tool that can be adapted to evaluating knowledge, attitudes, and behavior, and, ultimately, client outcomes in EBP (table 18.2).

Table 18.2 Evaluating EBP Educational Interventions—Adapting Kirkpatrick's Hierarchy

Taxonomy/hierarchy	Description and measurement
Participation or completion	Attendance at and views on the learning experience (e.g., course evaluation)
Modification of attitudes	Change in attitudes or perceptions toward EBP (e.g., subjective reaction, or satisfaction of participants with course, difference between pre- and postcourse attitude questionnaire)
Modification of knowledge or skills	Change in EBP knowledge or skills (e.g., difference in scores pre- and postcourse)
Massage therapists' behavior	Transfer of learning to the workplace or integration of new knowledge and skills leading to modification of behavior or performance (e.g., difference in performance after the teaching as shown by more evidence-informed treatment planning and communication with clients as noted in clinical records, in simulated clinical experiences, or in oral/practical examination)
Change in delivery of care and health outcomes	Changes in the delivery of care attributable to the educational intervention (e.g., client satisfaction questionnaires, practice audit showing compliance with EBP criteria in client health records)

Adapted, by permission, from S.M. Malick et al., 2010, "Is evidence based medicine teaching and learning directed at improving practice?" *Journal of The Royal Society of Medicine* 103: 231-238.

INTERPROFESSIONAL EDUCATION FOR AN INTEGRATED HEALTH CARE SYSTEM

Preparing students and professionals to more fully participate in an evidence-informed, integrated health care system and on diverse health care and research teams also requires changes in MT curricula and instructional methods. Interprofessional education (IPE) consists of occasions when two or more professionals learn from, with, and about each other (CAIPE 2002). Its purpose is to help professionals develop the skills necessary for collaborative, patient-centered practice (Oandasan and Reeves 2005; CIHC 2009).

As is the case for health professionals' education, massage therapists are traditionally educated within a professional silo that has little or no contact with other health disciplines. Any development of team skills or experience with interprofessional communication is largely delivered as theory in the classroom or practiced in the form of role play. It is not known to what extent MT educational programs are developing IPE curricula or teaching and evaluating interprofessional team skills. Given that the majority of massage therapists in the United States and Canada work as sole practitioners or in group practices where team coordination of client care is not an expectation of practice (American Massage Therapy Association 2010), IPE may be viewed as irrelevant to career success. In the near future, as increasing numbers of massage therapists find opportunities to work in group and integrated practices, sports clinics, hospitals and hospices, and elder care settings, such a view could be problematic. Interprofessional education will also prepare massage therapists to more fully participate on interdisciplinary research teams, which will promote the development of robust, clinically relevant research.

Innovative strategies in teaching and evaluating IPE at the undergraduate level include scheduling common classes and clinics with students from different disciplines to ensure that they learn with, from, and about each other. Effective evaluation strategies include the use of team clinical examinations, such as The Team Objective Structured Clinical Examination, in which interprofessional teams of six or seven students are tested in a simulated setting with a trained client. Together, they must create a collaborative, evidence-informed treatment plan (Marshall et al. 2009). Online education gaming and simulation also hold promise as creative and cost-effective ways of training diverse student health care professionals in interprofessional communication (Atack et al. 2009).

CONDUCTING RESEARCH IN MASSAGE THERAPY EDUCATIONAL INSTITUTIONS

Massage therapy schools with busy student clinics hold great potential for the advancement of MT research. Increasing participation in the student case report competition held by the Massage Therapy Foundation (MTF) is a case in point. Similarly, schools wanting to build research capacity can look to the Massage Therapy Research Consortium (MTRC) as an interesting model. The MTRC was created to advance massage therapy education and practice and to enhance public health by collaboratively building research capacity in several MT schools in North America and by fostering partnerships with research scientists. The Consortium acts as a network for participating schools, providing opportunities to learn, share experiences and expertise, and support the research endeavors of the schools. Recent research activities include a qualitative study of how clients of student clinics describe the effects of MT, a taxonomy of MT that facilitates a range of research-related functions, and a study of low back pain exploring two types of MT interventions that builds on the work of Cherkin and colleagues (2001), the outcomes of which have been recently published (Cherkin, Sherman, Kahn et al. 2011).

Research capacity in MT schools depends on many factors, including the level of embedded evaluation and research culture, financial stability, salaried teachers, teacher training, and access to research resources, such as computers, the Internet, and libraries (Dryden et al. 2004). It is also subject to market forces, such as profitability, graduate employment rate, competition among schools, and student preference for shorter, more affordable programs. For all these reasons, research-literacy education may be seen as nice to have but not essential, especially in tough economic times and when research-literacy competencies are not an important part of certification and licensure exams. Teaching research literacy and building research capacity requires investments in teacher training and infrastructure resources, as well as a belief in the value of evidence-informed practice for the future of the profession.

SUMMARY

This chapter explores educational strategies that support increased safety and efficacy for clients and encourage increased interprofessional collaboration. Educating competent, ethical therapists is an integral component of professional responsibility. This will increasingly require curricula that include research literacy and research capacity, improved teacher education, and instructional delivery that enhances evidence-informed, clinical–decision making skills and collaborative, client-centered practice. In the past 10 years, the MT field has made considerable headway in integrating research into education and clinical practice, but this trend needs to continue to ensure that the educational preparation of massage therapists will meet the needs of a rapidly changing and increasingly integrated health care system.

Critical Thinking Questions

1. Why are research-literacy skills fundamental to safe and effective clinical practice?
2. What are some of the most effective ways of teaching research literacy and evidence-based practice in educational settings? With undergraduates? With professionals?
3. Why is interprofessional education important to the development of the massage therapy profession?
4. In what ways can technology advance the education of health professionals in research literacy and evidence-based practice?

REFERENCES

Achilles, R., and T. Dryden. 2002. *Research literacy for complementary and alternative health care (CAHC) practitioners. Phases I & II final report.* Human Resources Development Canada, Office of Learning Technologies in the Workplace. www.hrsdc.gc.ca.

American Massage Therapy Association. 2010. Massage therapy industry fact sheet. www.massagetherapy.org/pdf/2010%20Massage%20Therapy%20Industry%20Fact%20Sheet%202010.pdf.

Andrade, C.K. and P. Clifford. 2008. *Outcome-based massage: From evidence to practice.* Philadelphia: Lippincott, Williams and Wilkins.

Atack, L., K. Parker, M. Rocchi, J. Maher, and T. Dryden. 2009. The impact of an online course in disaster management competency and attitude towards interprofessional learning. *J Interprof Care* 23(6): 586-598.

Atack, L., S. Shipwright, D. Mallory, and P. Demacio. 2010. Citizen researcher. In *Proceedings of world conference on educational multimedia, hypermedia and telecommunications 2010* (3264). www.editlib.org/p/35107.

Barnes, P.M., B. Bloom, and R.L. Nahin. 2009. Complementary and alternative medicine use among adults and children: United States, 2007. *Natl Health Stat Report* 12: 1-23.

CAIPE. 2002. Centre for the advancement of interprofessional education. www.caipe.org.uk/about-us/defining-ipe.

Canadian Interprofessional Health Collaborative (CIHC). 2009. The national interprofessional competency framework. www.cihc.ca/files/curricula/CIHCComp_OntarioRetreat_May2809.pdf.

Canadian Interdisciplinary Network for Complementary and Alternative Research (IN-CAM). www.incamresearch.ca/index.php?home&lng=en.

Cherkin, D.C., K.J. Sherman, J. Kahn, R. Wellman, A. Cook, E. Johnson, J. Erro, K. Delaney, and R.A. Deyo. 2011. "A comparison of the effects of 2 types of massage and usual care on chronic low back pain." *Ann of Intern Med* 155: 1-9.

Cherkin, D.C., D. Eisenberg, K.J. Sherman, W. Barlow, T.J. Kaptchuk, J. Street, and R.A. Deyo. 2001. Randomized trial comparing traditional Chinese medical acupuncture, therapeutic massage, and self-care education for chronic low back pain. *Arch Intern Med* 161(8): 1081-1088.

Cohen, M.H., and K.J. Kemper. 2005. Complementary therapies in pediatrics: A legal perspective. *Pediatrics* 115(3): 774-780.

College of Massage Therapists of Ontario (CMTO). 2010. Quality assurance programme. www.cmto.com/member/CEUNewGuide.htm.

Consortium of Academic Health Centres for Integrative Medicine (CAHCIM). www.ahc.umn.edu/cahcim/home.html.

Coomarasamy, A., and K.S. Kahn. 2004. What is the evidence that postgraduate teaching in evidence based medicine changes anything? A systematic review. *BMJ* 329: 1017.

Das, K., S. Malick, and K.S. Khan. 2008. Tips for teaching evidence-based medicine in the clinical setting: lessons from adult learning theory. Part I. *J R Soc Med* 101: 493-500.

Dryden, T., and R. Achilles. 2003. *Massage therapy research curriculum kit.* Evanston, IL: Massage Therapy Foundation.

Dryden, T., B. Findlay, H. Boon, S. Mior, M. Verhoef, and A. Baskwill. 2004. *Research requirement: Literacy amongst complementary and alternative health care practitioners—phase I & phase II.* Ottawa, ON: Health Canada. www.hc-sc.gc.ca/sr-sr/pubs/nhp/research_literacy-eng.php.

Esmail, N. 2007. Complementary and alternative medicine in Canada: Trends in use and public attitudes, 1997-2006. In *Public policy sources,* ed. K. McCahon. Vancouver, BC: Fraser Institute.

Field, T. 2006. *Massage therapy research.* Edinburgh: Churchill Livingstone.

Finch, P.M., 2007. The evidence funnel: Highlighting the importance of research literacy in the delivery of evidence informed complementary health care. *J Bodyw Mov Ther* 11: 78-81.

Gowan-Moody, D., and A. Baskwill. 2005. *Report on policy issues concerning the regulation of massage therapy in Canada.* The Federation of Massage Therapy Regulatory Authorities of Canada (FOMTRAC). www.saskmassagetherapy.com/doc/fomtracreport.pdf.

Grant, K.E., J. Balletto, D. Gowan-Moody, D. Healey, D. Kincaid, W. Lowe, and R. Travillian. 2008. Steps toward massage therapy guidelines: A first report to the profession. *Int J Ther Massage Bodywork* 1(1): 19-36.

Higher Ed Café. 2010. College students think smart phones r gr8! www.odassoc.com/higheredcafe/content/college-students-think-smart-phones-r-gr8.

Hymel, G.M. 2003. Advancing massage therapy research competencies: Dimensions for thought and action. *J Bodyw Mov Ther*7(3): 194-199.

———. 2006. Research methods for massage and holistic therapies. Edinburgh: Mosby.

IN-CAM outcomes database. www.outcomesdatabase.org.

International Journal of Therapeutic Massage and Bodywork: Research, Education, and Practice (IJTMB). 2010. www.ijtmb.org.

Integrative Health Care Policy Consortium (IHPC). http://ihpc.info.

International Research Congress on Integrative Medicine and Health (IRCIMH). 2010. www.imconsortium-congress2012.org.

International Society for Complementary Medicine Research (ISCMR). www.iscmr.org.

Kelly, M., K. Hardwick, S. Motitz, M.J. Kelner, B. Rickhi, and H. Quan. 2005. Towards integration: The opinions of health policy makers on complementary and alternative medicine. *Evid-Based Integr Med* 2(2): 79-86.

Lee, M.Y., R. Benn, L. Wimsatt, J. Cornman, J. Hedgecock, S. Gerik, J. Zeller, M.J. Kreitzer, P. Allweiss, C. Finklestein, and A. Haramati. 2007. Integrating complementary and alternative medicine instruction into health professions education: Organizational and instructional strategies. *Acad Med* 82(10): 939-945.

Malick, S.M., J. Hadley, J. Davis, and K.S. Khan. 2010. Is evidence based medicine teaching and learning directed at improving practice? *J R Soc Med* 103: 231-238.

Marshall, D., P. Solomon, M. Howard, A. Taniguchi, A. Boyle, K. Eva, P. Hall, L. Casimor, L. Weaver, and W. Jelly. 2009. The team objective structured clinical examination (TOSCE): Assessment tool of team and interprofessional competencies in primary care. www.cabhalifax2009.dal.ca/Files/Presentations_by_Sur/Marshall,_Denise_-_The_TOSCE_Workshop.pdf.

Massage Therapy Foundation. 2010a. Available grants. www.massagetherapyfoundation.org/AvailableGrants.html.

———. 2010b. Massage therapy research agenda. www.massagetherapyfoundation.org/massageagenda.html.

———. 2010c. Research conferences. www.massagetherapyfoundation.org/conferencesofinterest.html.

———. 2010d. Research database. www.massagetherapyfoundation.org/researchdb.html.

———. 2010e. Student case report contest. www.massagetherapyfoundation.org/contest.html.

———. 2010f. Practitioner case report contest. www.massagetherapyfoundation.org/PractitionerContest.html.

Massage Therapy Research Consortium. 2010. Participating schools. www.massagetherapyresearchconsortium.com/htm/schools.html.

Menard, M.B. 2009. *Making sense of research: A guide to research literacy for complementary and alternative therapists.* 2nd ed. Toronto, ON: Curties-Overzet.

Millbank Memorial Fund. 1998. Enhancing the accountability of alternative medicine. www.milbank.org/mraltmed.html.

National Centre for Complementary and Alternative Medicine (NCCAM). 2010. http://nccam.nih.gov/health/decisions/credentialing.htm.

New Zealand Massage Therapy Research Network (NZMTRN). http://nzmtrc.sit.ac.nz/

Oandasan, I., and S. Reeves. 2005. Key elements in interprofessional education. Part 1: The learner, the educator and the learning context. *Journal of Interprofessional Care* Supplement 1: 21-38.

Pediatric Complementary and Alternative Medicine Research and Education Network (PedCAM). www.pedcam.ca.

Porcino, A., and C. McDougall. 2009. The integrated taxonomy of health care: Classifying both complementary and biomedical practices using a uniform classification protocol. *Int J Ther Massage Bodywork* 2(3): 18-30.

Rich, G.J. 2002. *Massage therapy: The evidence for practice.* Edinburgh: Mosby.

Sackett, D.L., W.M. Rosenberg, J.A. Gray, R.B. Haynes, and W.S. Richardson. 1996. Evidence based medicine: What it is and what it isn't. *BMJ* 312: 71-72.

Sherman, K.J., D.C. Cherkin, J. Kahn, J. Errol, A. Hrbek, R.A. Deyo, and D.M. Eisenberg. 2005. A survey of training and practice patterns of massage therapists in two U.S. states. *BMC Complem Altern Med* 5: 13.

Straus, S.E., W.S. Richardson, P. Glasziou, and R.B. Haynes. 2005. *Evidence-based medicine: How to practice and teach EBM.* 3rd ed. Edinburgh: Churchill Livingstone.

The Interprofessional Care Strategic Implementation Committee (IPCSIC). 2010. Implementing interprofessional care in Ontario: Final report of the interprofessional care strategic implementation committee. www.healthforceontario.ca/upload/en/whatishfo/ipcproject/hfo%20ipcsic%20final%20reportengfinal.pdf.

Verhoef, M.J., and S.A. Page. 1998. Physicians' perspectives on massage therapy. *Can Fam Physician* 44: 1018-1024.

Verhoef, M.J., and R. Brundin-Mather. 2007. A national approach to teaching complementary and alternative medicine in Canadian medical schools: The CAM in UME project. *Proc West Pharmacol Soc* 50: 168-173.

Integrating Research in Clinical Practice

Janet R. Kahn, PhD, LMT

As many authors have noted, including several contributors to this book, the clinical research community is showing an unprecedented interest in therapeutic massage. Simultaneously, increased interest in research is being seen in massage therapy clinicians, educators, and clients. This chapter addresses why and how to responsibly use research in clinical practice. Along the way, it should help lay to rest some conversations that have distracted massage therapists and other related professionals from putting our best foot forward.

EVIDENCE-BASED PRACTICE VERSUS HUMANISTIC CLIENT CARE

In a world replete with false dichotomies, perhaps none has hurt the massage profession as much as the notion that science takes the heart right out of care. This concern has been expressed by many massage therapists over the years. In this view, the term evidence-based practice (EBP) conjures visions of a distant and dispassionate authority laying down the rules of practice, including what will and will not be compensated, which are based on research done by scientists who never meet massage clients. Many clinicians ask how someone who does not work with or know patients and who does not deal with the complexity of the therapy situation could possibly determine what is best. The often unspoken end of that argument is that since only massage therapists can know what their clients need, they shouldn't have to bother with the cold, hard, and detached evidence base, which cannot hold a candle to the warm, deep knowing that comes through their hands. This concern is not unique to massage therapists; it has also been articulated by a sister profession, nursing, where some have claimed that "the notion that we should or perhaps even could base our practice on 'generalizable evidence' demolishes our traditional practice. Such worldviews urge us to swap our ideas of crafting care around the unique complexity of the individual, for a generalization about what worked for most people in a study" (Barker 2000, 332).

Having been a practicing massage therapist for well over 30 years, I value this direct knowing, or *tacit knowledge,* as some have called it (Thornton 2006), which develops from years of experience. Yet arguments that put these two kinds of knowledge in competition do not serve massage therapists or their clients. The key is to look for synergy. The false aspect of the perceived dichotomy between

best research evidence

▸ The subset of clinically relevant research of the highest quality that can be used to improve practice.

clinical expertise

▸ The ability, acquired through training and experience, to accurately identify the health status of patients, along with the potential risks and benefits of appropriate interventions.

patient values

▸ The preferences, concerns, and expectations that are important to an individual patient in a clinical encounter.

EBP and direct knowing is that it corrupts the original notion of EBP. Sackett and colleagues (2000) offered a three-part structure for EBP, noting that "evidence-based medicine is the integration of best research evidence with clinical expertise and patient values." Best evidence is to be weighed with the practitioner's clinical expertise and each patient's values to determine the most appropriate course of treatment for that patient. This view of EBP takes nothing away from clinicians; rather, it requires that they learn to evaluate and bring evidence into the equation.

In addressing the medical profession, Sackett and others (1996) defined the three critical components of EBP. *Best research evidence* is clinically relevant research that can improve practice, including the potential to "invalidate previously accepted diagnostic tests and treatments and replace them with new ones that are . . . more accurate, more efficacious, and safer." *Clinical expertise* is the capacity "to use our clinical skills and past experience to identify each patient's unique health state and diagnosis, [and the] individual risks and benefits of potential interventions." Finally, *patient values* are "the unique preferences, concerns, and expectations each patient brings to a clinical encounter" (Sackett et al. 1996, 3). It remains for us to translate these criteria to the world of therapeutic massage.

WHAT IS BEST EVIDENCE?

Bringing the evidence of systematic investigation to bear on clinical care improves practice because it has been shown repeatedly that accumulated experience is not enough. Long experience, when unchecked by objective forms of evidence, can lead to stubborn habits and overconfidence. Too frequently, clinicians make inaccurate assessments of a client's condition and suboptimal choices about course of treatment (Gray 2002). Assessments and treatment are both shown to improve when aided by research (Paley 2006).

The relative value of research is often portrayed as a pyramid of publication types, resting on case reports at the bottom and moving upward through clinical trials, randomized controlled trials (RCTs), systematic reviews, and meta-analyses (Sackett et al. 1996). Some have argued that this represents too rigid a view, and that the value of evidence is more specific to the situation. Jonas (2001) proposed an *evidence house,* with rooms for different types of information and purposes from clinical care, to policymaking, to understanding mechanisms of action, and so forth. Finch (2007) proposed an *evidence funnel* with all types of qualitative and quantitative research, as well as untested theories and expert opinion. This funnel feeds nonhierarchically to the clinician, whose job is to identify what is most relevant and to combine this with client values and clinical expertise as stipulated by Sackett and colleagues 2000), ultimately rendering evidence-informed clinical care. How then shall clinicians become good relevance sorters? In the information age, this is surely one of the key skills that should be taught in massage schools (see chapter 18 for more information on integrating massage therapy research and education).

Yet relevance alone is insufficient. A critical goal in research design is to reduce the possibility of error, that is, the possibility that the results are inaccurate, or are attributable to a flaw in the study. Identifying and reducing error (its total elimination being impossible) is central to scientific method (Popper 1959; Mayo 1996). Best available evidence must have substantially reduced the probability of error.

ACCESSING AND USING RESEARCH TO HELP YOUR CLIENTS

In practice, literature is assessed to best serve a particular client. Acquiring the best available evidence can be a challenge in this field. In some cases, therapists may be unable to find any clinical research on massage for a particular condition. Nevertheless, to explore recommended search methods, let us start with a common problem for which massage research literature does exist: chronic back pain.

The Case of Mario

Mario, a 54-year-old man, presents with annoying but nondebilitating low back pain of 10- to 12-months duration that is unrelated to any injury or event that he can recollect. The low back pain is accompanied by intermittent mild sciatic pain. His physician has prescribed pain medication, which alleviates the pain for a short time only. A relative suggested that Mario try massage, and so he has come to massage therapist Quinn's office. Given Quinn's training, mindful presence, and skill level, Mario is likely to get a good massage. Further, Quinn has treated many people with back pain successfully, based on the feedback she has received from clients. Given her experience, she is inclined to do for Mario what she usually does: an assessment-based, tailored combination of Swedish, myofascial, and neuromuscular techniques, plus a demonstration of stretches for the piriformis and exercises to strengthen the abdominal muscles. This will be followed by the recommendation of weekly hour-long sessions over 4 weeks, with reassessment and a likely reduction to twice-monthly treatments for 2 months.

Search Strategies

What might best available evidence add to this picture? The first step is to articulate what therapists want to know. This will guide their search. Quinn's question is "What is the best kind of massage for chronic low back pain?" By beginning her search at the top of the pyramid, Quinn has the potential to locate systematic reviews. High-quality systematic reviews save time because experts have already identified, evaluated, and synthesized all relevant studies, according to clearly stated criteria, that address the topic. One of the best sources for such reviews is the database of the Cochrane Collaboration (www.cochrane.org/cochrane-reviews). To the good fortune of the massage profession, this database has a branch for complementary and alternative medicine (CAM). Beginning here, Quinn can wait to search for individual RCTs or other forms of research until after she has examined any systematic reviews. At that point, she may want to address more specific aspects of her central question that still remain unanswered.

In the search field on the Cochrane Collaboration webpage, Quinn types "massage AND back pain." She capitalizes the word *and* because a rule of database-search technique is that the words *and, or,* and *not* should only be used to show relationships between other words or phrases in the search. Therefore, they must be written in capital letters to indicate their role to the computer. These relational words are called *Boolean terminology* after George Boole, the 19th-century mathematician and logician. The words function just as you would suppose. In the present case, *and* narrows the search to show only those results that relate to both massage and back pain.

Boolean terminology

▸ The relational words *and, or,* and *not,* which can be used to manage the results that are obtained from a database search.

In response to the terms "massage AND acupuncture," Quinn finds a 2009 review by Furlan and colleagues (2009). Examination of the abstract is informative. A systematic review must report the criteria for the search, the databases that were searched (in this case, MEDLINE, EMBASE, and CINAHL, from their beginning to May 2008, and the Cochrane Central Register of Controlled Trials, HealthSTAR, and dissertation abstracts up to 2006), the number of qualifying clinical trials found (13 randomized trials with a total of 1,596 participants), the authors' assessment of the quality of the studies (8 had high risk of bias and 5 had a low risk), and their findings: "Massage was more likely to work when combined with exercises [usually stretching] and education. The amount of benefit was more than that achieved by joint mobilization, relaxation, physical therapy, self-care education, or acupuncture. It seems that acupressure or pressure point massage techniques provide more relief than classic (Swedish) massage, although more research is needed to confirm this."

Abstracts typically also include information about any adverse events resulting from massage in these trials. In this case, no serious adverse events occurred, but some participants reported posttreatment soreness and allergic responses to massage oils. Systematic reviews finish with a summary statement. In this case, it states "in summary, massage might be beneficial for patients with subacute (lasting 4 to 12 weeks) and chronic (lasting longer than 12 weeks) nonspecific low back pain, especially when combined with exercises and education" (1).

Quinn now considers how to use this information. Perhaps she will add exercise recommendations to her approach with Mario even beyond the abdominal strengthening. Perhaps she will feel increased confidence in her planned treatment. To further her search, Quinn might look at the types of massage used in the studies rated as good. She could also explore other reviews. Synopses of related reviews appeared in response to her original query of "massage AND back pain." One, for instance, explored use of superficial heat or cold for low back pain, which could apply to Quinn's work with Mario. Also, since the first systematic review had summarized RCTs published by 2008, Quinn might see if some more recent trials are available.

Databases

A number of databases that have somewhat different purposes and strengths may interest massage therapists. In addition to PubMed, covered in the following section, other useful databases include the Cumulative Index to Nursing and Allied Health Literature (CINAHL at www.ebscohost.com/cinahl); EmBase (www.embase.com), a comprehensive medical and pharmacological database with indexed records from more than 7,000 peer-reviewed journals; and SportDiscus (www.sirc.ca/products/sportdiscus.cfm).

PubMed (www.pubmed.gov), the world's preeminent source of health sciences literature, is at everyone's fingertips through the Internet. PubMed includes MEDLINE, a database containing over nine million references from peer-reviewed journals. Although maintained by the U.S. National Library of Medicine (NLM), MEDLINE contains journals of quality from around the world. PubMed also includes citations to some journals not indexed by MEDLINE, and provides links to the increasing number of full-text articles being provided by publishers. Although MEDLINE's indexed journals only go back to the mid-1960s, a recent PubMed search for literature by Cyriax produced citations going back to 1945 for author James Cyriax and to 1917 for author E.F. Cyriax.

The Massage Therapy Foundation maintains a research database (www.massagetherapyfoundation.org/researchdb.html). Importantly, this database includes citations to journals not indexed in MEDLINE. Some are peer-reviewed (e.g., *Journal of Soft Tissue Manipulation*) and some are not (e.g., *Massage and Bodywork, Massage Magazine, Massage Therapy Journal*). You can also access PubMed from the Massage Therapy Foundation's website.

Back to Massage Therapist Quinn

Quinn is still looking for literature to inform her treatment of Mario's back pain. More specifically, she wants to determine if studies of massage for chronic back pain have been published since 2008, the cutoff date in the Cochrane Review. Quinn goes to PubMed and limits her search. An unlimited search for "massage AND chronic low back pain" yields 68 citations. However, by instructing PubMed to limit the results to clinical trials, meta-analyses, practice guidelines, randomized controlled trials, and reviews, Quinn reduces the yield to 42 citations. If she further limits this to publications from January 1, 2009 onward, the search yields three relevant studies, including one (Thompson et al. 2009) that is directly available in full-text format.

Designing an effective search involves both science and art. PubMed itself provides helpful tutorials that can be accessed in the left-hand column on the website's homepage. Therapists can find a virtual cornucopia of information on everything from learning which terms to use in their search (MeSH, or medical subject headings, are the NLM's controlled vocabulary used for indexing literature) to how to store their searches on the site's server or download them. In addition, a helpful article by Beatriz Vincent and colleagues (2006) is retrievable online at www.TheOncologist.com/cgi/content/full/11/3/243.

A Third Criterion

As an experienced and competent therapist, Quinn likely brings at least a minimal level of clinical expertise to the pursuit of evidence-influenced practice. Having searched the literature and found both a systematic review of massage for chronic back pain and a recent RCT, Quinn's final step is to decide whether this evidence applies to Mario (or to her other clients with chronic back pain). Why would it not apply? Straus and Sackett write that "rather than demanding that our patient meet all the inclusion criteria of the study under consideration, it is suggested that we ask if our patient is so different from those included in the study that its results cannot be applied to him." (1999, 29) In the case of Mario, Quinn considers whether the duration of chronicity was decidedly different from the study participants, or whether sciatica had been an exclusion criterion for the studies, since these things might influence treatment response. Yet, such differences between particular clients and a study population can simply become a consideration in therapists' valuation of the evidence to their situation, not necessarily a reason to completely reject it.

If Quinn decides that Mario is similar enough to the subjects in the study for the evidence to be relevant, it does not mean she must now perform the precise protocol from the study. This is because the next question asked in EBP is whether the treatment described in the evidence is feasible for Mario. Perhaps it involves coming for treatment twice per week. Is he willing and able to do this? If it involves an exercise regimen, is he willing and able to carry one out? Feasibility and likelihood of compliance are critical issues that must be considered. A regimen that is not or cannot be followed does not constitute an improvement in care. Thus, Quinn needs to explore these issues with Mario, along with any others that may help assess the fit between his values and the proposed protocol. Finally, Quinn must also consider whether there would be any increased risk for Mario in following a new protocol based on the findings of her search.

COMPARATIVE RESEARCH

Although this chapter examines the ways that systematic reviews and RCTs can be used to improve practice, additional types of research that may be helpful are coming to the world of massage. The systematic review Quinn found gave recommendations that she could compare with her practices, but assessing that comparison was left to her clinical judgment. That situation holds potential for bias, since it is likely that Quinn, like so many of us, has a more vivid recall of her successes than of treatments that did not prove useful.

Additional forms of comparative research could help massage therapists develop more evidence-informed practices. These include comparative-effectiveness research (CER) within and between disciplines, as well as dose-response research. CER refers to studies that make direct comparisons between different treatment approaches to the same condition. The recent increase in interest and funding for CER is a promising sign, and many are hopeful that CAM treatments will be compared with those of conventional medicine.

An example of a treatment comparison pertinent to the massage profession is a large-scale comparison of three different treatments for chronic low back pain. Cherkin and colleagues (2001) randomized 262 participants to receive acupuncture, massage therapy, or self-care education, and followed up to assess their progress at 4-, 10-, and 52-week intervals. At the 10-week interval, massage therapy was significantly outperforming both acupuncture and self-care education in the reduction of bothersome symptoms. It was also outperforming acupuncture for reduction of disability. Massage therapy continued to outperform acupuncture, but not self-care education, in both of those domains at the 52-week interval (figure 19.1). Further, participants in the massage therapy group used the fewest medications and had the lowest costs for subsequent care. Quinn will need to decide whether, and how, data from that study should influence her practice.

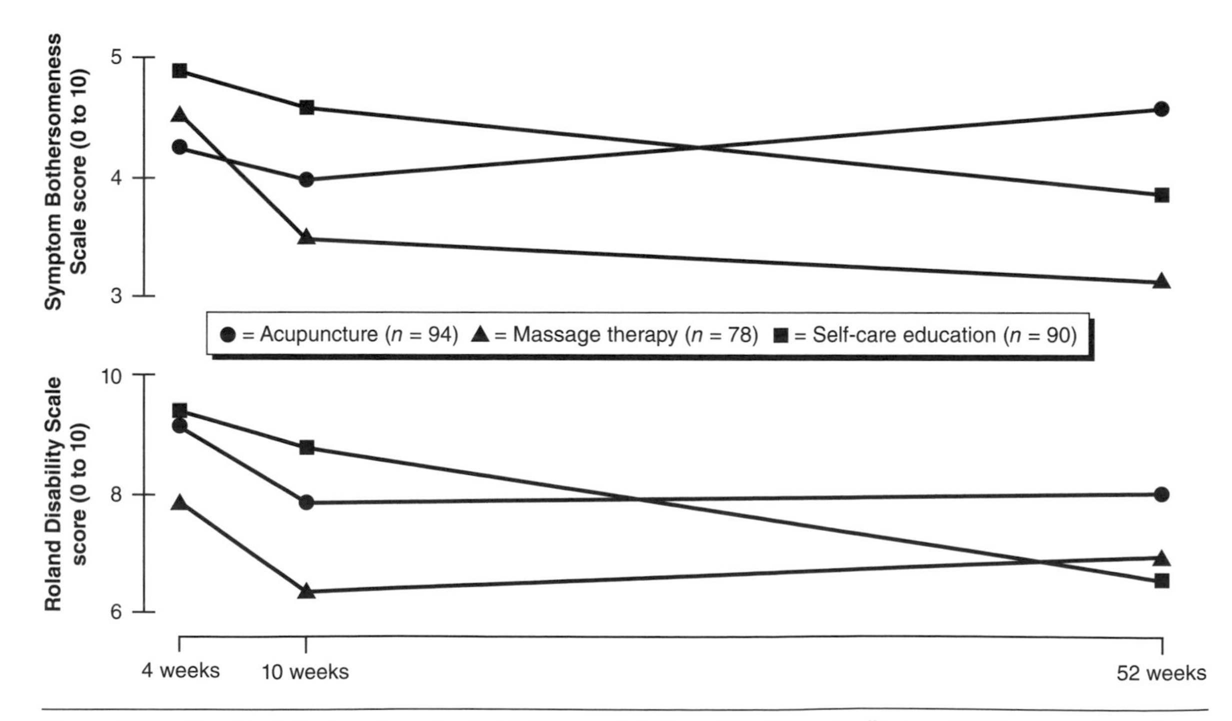

Figure 19.1 Graphical display of unadjusted follow-up data from Cherkin and colleagues' 2001 comparison of acupuncture, massage therapy, and self-care education for chronic low back pain.

Dose-response studies are standard in pharmaceutical research but are new to massage. The goals are to find a minimal dose that yields an effect and an optimal dose for maximum effect with minimal side effects. Recall that Quinn's pattern was to see clients weekly for 4 weeks, then biweekly for another 8 weeks. Based on her clinical expertise, she felt this was a good pattern. Yet, her clinical experience cannot be scientific evidence unless she keeps standardized records of treatment that related frequency and duration of sessions to outcomes. Dose-response studies have the potential to improve the practice of massage by answering a very important question about treatment patterns: whether frequency and duration of treatment influence outcome, and if so, in what patterns.

RECOMMENDATIONS FOR MASSAGE THERAPISTS

Communication between massage therapists and researchers, through direct conversation as well as through the literature itself, is increasing. Massage therapists can take steps to further this communication. Therapists must weave research awareness and the kind of critical thinking it promotes into their everyday lives. MT schools must address this matter in training the next generation of practitioners. For massage therapists already in practice, many possibilities exist, beginning with the increased access to online and in-person courses in research literacy.

Forging Partnerships

Translational research has typically referred to information flowing from the laboratory or clinical trial site to the bedside, or in this case, the massage table. In fact, information needs to flow in both directions. It has been a legitimate critique of much massage research that the treatments tested bore little relationship to what many clinicians actually do. This makes it too easy for massage therapists to read a study and disregard it, thinking "of course that didn't work; that is not what I do with my clients." This reinforces the tendency to favor presumed clinical expertise over evidence.

The goal of massage therapists must be to seek the heightened quality of care that can come when the best available evidence is paired with clinical expertise and patient values. Yet the best available evidence should also be the best possible evidence. It must include the design of research protocols reflecting typical care and best care, so that the data yielded are highly relevant to practice. The information that comes from clinical expertise must flow from the treatment room to the research institute, informing study design. It can also flow in human form. Indeed, more massage therapists are being brought into the research process to provide expert consultation on protocol design, learning themselves how research is conducted in the process. It can flow in written form, as more massage therapists publish case reports (see chapter 20) and opinion pieces that help the clinical and research communities improve MT research design. Most importantly, as research increasingly reflects current clinical practice, it will yield evidence that clinicians readily recognize as relevant to their professional development and their clients' well-being.

SUMMARY

This chapter explores the false dichotomy that is currently encountered often in the MT profession—specifically, that evidence-based practice (rooted in science), and the ways that practitioners understand their patients and practice through experience (more of an art) are fundamentally incompatible. Sackett's broader concept of evidence-based practice correctly views these important sources of information as compatible, integrating the best research evidence with clinical expertise and patient values to optimize care.

Critical Thinking Questions

1. How does Sackett's definition of EBP address the false dichotomy between evidence-based practice and practitioners' tacit knowledge?
2. What is meant by *best evidence?*
3. How is designing an effective search for best evidence both a science and an art?
4. How can comparative research help massage therapists develop more evidence-informed practices?
5. What is *translational research,* and why is it necessary?

REFERENCES

Barker, P. 2000. Reflections on caring as a virtue ethic within an evidence-based culture. *Int J Nurs Stud* 37: 329-336.

Cherkin, D., D. Eisenberg, K.J. Sherman, W. Barlow, T.J. Kaptchuk, J. Street, and R.A. Deyo. 2001. Randomized trial comparing traditional Chinese medical acupuncture, therapeutic massage, and self-care education for chronic low back pain. *Arch Intern Med* 161: 1081-1088.

Cherkin , D.C., K. Sherman, J. Kahn, J. Erro, K. Delaney, A. Cook, and R. Deyo. 2009. A randomized trial comparing relaxation massage, focused structural massage, and usual care for chronic low back pain. *Altern Ther Health Med* 15 (3): S99-S100.

Chou R., A. Qaseem, V. Snow, D. Casey, J.T. Cross Jr., P. Shekelle, and D.K. Owens. 2007. Diagnosis and treatment of low back pain: A joint clinical practice guideline from the American College of Physicians and the American Pain Society. *Ann Intern Med* 147: 478-491.

Finch, P. M. 2007. "The evidence funnel: Highlighting the importance of research literacy in the delivery of evidence informed complementary health care." *J Bodywork Mov Ther* 11(1): 78-81.

Furlan, A.D., M. Imamura, T. Dryden, and E. Irvin. 2009. Massage for low-back pain. *Spine* 34: 1669-1684.

Gray, G.E. 2002. Evidence-based medicine: An introduction for psychiatrists. *J Psychiatr Pract* c(1): 5-13.

Jonas, W.B. 2001. The evidence house: How to build an inclusive base for complementary medicine. *Western J Med* 175(2): 79-80.

Mayo, D.G. 1996. *Error and the growth of experimental knowledge*. Chicago: University of Chicago Press.

Paley, J. 2006. Evidence and expertise. *Nurs Inq* 13(2): 82-93.

Popper, K. 1959. *The logic of scientific discovery*. London: Hutchinson.

Sackett, D.L., W.M.C. Rosenberg, J.A.M. Gray, R.B. Haynes, and W.S. Richardson.1996. Evidence-based medicine: What it is and what it isn't. *Brit Med J* 312: 71-72.

Sackett, D.L., S.E. Straus, W.S. Richardson, W. Rosenberg, and R.B. Haynes. 2000. *Evidence-based medicine: How to practice and teach EBM.* Edinburgh: Churchill Livingstone.

Straus, S.E. and D.L. Sackett. 1999. Review on evidence-based cancer medicine: Applying evidence to the individual patient. *Ann Oncol* 10: 29-32.

Thompson, J.M., R. Chiasson, P. Loisel, L.C. Besemann, and T. Pranger. 2009. A sailor's pain: Veterans' musculoskeletal disorders, chronic pain, and disability. *Can Fam Physician* 55(11): 1085-1088.

Thornton, T. 2006. Tacit knowledge as the unifying factor in evidence-based medicine and clinical judgement. *Philos Ethics Humanit Med* 1: 2.

Vincent, B., M. Vincent, and C.G. Ferreira. 2006. Making pubmed searching simple: Learning to retrieve medical literature through interactive problem solving. *Oncologist* 11: 243-251.

chapter

20

Clinical Case Reports

Michael D. Hamm, LMP, CCST

At once the most humble and specific of all methods of research, the clinical case report (CR) has great potential to transform the practice of massage therapy (MT) (Chaitow 2006). Reading and writing CRs helps practitioners and student massage therapists improve professional communication and client care. This chapter presents an overview of CRs, including their value for improving clinical practice and contributing to the ongoing development of a rich and diverse body of research in MT.

THE VALUE OF CASE REPORTS

> Always note and record the unusual . . . Publish it.
>
> Place it on permanent record as a short, concise note.
>
> Such communications are always of value.
>
> *Sir William Osler (Wright and Kouroukis 2000, 429)*

Although MT research is still in its infancy, there has been dramatic growth in recent years (Moyer, Dryden, and Shipwright 2009), primarily in the form of clinical trials and descriptive studies. However, the number of published CRs conducted by massage therapists is still very small. All are recent, and all examine the use of MT for specific conditions. Finch and colleagues (2007) measured changes in pedal plantar pressure in a client with diabetic neuropathy. Eisensmith (2007) used MT to relieve the symptoms of temporomandibular dysfunction, and Zalta (2008) focused on treating patellofemoral pain syndrome following surgical reconstruction of the anterior cruciate ligament (ACL). Hamm (2006) investigated MT for the concurrent treatment of scoliosis, costovertebral dysfunction, and thoracic outlet syndrome, and LeMoon (2008) used the case of an undiagnosed lumbar-disc herniation to examine her own clinical reasoning process. Most recently, Chunco (2011) explored the effects of massage on pain, stiffness, and fatigue associated with ankylosing spondylitis.

CRs such as these are valuable in several ways (figure 20.1). Obviously, each is an initial exploration of whether massage therapy may benefit a particular condition, which can set the stage for further research. CRs also maximize *ecological validity* in that they represent treatment as it is conducted in real life, as opposed to the more artificial conditions that are usually imposed in a larger scale study. In addition, CRs develop critical thinking and research skills in the practitioners who undertake them. They also elevate the profession by adding to the evidence base, demonstrating that the profession is

ecological validity

▸ The extent to which the details of a research study resemble the way an intervention is conducted in real life.

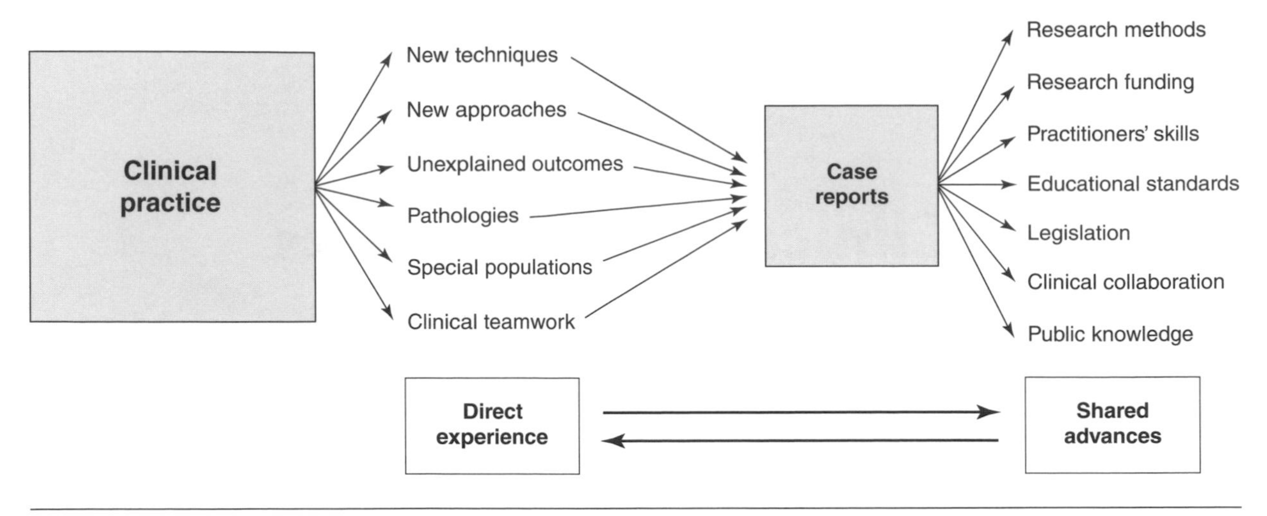

Figure 20.1 The ideal mechanism for case reporting.

capable of critical self-examination and making the results available to all health and wellness professions.

Given these valuable benefits, why have there been so few CRs? While practical obstacles can exist, such as a shortage of time or lack of access to resources for completing research, as well as systemic disadvantages in the form of limited research literacy and training within the profession (Menard 2003), the essential obstacle is a MT culture that is unaccustomed to scientific discourse. Students and practicing therapists may perceive science as dismissive of clinical intuition and artistic sensibility, and they may feel intimidated by the process of writing for publication (Hamm 2010). This must change. Massage therapists need to generate high-quality CRs with far greater frequency, which will help the broader research and health care communities gain an accurate understanding of MT.

An especially exciting development is the establishment of two separate annual case report competitions sponsored by the Massage Therapy Foundation. Full details on their student case report competition and practitioner case report competition are available on the foundation's website (www.massagetherapyfoundation.org).

WHAT IS A CASE REPORT?

A CR is a standardized format that clinicians in any health care field can use when reporting interesting and clinically relevant phenomena to their peers. This can include unexpected outcomes, unforeseen difficulties, safety issues, and new techniques. Once published in an academic or trade journal, CRs are read by researchers seeking information and ideas to incorporate into their own studies; teachers, students, and fellow clinicians in pursuit of the latest clinical knowledge; and members of the public acquiring information about treatment for their own or a loved one's condition. A well-conducted CR can provide rich and specific information, generate new hypotheses for research, call established theory into question, draw awareness to rare cases, and describe the clinical–decision making process in detail.

Given the sometimes insular nature of many MT practices, most massage therapists seeking to advance their skills have relatively few opportunities to gain insight about how their colleagues practice. A CR provides this otherwise rare opportunity, which may be its greatest benefit. In addition, the research literature reviewed in a CR provides unique and up-to-date information on the relevant condition, population, or treatment. It also allows the reader to visualize the clinical setting, the methods employed, and the process by which clinical decisions were made. Other reasons for regularly reading CRs include the following:

- Learning new strategies for working with specific conditions.
- Increasing awareness of how MT can interact with drugs or other therapies.
- Enhancing knowledge of specific MT techniques.
- Gaining familiarity with a range of assessment methods.
- Improving skills in clinical decision making.

Similarly, the process of writing and submitting a CR for publication can potentially bring rewards to the massage therapist in the form of career advancement, collaboration with other health professionals, and improved clinical decision making.

PREPARING A CASE REPORT

Case reports can be completed *prospectively,* meaning they are planned in advance of treatment delivery, or *retrospectively,* when they are based on chart notes and related data for treatment that has been completed. A prospective CR allows the clinician to tailor the study's design to the subject at hand. This can be quite advantageous; for example, the clinician can build in baseline and follow-up periods that have the potential to best illustrate the effectiveness of the treatments under investigation.

The following suggestions are offered to help make CR preparation more efficient and complete.

prospectively

▸ Done in accordance with or in expectation of the future; a case report completed prospectively is planned and started before clinical data have been collected.

retrospectively

▸ Done in accordance with the past; a case report completed retrospectively is undertaken after clinical data have been collected.

Finding a Case

A good CR begins with a compelling case. This may involve identification of a specific condition or population that you wish to address in a CR. Consulting with colleagues, clients, or mentors to learn about specific opportunities for access to the condition or population can be useful. However, most clinicians already have interesting cases worthy of a CR among their existing clients. Whichever approach turns out to be most appropriate for your specific interests and circumstances, be sure to select a case has the potential to be clinically interesting, both for you and for other members of the profession. Just as important, be sure that the client you invite to be a CR participant is someone who is reliable enough keep appointments and follow treatment guidelines. Perfect reliability is not necessary, since CRs take place in and are meant to reflect the real world, but a highly unreliable participant will prevent the CR from having the structure necessary to provide interesting and useful information.

Asking a Good Question

A well-crafted research question is the key to an effective study (Cassidy 2002). The research question often begins with curiosity on the part of the author, and is refined through preliminary research and reflection. Key points to keep in mind are that the CR needs to be grounded in the existing literature, representative of real-life practice, and specific enough to be described and quantified.

When forming a research question, consider its scope. A question such as "Does MT work for fibromyalgia?" is too broad to be effectively addressed by a case study. It does not specify what type of MT is being applied, which symptoms of fibromyalgia are being examined, or what *work* means in this context. Questions for CRs need to be clear and specific (Ernst 2002).

To create an appropriate research question, start with a brief literature search on your topic. A literature search applied to our example would reveal that depression and fibromyalgia are comorbid; that is, they frequently present simultaneously. The literature would also reveal that relaxation and Swedish forms of MT have been shown to reduce depression and improve quality of life in persons with fibromyalgia. Based on these findings, a more refined research question for a CR might ask "Does Swedish relaxation massage reduce depressive symptoms in a client with fibromyalgia?"

Designing a Treatment Series

A CR can chronicle a single session or can span an extended series of treatments. Similarly, it can focus on a single modality for treatment or on a combination of treatments. Regardless of session length and frequency, it is helpful to have a baseline measurement period prior to treatment and a posttreatment measurement period. However, logically, this may only be feasible when conducting a prospective study. The client who is the subject of the CR should be asked not to make major lifestyle changes during the study, such as starting new medications or physical activities, unless medically necessary. Minimizing such changes, when possible, strengthens the potential of the CR to reach more definitive conclusions concerning the effects of treatment. However, we must also recognize and accept that CRs document treatment that takes place in the real world, and not in the sterile, controlled conditions of the laboratory.

Collecting Data

The process of collecting data need not be complicated. Consider which quantitative and qualitative measures would be both *feasible* and *relevant*. Much of the most important data are already collected by massage therapists as part of ordinary practice, including chart notes, impressions gathered from palpation, and clients' feedback. Nevertheless, it may also be helpful to formalize some assessments by means of surveys or other instruments; table 20.1 offers some suggestions. Assistance from other healthcare professionals, who can lend their expertise, equipment, or facilities, can also be very useful in assisting the process of data collection. Be prepared to include both quantitative assessments and qualitative observations.

feasible

▸ Able to be accomplished or achieved.

relevant

▸ Connected, appropriate, or salient to a given topic.

Enlisting Peers and Trusting Common Sense

Before proceeding with treatment, consider seeking a review of your plan from a trusted colleague. Does the study design make sense to them? Is the description of methods clear enough that they could carry out a similar study? Do they have additional ideas for research literature that should be consulted or clinical procedures that should be implemented? Hearing their input early in the process can save time and effort and can result in a higher quality CR. Finally, common sense is important; if a report is careful, thoughtful, and compelling, it is likely to be valuable (McCarthy and Reilly 2000).

Table 20.1 Possibilities for Measurement

Type of measure	Examples
Functionality	• Tracking a standardized exercise regimen (e.g., changes in weight, reps, range of motion [ROM], walking speed) • Muscle testing, dexterity testing • Gait assessment
Pain	• Visual analog scale: (e.g., no pain to unbearable pain) • Descriptive pain scale (e.g., mild, moderate, or severe?) • Numerical pain scale (e.g., 1 to 10) • Recording onset time or duration of pain during some regular activity (e.g., typing at a keyboard)
Sleep	• Hours per night? • Number of times woken up? • Quality of sleep (e.g., poor to excellent)
Visual/palpatory assessment	• Position of bony landmarks (estimated or measured with precise tools) • Visual or palpatory observation of tissue quality • Cataloging locations of trigger points • Assessment of joint ROM (estimated or measured with precise tools)
Imaging	• Photographs • X-rays, MRIs, CT scans
Qualitative questionnaires	• Ask about client's desires or expectations ("What do you hope to get out of this?") • Ask about mood or motivation ("How is your mood today?") • Ask about perceived effectiveness ("Do you think this is helping?")
Standardized outcomes/ measures (Kania et al. 2009)	• IN-CAM Outcomes Database • Patient-Reported Outcomes Measurement Information System (PROMIS) • Patient-Reported Outcome and Quality-of-Life Instruments Database (PROQOLID)

TELLING A STORY: THE CONTENT OF A CASE REPORT

Writing a CR can seem daunting. What background information is necessary? How detailed should the methods section be? What kind of language is best? These questions are easier to answer when you have a clear understanding of the likely audience for your CR. Imagine describing a massage treatment to healthcare professionals, such as nurses or physicians. They are not trained in MT, but they are familiar with anatomy, physiology, and client care. Consider the details they would want and need to know to best understand the case, and be sure to include them.

Keep in mind that a CR is similar to a conversation; essentially, it is a structured form of storytelling (see table 20.2). Set out to command attention, use clear language, and earn the audience's trust and interest.

Table 20.2 Science as Conversation

Structure	Conversation goal	Content
Abstract	"Here's why you should hear me out."	• Quick overview of background, methods, results, and conclusion • Keywords (for database searching)
Introduction	"Here's what you need to know first."	• Setting the plot: Why is this intriguing? • Balanced, relevant literature review • Why and how is massage expected to help? • Rationale for treatment/assessment choices
Methods	"Here's what I decided to do."	• Careful, comprehensive client profile • Detailed description of treatment plan, including modalities, assessments, and session frequency and timing.
Results	"Here's what happened."	• Narrative summary of treatment sessions: What changes occurred? Was the treatment plan altered? Why? • Organized display of assessment results • No raw data, no interpretation
Discussion	"Here's what I think it means, and where we should go from here."	• Connect results back to introduction • Speculate on why the treatment worked (or didn't work) • Implications for massage profession? • Ideas for future studies?
References	"Here's why you should trust me."	• Keep track of sources throughout research • Format to the journal's specifications • Are the citations truly relevant and useful?

CRs have the same basic structure as other research articles, but also have some unique features. What follows is an overview of the major sections.

Introduction

The introduction gives the reader the necessary background information needed to understand the current study's methods, evaluate the client's clinical condition, and interpret the significance of the results. It is essential to include a review of the relevant literature in this section. As you decide which sources and information to include, consider the following questions. What information would a fellow clinician need to treat this client? What consensus or controversies exist related to the condition, the specific population, or the MT modalities being investigated? How does this background data support the research question? An effective introduction is thorough but is not necessarily exhaustive. By the end of the introduction, a CR reader should have a clear sense of what is known, what remains to be discovered, and why the topic matters. These, in turn, lead logically to the research question itself, which should be explicitly stated for the sake of clarity.

Methods

The methods section should provide enough detail that a skilled colleague could carry out a similar study. This means including a well-rounded profile of the client, a lucid description of the treatment plan and any deviations from that plan, and a clear account of the measurements used. Basic details are important. At a minimum, be sure to indicate session length and frequency, the specific modalities applied, when and how measurements were taken, relevant details of the participant's health history, and the goals of treatment.

BOX 20.1
Description of Massage Techniques

An often overlooked aspect of massage CRs is a sufficiently detailed description of technique (Moyer, Dryden, and Shipwright 2009). In much of the research literature, massage is treated as a uniform practice, yet any practicing therapist knows that an immense variety of applications can be made in a single massage session. Detailed descriptions of massage applications make for a better definition of massage, better research methods, and a better-informed health care world.

Examples of Methods to Discuss in a CR

- Which body regions were the focus of the massage, and approximately how much time was spent on each region?
- Which structures were specifically targeted? (Muscles, fascia, bones, viscera, nerves?)
- What was the intention behind the overall treatment approach? To create more mobility and functionality? To reduce stress and pain? To foster body awareness or trauma recovery?
- Were any aspects of communication with the patient worth mentioning?
- Were there important elements in the therapist's body mechanics or hand shape?

Results

A good treatment summary is concise and is more detailed on key points. Special attention should be paid to those aspects of MT that are frequently underrepresented in the literature. These include the utterances and behaviors of the client, as well as the author's qualitative observations. In addition to your narrative summary of the results, you should also consider graphical, tabular, and quantitative methods for presenting your findings effectively. These approaches, when done well, allow for efficient use of journal space and can add to the clarity and interpretability of your results. Finally, keep in mind that it is essential to avoid prejudging the data. A good results section is balanced, pertinent, and compelling, but does not contain your conclusions. These belong in the discussion section.

Discussion

The discussion section is your opportunity to offer an interpretation of results. It is important to restate the research question and to make a balanced appraisal of any conclusions to be drawn from the results. Keep in mind that an individual

CR cannot definitively prove anything by itself, nor is that its purpose. Authors can and should report their hunches, assert likelihoods, and otherwise opine on what happened, but they should avoid the temptation to state these as proven fact (Gleberzon 2006).

This section also presents the opportunity to reflect on the study's design and execution. Were there unforeseen challenges? Could certain methods have been improved? In hindsight, how effective was the clinical approach? What kinds of studies or questions would be most appropriate for future research? Discussion of such issues shows that you have been thoughtful in completing your research. It can guide future clinicians in most effectively contributing to the base of research evidence.

Finally, you may want to take the opportunity to place your findings into the context of the profession or health care in general. If appropriate, you might indicate how you think the MT profession could employ your CR's techniques or clinical approaches in similar cases. You could also outline the lessons your CR offers to health care, MT educators, or the public.

MT AND HYPOCHONDROPLASIA: AN EXAMPLE

A recent CR by Amy Axt Hanson (2010) that examined MT to improve mobility in a client with hypochondroplasia (dwarfism) was awarded first place in the Massage Therapy Foundation's 2009 student case report competition. This excellent example of this form of research is included at the end of this chapter as a supplement (see pages 243-253).

The subject of this case report is compelling. Because there was no previous MT research with this population, it fills an important gap in the professional literature. Hanson makes effective use of the wealth of information on common physical limitations associated with this condition. She describes the different types of dwarfism as well as secondary conditions, such as spinal stenosis, reduced mobility, and compartment syndromes. She goes on to describe her client's symptoms, including fascial restriction in the legs, muscle fatigue, and neuropathy in the feet, and hypothesizes that "fascial adhesions or inelasticity could be compressing nerves and blood vessels in [the client's] lower legs, creating or exacerbating her symptoms, and a series of sessions were planned in which myofascial techniques would be used along with other massage techniques" (173).

The sections that follow contain appropriate methodological detail, including MT techniques that are carefully described and referenced when possible. Treatment goals are clearly articulated, and the client's range of motion (ROM) and fascial mobility are assessed and reported. Hanson maintains the reader's interest and trust by being cautious in her conclusions while defending her clinical reasoning, stating "it is reasonable to assume that these improvements were due to the easing of fascial restrictions, but this can only be inferred because massage practitioners have no methods to quantitatively measure fascial restrictions" (175). The report ends with an extended discussion of MT treatment considerations, including recommendations pertaining to practical difficulties that may need to be addressed when administering MT to members of this population.

As is necessarily the case with CR research, the present example exhibits some limitations imposed by the need to accommodate real life. The primary measure of progress was walking distance, which was approximated in city blocks and self-reported by the client. A more rigorous measure of functionality, such as monitored treadmill walking, may have served to strengthen the study, though this must be balanced against the investment of time and energy that is being made by the client. In addition, inclusion of a chronological table and a body diagram could have improved the description of the treatment strategy.

FUTURE DIRECTIONS

CRs have transformative potential both within and outside of the profession. In addition to generating CRs, massage therapists should strive to utilize CRs already in existence. Educational programs should begin to incorporate published CRs into their curricula, and should ensure that graduating MT students are equipped with fundamental research literacy and research capacity skills (Hamm 2010). With increasing numbers of published and accessible CRs, practitioners will not need to rely entirely on weekend workshops and conventions to learn from one another.

It is easy to state that more MT CRs should be read and published, but it is challenging to imagine how we can best accomplish this as a profession. What compels a practitioner to seize a particular case and do the considerable work of reporting it? Ultimately, scientific curiosity must become more embedded in MT values and clinical practice. Transforming the culture of scientific inquiry in MT will drive more discussion, more reflection, more publications, and more changes in professional behavior in the service of better health for all.

SUMMARY

Though there are currently only a few published massage therapy case reports, their quantity can be expected to increase as the profession becomes increasingly evidence based. In addition to strengthening the profession's evidence base, case reports have the potential to explore interesting and important research questions in real-world clinical settings, to elevate the status of the profession, and to disseminate findings across the larger spectrum of health and wellness professions. Whether it is by reading them or conducting them, massage therapists should now be informing their practice with case reports.

Critical Thinking Questions

1. List and describe the ways that case reports are valuable to the profession of massage therapy.
2. What is *ecological validity,* and how does the concept relate to case reports?
3. What are some of the obstacles that may have prevented massage therapists from conducting case reports?
4. What are some of the specific things that can be learned from reading case reports?
5. Explain the difference between a case report conducted *prospectively* and one conducted *retrospectively.*
6. Based on your clinical experience, what is a research question you might like to address with a case report? What methods of assessment might you use?

REFERENCES

Cassidy, C.M. 2002. *Methodological issues in investigations of massage/bodywork therapy*. Evanston, IL: AMTA Foundation.

Chaitow, L. 2006. Editorial: The 'humble' case-study. *J Bodyw Mov Ther* 10(1): 1-2.

Chunco, R. 2011. The effects of massage on pain, stiffness, and fatigue levels associated with ankylosing spondylitis: A case study. *Int J Ther Massage Bodywork* 4(1): 12-17.

Eisensmith, L. 2007. Massage therapy decreases frequency and intensity of symptoms related to temporomandibular joint syndrome in one case study. *J Bodyw Mov Ther* 11(3): 223-230.

Ernst, E. 2002. Evidence-based massage therapy: A contradiction in terms? In *Massage therapy: The evidence for practice,* ed. G.J. Rich, 11-25. Edinburgh: Harcourt.

Finch, P., A. Baskwill, F. Marincola, and P. Becker. 2007. Changes in pedal plantar pressure variability and contact time following massage therapy: A case study of a client with diabetic neuropathy. *J Bodyw Mov Ther* 11(4): 295-301.

Gleberzon, B.J. 2006. A peer-reviewer's plea. *J Can Chiropr Assoc* 50(2): 107-109

Hamm, M. 2006. Impact of massage therapy in the treatment of linked pathologies: Scoliosis, costovertebral dysfunction, and thoracic outlet syndrome. *J Bodyw Mov Ther* 10(1): 12-20.

———. 2008. *Clinical case reports for bodyworkers.* Golden, CO: Massage and Bodywork.

———. 2010. Case report: A year in the life of a massage research curriculum. Paper submitted to the Highlighting Massage Therapy in CIM Conference, Seattle, Washington, May 13-15.

Hanson, A.A. 2010. Using massage to improve mobility in a client with hypochondroplasia (dwarfism): A case report. *J Bodyw Mov Ther* 14(2): 172-178.

Kania, A., M.J. Verhoef, T. Dryden, and M.A. Ware. 2009. IN-CAM outcomes database: Its relevance and application in massage therapy research and practice. *Int J Ther Massage Bodywork* 2(1): 8-16.

LeMoon, K. 2008. Clinical reasoning in massage therapy. *Int J Ther Massage Bodywork* 1(1): 12-18.

McCarthy, L., and K. Reilly. 2000. How to write a case report. *Fam Med* 32(3): 190-195.

Menard, M.B. 2002. Methodological issues in the design and conduct of massage therapy research. In *Massage therapy: The evidence for practice,* ed. G.J. Rich, 27-41. Edinburgh: Harcourt.

———. 2003. *Making sense of research: A guide to research literacy for complementary practitioners.* 2nd ed. Toronto, ON: Curties-Overzet.

Moyer, C.A., T. Dryden, and S. Shipwright. 2009. Directions and dilemmas in massage therapy research: A workshop report from the 2009 North American research conference on complementary and integrative medicine. *Int J Ther Massage Bodywork* 2(2): 15-27.

Wright, S.M., and C. Kouroukis. 2000. Capturing zebras: What to do with a reportable case. *Can Med Assoc J* 163(4): 429-431

Zalta, J. 2008. Massage therapy protocol for post-anterior cruciate ligament reconstruction patellofemoral pain syndrome: A case report. *Int J Ther Massage Bodywork* 1(2): 11-21.

MASSAGE THERAPY FOR HYPOCHONDROPLASIA: IMPROVING MOBILITY IN A CLIENT WITH HYPOCHONDROPLASIA (DWARFISM): A CASE REPORT[1]

Amy Axt Hanson, LMP

Keywords

- myofascial release
- muscle fatigue
- achondroplasia
- structural bodywork
- climbing stairs
- compartment syndrome

Summary

A client with hypochondroplasia dwarfism and a medical diagnosis of spinal stenosis had found that her ability to walk had decreased over the past 7 years from easily walking 6 miles (10 K) to now needing to rest every half block (171 ft/52 m) due to muscle fatigue. Such weakness is consistent with nerve impingement due to spinal stenosis, which would not be improved by massage. However, during a preliminary assessment, it was found that both lower legs had severe fascial adhesions, possibly compressing lower leg blood vessels and nerves. It was hoped that by using myofascial massage techniques to relieve the adhesions, her mobility would improve over the course of 8 sessions. Myofascial massage techniques showed positive results in reducing adhesions, improving circulation, and increasing the distance the client could walk before resting to 2 blocks (686 ft/209 m). Working with this client showed that Licensed Massage Practitioners (LMPs) can easily accommodate clients of very short height.

Introduction

Clients of very short height are a surprisingly large group, with a study done in 2003 by the advocacy group Little People of America finding that 1 in 277 US adults, or roughly a million people, were 4 feet 10 inches/147 cm or shorter. Most were thought to simply have a family history of short height. Although exact numbers of dwarfs are unknown, they are estimated to account for more than 200,000 people in the US (Adelson, 2005a). That figure seems to be low even for a baseline: the same study found that roughly 169,000 people in the US were 4 ft, 6 in/137 cm or shorter, a height likely tied to a medical cause (Adelson, 2005a). To be considered a dwarf, a client must be 4 ft, 10 in or shorter due to a medical condition that limits growth. Those medical conditions identified to date include faulty mechanisms of cartilage and bone development, pituitary or thyroid hormone deficiencies,

[1]Reprinted from *Journal of Bodywork & Movement Therapies*, Vol. 14, A.A. Hanson, "Improving mobility in a client with hypochondroplasia (dwarfism): A case report," pgs. 172-178, Copyright 2010, with permission of Elsevier.

absent or incomplete chromosomes, genetic syndromes, malnutrition, extreme emotional neglect or abuse, and chronic diseases of the kidney, heart, liver, or gastrointestinal tract (Adelson, 2005b).

The client in this report was diagnosed with the bone growth disorder hypochondroplasia (literally 'under cartilage molding'), which produces defective conversion of cartilage into bone due to point mutations in the same fibroblast receptor protein linked to achondroplasia (literally 'no cartilage molding') (Francomano, 2005a; Hall, 2005). Hypochondroplasia is considered to be a less severe form of achondroplasia (Beighton, 1993; Francomano, 2005b; Greenfield, 1990a; Greenspan, 2000a). Achondroplasia is the most commonly diagnosed form of dwarfism, appearing in 1 of every 15,000-40,000 live births, and is thought to account for half of all cases of dwarfism (Francomano, 2005c; Greenfield, 1990a). The prevalence of hypochondroplasia is unknown but thought to be similar to achondroplasia, only less frequently diagnosed since body changes are milder and likely to be overlooked (Francomano, 2005c,d).

Typical presentation of hypochondroplasia and achondroplasia includes normal trunk length but disproportionately short arms and legs. Hands and feet are broad and short (Francomano, 2005b,e; Spranger et al., 2002). Much is known about hypochondroplasia and achondroplasia from X-ray studies of skeletal features, with several issues being pertinent to discussions of mobility, including lumbar hyperlordosis, a squared, shortened ilia, a more horizontally tilted sacrum, short femoral neck, mild genu varum (bowed legs), and a reduced greater sciatic notch (Beighton, 1993; Bogumill and Schwamm, 1984; Francomano, 2005c,e; Greenfield, 1990b; Greenspan, 2000b; Spranger et al., 2002). These clients tend to have shorter than average pedicles, the bridges between vertebral bodies and the arch holding the transverse and spinous processes. With smaller than average vertebral and intervertebral foramina, any further narrowing due to injuries, herniated disks, bone spurs, or cartilage aging can produce pain, numbness, and weakness in the extremities, particularly the legs (Beighton, 1993; Francomano, 2005c; Greenfield, 1990b; Greenspan, 2000c; Spranger et al., 2002). According to orthopedic surgeon Dr. Steven E. Kopits, who specialized in dwarfism, 'with progression of the severity, the patients have to make obligatory stops at periodic distances during gait because of numbness, pain, and weakness of the lower limbs' (Kopits, 1976a). This accurately describes the client in this study, who was limited in the distance she could walk before having to stop and rest due to muscle weakness in her legs. In addition, she found climbing stairs difficult, and had to bring both feet to each step. After sitting at her desk for 4 or more hours, and on waking in the morning, various areas of her feet and toes tingled, which could be relieved by dorsiflexing and plantar flexing her feet, or by walking.

During assessment it was discovered that the client had severe fascial restrictions in both lower legs, and the skin of her lower legs and feet felt significantly cooler to the touch than her thighs or arms. Fascial adhesions are considered to be a potential cause of blood and nerve flow impingement (Archer, 2007a; Travell and Simons, 1993). Layers of fascial connective tissue are found most superficially as a body stocking under the dermis, and also more deeply wrapping groups of muscles (compartments), each named muscle, each inner bundle (fascicle) within a muscle, and each individual muscle cell (fiber). Fascia separates various functional groups yet holds them together (Smith, 2005a). In the lower leg, deep fascia divides muscles into anterior, lateral, deep posterior, and superficial posterior compartments, with major bundles of nerves, arteries, veins, and lymph vessels running between compartments, within compartments, and underneath the superficial fascial layer (see figure 20.2).

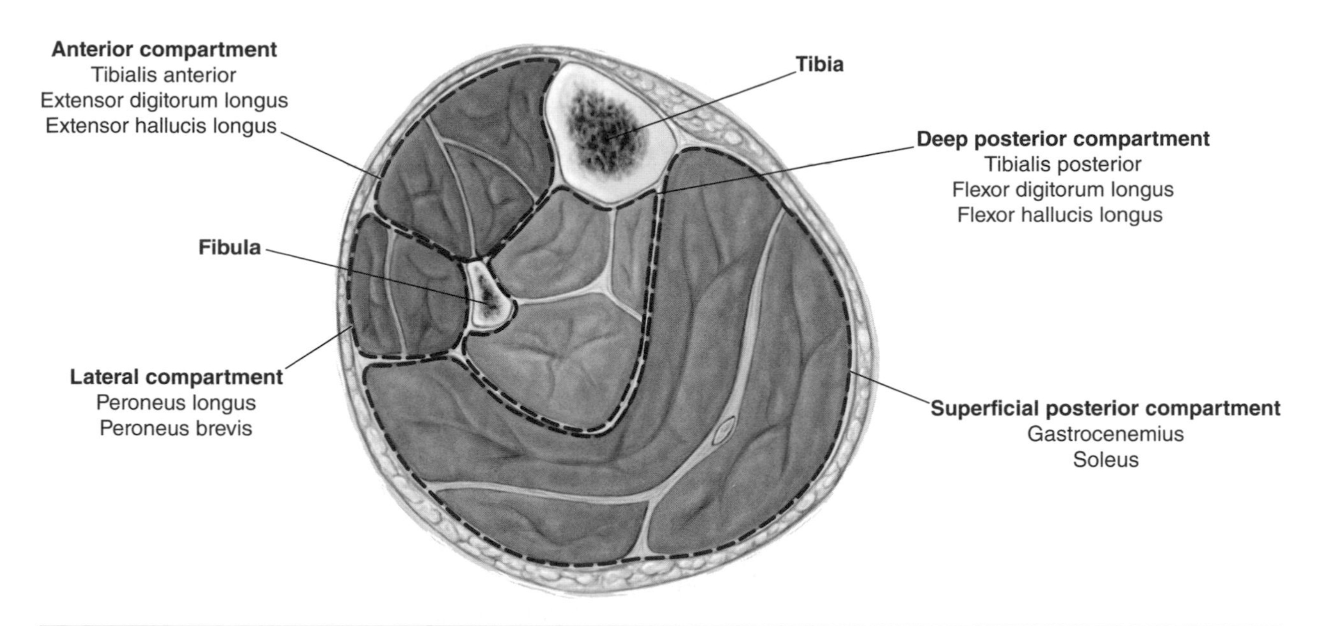

Figure 20.2 Cross-section of the lower leg showing the major fascial divisions grouping muscles into the anterior, lateral, deep posterior, and superficial posterior compartments.

These nerves, blood, and lymph vessels can become compressed due to contraction of surrounding muscles, from inelasticity in the fascial wrapping, or from a gluing together of fascial septa on either side of the nerves and vessels. Collagen fibers can lose elasticity and/or become bonded to collagen fibers in adjacent fascial layers from disuse, dysfunctional use, aging, or injury (Smith, 2005b). These adhesions, if severe enough, can produce muscle fatigue and pain, and at the most extreme, produce compartment syndrome in which underlying muscle tissue degenerates (Travell and Simons, 1993).

In participating in this study, the client's primary interest was to see whether massage could increase the distance she could walk before the onset of muscle fatigue. She was unconcerned with the tingling in her feet, and had no expectation of any other changes. It was suspected that fascial adhesions or inelasticity could be compressing nerves and blood vessels in her lower legs, creating or exacerbating her symptoms, and a series of sessions were planned in which myofascial techniques would be used along with other massage techniques. It was not known whether there might be undiagnosed cardiovascular issues; improvements could also be limited by spinal stenosis, a true neurological condition that produces pain and weakness in the legs (Mayo Clinic, 2008).

Methods

Profile of client

A 63-year-old librarian was, at 4 ft, 4 in (132 cm), the only member of her family with hypochondroplasia. Her ability to walk had been normal until her 40s, allowing her to participate in 10-km (6-mile) fundraising walks. She was diagnosed with spinal stenosis 13 years ago and started experiencing muscle weakness in her legs 7 years ago, which had progressed to where she could only walk half a block (171 ft/ 52 m) before having to stop and rest for several minutes. Muscle weakness only occurred when walking, and was not associated with any pain or burning in her legs or lower back, although occasionally she felt tingling in her feet and toes at this time. She was not able to link the fatigue to any specific muscle or group of muscles. When she forced herself to keep walking, her leg muscles no longer functioned and she fell. Use of a cane as a mobility aid did not improve her muscle fatigue or distance, but helped her walk faster and feel more balanced.

Tingling in her toes and feet had become more pronounced over the past 5 years, especially when she woke up in the morning or sat at her desk at work for 4-5 h. She had not noticed a pattern to the tingling, which occurred in her toes, heels, and various areas of her feet (lateral, medial, and superior sides). The tingling was relieved by dorsiflexing and plantar flexing her foot, or by walking, and disappeared within 5 min.

The client had a positive attitude toward life, adapting to her increasing limitations with good humor. She often used a cane when walking at work, home, and shopping, and for longer distances used a mobility scooter. She felt that her mobility would be improved by losing weight, and had been following a nationally franchised weight-reducing program for 3 years, losing 38 pounds (17 kg) to bring her to a current weight of 163 pounds (73 kg).

The client had never received massage of any kind. She received physical therapy for low back pain 13 years ago for a term of 2 months. At that time, she had steroid injections to relieve low back pain caused by spinal stenosis. She also performed stretching exercises for her legs and back, and felt that it helped improve her mobility, but also felt that reduced pain from her steroid injections was more important in improving her mobility. At the outset of the study, she had no pain in her legs or low back, but sometimes felt tightness down the posterior muscles of her leg, especially when walking and climbing stairs. This tightness required her to bring both feet up to each stair before tackling the next.

On initial assessment, the client was found to have fascial tension in both lower legs to the extent that skin moved very little in any direction. Muscles of the anterior and lateral compartments felt tight. She had light to moderate range of motion (ROM) limitations in all planes of the hips, knees, and ankles, with no limitation in knee extension. Of note was a moderate-plus limitation in dorsiflexion and plantarflextion of her ankles. Hip flexion had a firm active end point at 90 degrees, with no further gain in ROM on passive movement.

The client stood with light lateral rotation of both femurs, low medial arches, lumbar hyperlordosis, and no other significant postural deviations. On initial assessment, her lower legs, feet, and toes felt significantly cooler in temperature than her thighs. She had no significant tension in the muscles of her lower leg posterior compartments, anterior thighs, or posterior thighs.

The client was very interested to see if massage could improve her ease of movement and flexibility to the extent that it might increase her walking distance from half a block to two blocks between rest stops. She had no other goals for this study, but the author was interested to see whether easing the client's myofascial restrictions might be accompanied by an increased ROM and reduction in the tingling of her toes and feet.

Treatment plan

Eight massage sessions were conducted over the course of 15 weeks, with each session lasting 1.5 h (plus additional time for assessment). The time between massages averaged 14 days, ranging from 11 to 21 days. Two weeks after session 8, final information was gathered on walking distance.

Session 1 used whole-body Swedish massage and deep tissue techniques (focused work on deeper muscles, both with-fiber and cross-fiber, with the intent to release longstanding adhesions) for assessment, palpation, and to introduce the client to massage.

Techniques in sessions 2-6 included prone broad-plane, linear shift, and horizontal-plane myofascial release techniques (Archer, 2007b) to the posterior compartment, plus Swedish and deep tissue techniques to posterior lower leg, hamstrings, iliotibial band, gluteals, and back. Supine techniques included broad-plane, linear shift, and horizontal-plane myofascial release to anterior and lateral lower leg, plus Swedish and deep tissue techniques to anterior lower leg and quadriceps. Sessions 7 and 8 used the more specifically targeted, heavier-pressure techniques of structural bodywork using the finger chisel, dorsum of hand, and octopus-hand strokes intended to produce myofascial release of heavy adhesions and deep structures (Smith, 2005c). With the client standing and slowly flexing her knees, greater pressure was directed to the extensor retinaculum, anterior valley, and gastrocnemius/soleus. A small structural ball was placed under each medial arch with knee flexion while the client was standing. With the client supine and dorsiflexing and plantar flexing her feet, greater pressure was directed to the flexor retinaculum, anterior and lateral compartments. Muscle rolling was employed to help release muscle group adhesions (Archer, 2007b). Session 8 also included horizontal-plane release just superior to and inferior to each knee (supine and prone), and traction release to each femur was employed in order to help release fascia of the ankle, knee, and hip joints (Archer, 2007c). Side-lying contract-relax stretches of the iliopsoas were conducted in sessions 2, 4, 5, 6, 7; direct iliopsoas massage was performed in session 3 (Archer, 2007d).

Hip and knee ROM were checked in sessions 2, 4, and 7; ankle ROM was checked at sessions 2, 4, 7, and 8. At the start of each session, the client reported the distance she could walk before symptom onset during the intervening two weeks. Results were encouraged to be average distances, not an unusual maximum for that time period. The client was assigned no stretching homework in order to monitor results from myofascial techniques alone.

Results

Improved functional outcomes

At the beginning of the series, the client's feet and lower legs felt significantly cooler in temperature than her thighs before massage; during and after massage sessions, her calves and feet felt noticeably warmer and often changed color from uniformly pale to showing patches of pink. By session 8, her legs and feet felt significantly closer to thigh and trunk temperature prior to massage. Similarly, fascial restrictions noted in session 1 that resisted skin movement in any direction were eased throughout the course of this study so that by session 8, the skin on the client's lower leg moved well in all directions.

During sessions 1 and 2, when the client lay prone, the tingling in her feet increased and became uncomfortable. Semi-side-lying alleviated this. On session 3, the client found she could lie prone comfortably, which lasted for all subsequent sessions.

After each session, the client reported a greater feeling of ease of movement in her lower legs, a feeling that she retained until the next session. At session 4, she reported that climbing stairs had become easier, as she could now ascend stairs with one foot per step. Previously, she had to bring both feet to each step before continuing.

During sessions 1-6, the client's ROM in her ankles (dorsiflexion and plantar flexion) were limited to a moderate-plus extent and did not change as a result of broad-plane myofascial techniques. After the more focused, deeper structural/ myofascial work conducted during session 7, ankle dorsiflexion and plantar flexion improved significantly to only a light limitation.

Structural myofascial work done in session 8 raised the medial arches of her feet.

Walking distances before stopping were reported at the beginning of each massage session and are reported in Figure 20.3. Blocks were converted to feet/ meters after the client walked with the author and pointed out where she usually had to stop. Distances were measured with a 25-foot carpenter's measuring tape. At the study's outset, the client could only walk half a block (171 ft/52 m) before having to stop. Swedish techniques performed at session 1 allowed the client to walk three-quarters of a block (257 ft/ 78 m) before having to stop. No distance improvements were noted in conjunction with the broad-plane myofascial techniques performed during sessions 2 through 4. Broad-plane myofascial work done at session 5 resulted in an improvement to 1 block (343 ft/104 m) before stopping; the same work done at session 6 resulted in her ability to walk 1.5 blocks (514 ft/157 m) before stopping. Structural bodywork techniques in sessions 7 and 8 improved the client's ability to walk 2 blocks (686 ft/209 m) before having to stop. (A year after the initial work, the client continues able to walk 2 blocks before having to stop.)

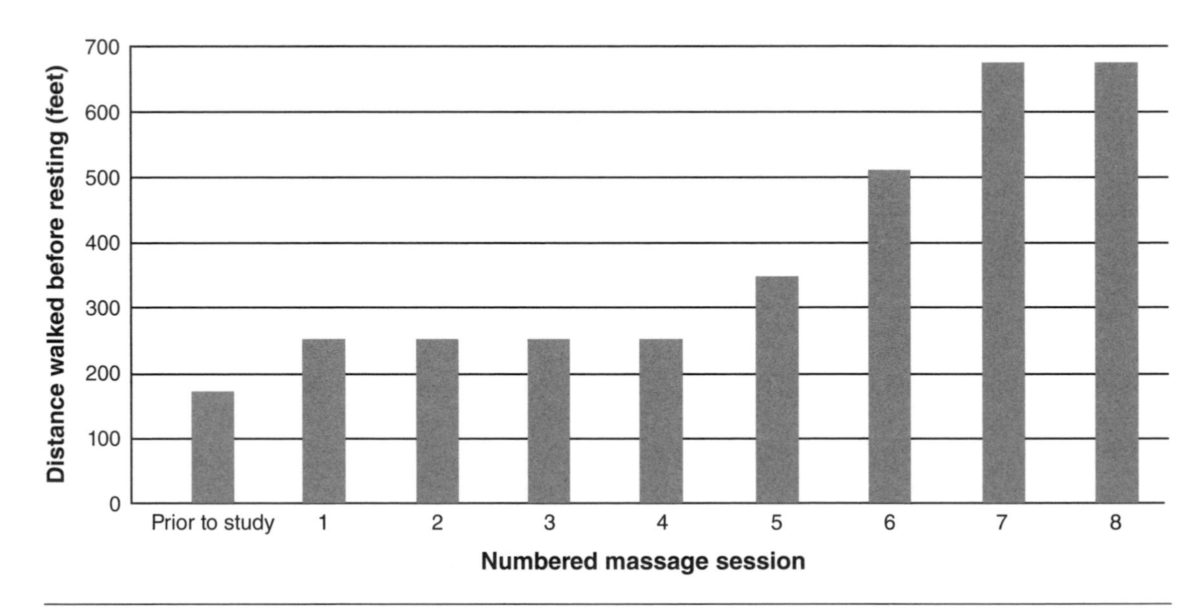

Figure 20.3 The average distance the client could walk before needing to rest prior to the study and in the two-week period after each numbered massage.

Unchanged functional outcomes

The tingling reported by the client in her toes and feet did not change during the course of this study, nor was there any change in the lateral rotation of her feet.

As a gauge of iliopsoas tension, the client had little femur extension beyond the frontal/coronal plane. This did not change with side-lying iliopsoas contract-relax stretches, or with direct iliopsoas massage. All other ROM limitations in her hips and knees were unchanged.

It is not known how much change in muscle tension was achieved in the anterior and lateral compartments of the lower leg during the course of this study due to incomplete attention by the student LMP.

Discussion

Adhesions of the intramuscular and superficial fascia can bring about decreases in circulation, leading in extreme cases to compartment syndromes and muscle necrosis (Travell and Simons, 1993). It was hypothesized that the client's muscle weakness may have been due in part to fascial tension in her lower legs that was constricting nerve or blood flow to her calves and feet. As her fascial restrictions were reduced, circulation improved as observed by skin color change and a feeling of warmth to the practitioner's hand (Smith, 2005d). Concurrent with this, the client reported steady improvements in ease of movement, stair-climbing ability, and walking distance. It is reasonable to assume that these improvements were due to the easing of fascial restrictions, but this can only be inferred because massage practitioners have no methods to quantitatively measure fascial restrictions.

It was hoped that ROM change would be seen at each session as an indication of fascial easing, but this client's ROM remained unchanged until session 7, when significant gains in dorsiflexion and plantar flexion occurred as a result of structural bodywork techniques. It is possible that these techniques are inherently more effective than lighter work, though it is also possible that the client responded well because her fascial restrictions had been released enough so that stronger work could be effective. The unchanged ROM limitations of her hips and legs may not have had a fascial origin, as it was later discovered that her initial assessment had been in comparison to LMP expectations learned from average-height clients. It may be that her "limitations" were in fact entirely within the normal range of motion for bone configurations inherent to the legs and hips of clients with hypochondroplasia.

Measuring progress via the large-scale measurement of walking distance was also problematic because although there was a gain after the first massage, there seemed to be no change for the following 3 massages, with improvements only being seen in the 2-week period following session 5. Future studies would be better served by having the client walk in place or walk on a treadmill until the point of muscle fatigue in order to more finely gauge progress. Having the client self-report her average walking distances also adds uncertainty to the data in that city blocks are not standard units, and can vary widely. A measure of confidence in the data was obtained by the fact that the client trevelled the same route every day between home and work, making it possible for stopping locations to be determined. There still remains the possibility that the client might have wanted to please the practitioner by reporting results greater than those actually obtained. The author would always ask about changes in mobility and symptoms, making the point of saying that 'no change is totally fine, too.' Since the client consistently reported no change in walking distance for many sessions, nor a reduction in foot or toe tingling throughout the course of the study, the author is more confident with this data.

The client's greater ease of climbing stairs was an unexpected bonus to the work, and may be another indication of fascial easing given the client's initial reports of feeling tightness down the back of her legs when climbing stairs. It improved her quality of life in that she sometimes had to climb a flight of stairs at work to reach certain books. In addition, her home has stairs to the basement and to the second floor, and she used a stepstool in the kitchen to reach the countertops.

The tingling in the client's toes remained an unresolved issue. It was hoped by the LMP that these symptoms could be reduced, but such was not the case, and it is considered that these may be a symptom of spinal stenosis or undiagnosed cardiovascular or neurologic issues.

Changes in our assumptions of normal

As the study progressed, the author found it refreshing to work with a client who allowed a re-examination of various assumptions of normality. For example, it is entirely normal for clients with hypochondroplasia and achondroplasia to have bone configurations that produce lumbar hyperlordosis that no amount of bodywork could change. Lumbar nerve difficulties are common due to their commonly shortened lumbar pedicles, and work to relieve false sciatica, while helpful, would not relieve symptoms of true sciatica. The author found it an interesting challenge to conduct the iliopsoas tension/length test (Thomas' test). Lack of tension in the iliopsoas is seen when the client's knee rests below horizontal, but a shorter leg length results in smaller angles below horizontal and potentially a more difficult test interpretation. Interestingly, predicting muscle issues by watching a client walk is impossible for clients with hypochondroplasia because normal posture and gait patterns have not been documented. Normal gait has been determined for achondroplasia, with data available as a master's thesis (Knudsen, 1993); it has been broadly described elsewhere as a 'characteristic waddling gait' (Greenspan, 2000d). Altered gait is expected due to significant differences in bone structures, including lumbar hyperlordosis, mild genu varum short neck of the femur, and hip changes including a more horizontal tilt to the sacrum.

Practical (office) considerations

No matter what the cause of a client's short height, LMPs will find they need to make only minimal changes in office equipment and routine to maximize client comfort. When lying supine, this client's lower legs were held in significant flexion by an 8-inch bolster or pillow; a 4-inch bolster (in this case, a rolled-up yoga mat) worked best (see Figures 20.4 and 20.5).

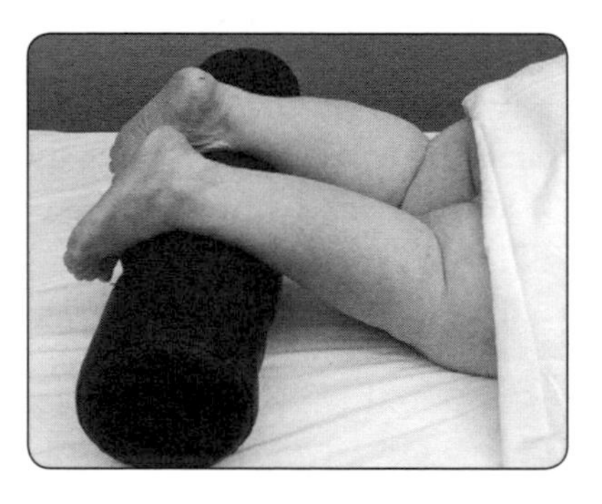

Figure 20.4 An 8-inch standard bolster held the client's lower legs in significant flexion.

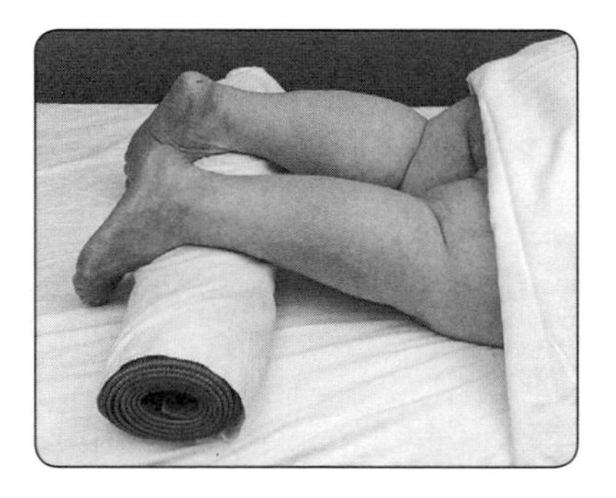

Figure 20.5 A 4-inch bolster (in this case, a rolled-up yoga mat) reduced flexion in the client's lower legs.

A low chair aided client comfort during intake and tests for true neurological conditions. Since this client was quite mobile, a footstool leading to an average-height chair helped her climb onto the table; later a set of folding stairs was used (see Figure 20.6).

Less-mobile clients may require an electric or hydraulic table. Stairs are usually a challenge and/or a barrier, so massage space must be wheelchair accessible (see figure 20.7).

Since short-height clients do not span the massage table as fully as do average-height clients, LMP body mechanics benefit by positioning them at the distal end

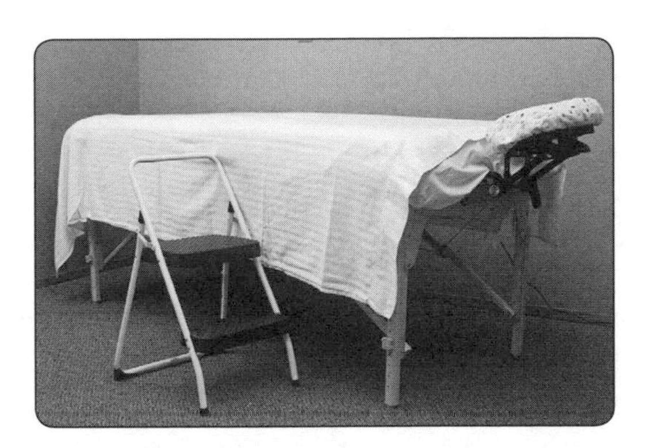

Figure 20.6 A set of folding steps can be used for clients to get up onto a fixed-leg table. This version has steps 8 and 10 inches (20 and 25 cm) high, which is still a challenge. An electric or hydraulic table eliminates problems for both clients and LMPs.

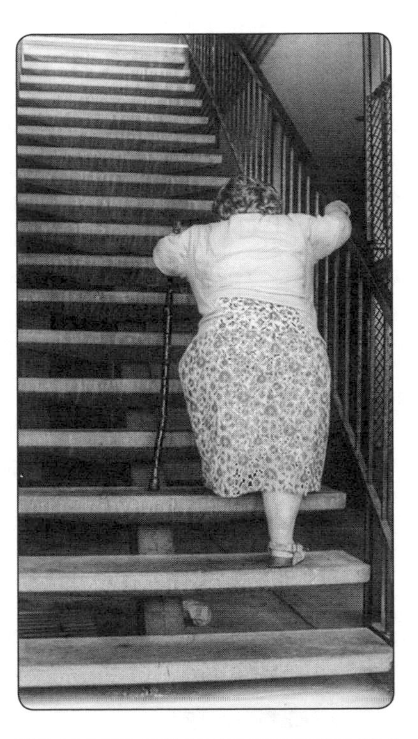

Figure 20.7 Stairs can be a challenge for even the most mobile dwarf clients, and a barrier to those in a wheelchair.

of the table when sessions include a substantial amount of lower extremity work (see figures 20.8 and 20.9).

Finally, to paraphrase orthopedic surgeon and dwarfism specialist Dr. Stephen E. Kopits (1976b) the challenge to LMPs is not to see the unusual bone structures of dwarfism as a problem. The only problem, and this is the case with all clients, comes from their long-term use patterns of these bones and muscles.

LMPs fortunate enough to work with this population will find that massage therapy offers the possibility of improving range of motion and ease of movement in a supportive, non-clinical, and body-neutral environment.

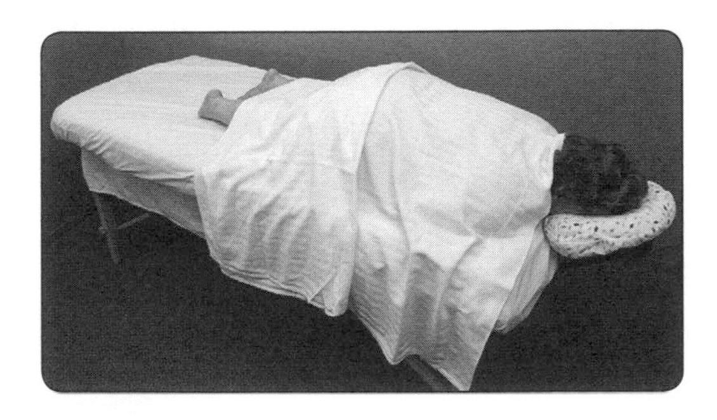

Figure 20.8 Dwarf clients do not span the massage table as fully as clients of average height.

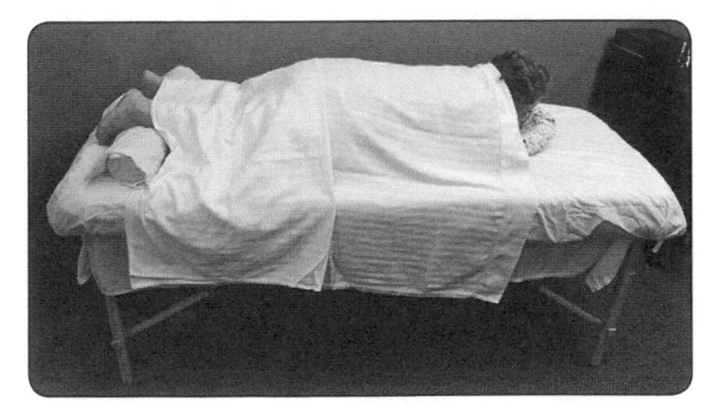

Figure 20.9 For significant amounts of foot and leg work, the client should be positioned at the distal end of the table to optimize LMP body mechanics.

Acknowledgments

The author is grateful to the client for her participation in this study, to Dr. John E. Hanson for his support and technical expertise, and to the teachers at Cortiva Institute- Seattle School of Massage Therapy for their insights, suggestions, encouragement, and education in medical massage therapy.

Case Report References

Adelson, B.M., 2005a. Dwarfism: Medical and Psychosocial Aspects of Profound Short Stature. The Johns Hopkins University Press, Baltimore, p. 22-23.

Adelson, B.M., 2005b. Dwarfism: Medical and Psychosocial Aspects of Profound Short Stature. The Johns Hopkins University Press, Baltimore, p. 17-20 & 287-297.

Archer, P., 2007a. Therapeutic Massage in Athletics. Lippincott Williams & Wilkins, Philadelphia, p. 232-234.

Archer, P., 2007b. Therapeutic Massage in Athletics. Lippincott Williams & Wilkins, Philadelphia, p. 164-174.

Archer, P., 2007c. Therapeutic Massage in Athletics. Lippincott Williams & Wilkins, Philadelphia, p. 171-172.

Archer, P., 2007d. Therapeutic Massage in Athletics. LippincottWilliams & Wilkins, Philadelphia, p. 134.

Beighton, P., 1993. McKusick's Heritable Disorders of Connective Tissue. Mosby-Year Book Inc, St. Louis, p. 578.

Bogumill, G.P., Schwamm, H.A., 1984. Orthopaedic Pathology: A Synopsis With Clinical and Radiographic Correlation. WB Saunders Co, Philadelphia, p. 43-49.

Francomano, C.A., 2005a. Hypochondroplasia. GeneReviews. Available from: http://www.ncbi.nlm.nih.gov/bookshelf/br.fcgi?bookZgene&partZhypochondroplasia, p. 4 [Internet][cited 2008 August 4].

Francomano, C.A., 2005b. Hypochondroplasia. GeneReviews. Available from: http://www.ncbi.nlm.nih.gov/bookshelf/br.fcgi?bookZgene&partZhypochondroplasia, p. 1 [Internet] [cited 2008 August 4].

Francomano, C.A., 2005c. Hypochondroplasia. GeneReviews. Available from: http://www.ncbi.nlm.nih.gov/bookshelf/br.fcgi?bookZgene&partZhypochondroplasia, pp. 6-7 [Internet]. [cited 2008 August 4].

Francomano, C.A., 2005d. Hypochondroplasia. GeneReviews. Available from: http://www.ncbi.nlm.nih.gov/bookshelf/br.fcgi?bookZgene&partZhypochondroplasia, pp. 6-7 [Internet][cited 2008 August 4].

Francomano, C.A., 2005e. Hypochondroplasia. GeneReviews. Available from: http://www.ncbi.nlm.nih.gov/bookshelf/br.fcgi?bookZgene&partZhypochondroplasia, pp. 2-3 [Internet][cited 2008 August 4].

Greenfield, G.B., 1990a. Radiology of Bone Diseases. JB Lippincott Co, Philadelphia, p. 276.

Greenfield, G.B., 1990b. Radiology of Bone Diseases. JB Lippincott Co, Philadelphia, p. 272-276.

Greenspan, A., 2000a. Orthopedic Radiology: A Practical Approach. Lippincott Williams & Wilkins, Philadelphia, p. 910.

Greenspan, A., 2000b. Orthopedic Radiology: A Practical Approach. Lippincott Williams & Wilkins, Philadelphia, p. 908-909.

Greenspan, A., 2000c. Orthopedic Radiology: A Practical Approach. Lippincott Williams & Wilkins, Philadelphia, p. 909-910.

Greenspan, A., 2000d. Orthopedic Radiology: A Practical Approach. Lippincott Williams & Wilkins, Philadelphia, p. 908.

Hall, B., 2005. Bones and Cartilage: Developmental and Evolutionary Skeletal Biology. Elsevier Academic Press, Amsterdam, p. 437.

Knudsen, M., 1993. Range of motion and flexibility of adults with achondroplasia [master's thesis]. Denton (TX), Texas Woman's University.

Kopits, S.E., 1976a. Orthopedic complications of dwarfism. Clinical Orthopaedics and Related Research 114, 158.

Kopits, S.E., 1976b. Orthopedic complications of dwarfism. Clinical Orthopaedics and Related Research 114, 154.

Mayo Clinic, 2008. Spinal Stenosis. MayoClinic.com Available from: http://www.mayoclinic.com/health/spinal-stenosis/DS00515 (accessed 11.03.08.). p. 1-2. [cited 2008 August 8].

Smith, J., 2005a. Structural Bodywork. Elsevier, London, p. 58-62.

Smith, J., 2005b. Structural Bodywork. Elsevier, London, p. 73-74, 84-89.

Smith, J., 2005c. Structural Bodywork. Elsevier, London, p. 135-141.

Smith, J., 2005d. Structural Bodywork. Elsevier, London, p. 136.

Spranger, J.W., Brill, P.W., Poznanski, A., 2002. Bone Dysplasias: An Atlas of Genetic Disorders of Skeletal Development. Oxford University Press, Oxford, p. 90.

Travell, J.G., Simons, D.G., 1993. Myofascial Pain and Dysfunction, The Trigger Point Manual, The Lower Extremities. Lippincott Williams & Wilkins, Philadelphia, p. 361-362, 443-444.

chapter

21

Writing Journal Articles

Paul Finch, PhD, DPodM

When I submitted my first paper for publication (many years ago now), I remember that the event was associated with a host of emotions—excitement, a sense of achievement, and, somewhat unexpectedly, fear and trepidation. I experienced the same emotions again when it actually appeared in print. The second paper I submitted was also accompanied by this set of emotions, but when that paper was rejected by a competitive, influential journal, I also felt disappointment and discouragement. Note, however, that the person who is never rejected is the person who never submits for publication. Accept this with equanimity, and you will have taken an important step on the path to being a published researcher or writer of scholarly work.

Regardless of whether the research in question is quantitative, qualitative, mixed method, a randomized clinical trial, a case study, or some other category of work, publication is the culmination of the process. It is a major way (although not the only way) in which the activities of researchers connect with the practice community. This connection is crucial to an evidence-informed, reflective approach to health care delivery (Finch 2007), the goal of which is to optimize treatment outcomes (Sackett et al. 2000). While the relationship between research- and evidence-informed practice is a pragmatic reason to publish, it is also true that writing about your work contributes to the development of your research skills. Writing demands a logical and disciplined approach that can be translated to the next research endeavor. Additionally, the work involved in searching the literature and constructing a paper in the context of existing research adds to your knowledge base, which will be the platform for subsequent research proposals (Rosenfeldt et al. 2000).

For these reasons, it is clear that the dissemination of findings through publication is fundamental to research. It can be challenging, satisfying, and rewarding. While the positives tend to easily outweigh the negatives, it can also be daunting and it is not without risk. Through research and publication, parts of the self are exposed, and this can be unsettling. Logically, the beginning of this exciting process is deciding the type of article you will write.

literature review

▸ A broad term for an overview of the available knowledge in a particular area.

narrative review

▸ A literature review that identifies and examines relevant studies, and attempts to reach a conclusion about the state of knowledge on a topic, based on the reviewer's interpretation of the relevant studies.

TYPES OF JOURNAL ARTICLE

While every journal has its own specific author guidelines, there are common categories to consider when writing a paper. The following list is not exhaustive, but should serve as an overview:

Literature reviews provide an overview of a particular research area and identify, compare, and contrast relevant studies. Subtypes of literature review include *narrative reviews, systematic reviews,* and *meta-analyses.*

systematic review

▸ A literature review that identifies and examines relevant studies and unpublished sources of data acquired by means of predetermined search criteria and strategies.

meta-analysis

▸ A literature review that identifies and examines relevant studies and unpublished sources of data acquired through predetermined search criteria and strategies, and then incorporates statistical analysis of study results to reach objective, quantitative conclusions.

research report

▸ An article that presents findings or theories based on data collected by the author.

brief communication

▸ A short-format article that presents a subject of interest, work in progress, or a summary of original research.

practice guideline

▸ A presentation of research evidence and clinical knowledge with recommendations for practice related to a particular condition.

commentary

▸ An article that adds context and detail to a topic or to another article.

editorial

▸ An article that presents the author's opinion or perspective of a situation or event.

Narrative reviews identify and examine relevant published studies, and attempt to reach to a conclusion about the state of knowledge on a topic based on the reviewer's reading and interpretation of those primary sources. Systematic reviews extend this approach by including additional sources of data, such as unpublished dissertations, acquired by means of a predetermined search strategy intended to further reduce the likelihood of a biased conclusion. Both of these forms of review can be thought of as providing a scholarly summary of what is known about a particular topic (Menard 2009). Meta-analysis is a refined form of literature review that incorporates statistical analysis of study results to reach one or more quantitative conclusions based on the available evidence (Rosenthal 1998).

Research reports present findings and theories based on data that the authors have collected themselves (as opposed to the previously mentioned reviews, in which the authors may be analyzing or reanalyzing data that have been collected by other researchers) that are relevant to the journal readership. By contrast, *brief communications* use a small amount of journal space to report subjects of topical interest, work in progress, or original research that is narrower in scope than the contents of a full-length research report.

Practice guidelines present an overview of research evidence and clinical knowledge and make recommendations for practice based on the best available evidence related to a particular condition. *Commentaries, editorials,* and *position papers* present a carefully argued and appropriately referenced point of view. *Book reviews* offer a critical perspective on a book, usually one that has just recently been published, relevant to the subject of the journal in which it appears.

These are generic categories of submission, and each has associated limits regarding word count, tables, and figures. Authors should consult the specific instructions of a journal they are targeting early in the writing process to avoid unnecessary rewriting. Examples of author guidelines for journals with clear relevance to MT research can be found in the *International Journal of Therapeutic Massage and Bodywork* (http://journals.sfu.ca/ijtmb/index.php/ijtmb/about/submissions#authorGuidelines), and the *Journal of Bodywork and Movement Therapies* (www.bodyworkmovementtherapies.com/authorinfo).

CHOICE OF JOURNAL

In addition to the type of article you decide to write, the journal you hope to be published in is an important consideration. The first question to be asked is whether the journal is peer-reviewed. Peer review is a process by which a submission is reviewed by a number of qualified professionals, selected by a journal editor, to determine if the submission meets the journal's standards for publication. In the case of research-based submissions, this will include a critique of the methods used to collect, analyze, and interpret the data. The reviewers inform the journal editor whether they find that the submission should be considered for publication or find that it should be rejected for one or more reasons. Submissions that are not rejected are almost never accepted for publication as they are, but are usually returned to the author with reviewers' feedback that can be incorporated during the revision process prior to publication. In general, scholarly work is best published in a peer-reviewed journal, although there are other factors to consider.

The first of these relates to the intended audience. Before proceeding, authors need to consider whom they hope to reach. Appleton and Ratnaike (2008) recommend that authors read some of the journals to which they might submit their work to gain a sense of the journals' scope and of the type of articles they publish.

Determining a journal's audience and the sort of article of interest to readers are also clearly relevant issues (Lee 2008).

A journal's format is also worth considering. Most print journals now have an electronic counterpart, but the same cannot be said in reverse. Thus, the question is not so much online or print, but whether a hard-copy publication is important. Beyond this, the question of access is also important. This means both access to the journal and, more broadly, to information. This raises the issue of barriers, which may be present at either end of the publication process. For the reader, barriers include the cost of subscription and physical access. From the author's point of view, cost can also be a barrier because some journals charge a publication fee. Increasingly, open-access online journals, such as the *International Journal of Therapeutic Massage and Bodywork,* are as close to barrier free as it gets, since access is possible from any computer with Internet capability. Ultimately, the author must decide how to weigh such factors to choose the most appropriate journal for potential publication.

position paper

▸ An article that presents a detailed theory, model, or set of opinions on a particular topic.

book review

▸ A critical appraisal of a book, usually one that has been recently published.

WRITING THE PAPER

When conducting research, it is never too early to begin planning and preparing the associated paper and considering which journal it might be submitted to. As noted by Keen (2007), it is important to identify the authors early, determine the order of authorship, and agree on the division of labor. If the endeavor is a solo project, the answers will be clear, but if it is not, upfront discussion will prevent problems later.

If you will lead the writing project, the demands of life must be organized to accommodate your writing. Writing is something that most authors find difficult to do in short snippets of time. Clarity of purpose and thought are required, and these necessitate dedicated periods of uninterrupted time. It is important to schedule a block of time when those around you know that you should not be disturbed. This takes discipline, but it will pay off in the long run.

Having carved out time to write, the challenge is to begin. This means opening the file, either electronic or hard copy, and putting something in it. A good starting point is to develop one page that captures the structure of the paper—that is, a list of section headings that can be subsequently developed to include subheadings and key points. Although this has a linear feel to it, the reality is that writing is an iterative process in which the different sections are written and refined in an interconnected fashion. The exact headings you use will be influenced by the type of paper you are writing, but the following list is general enough to be a useful beginning:

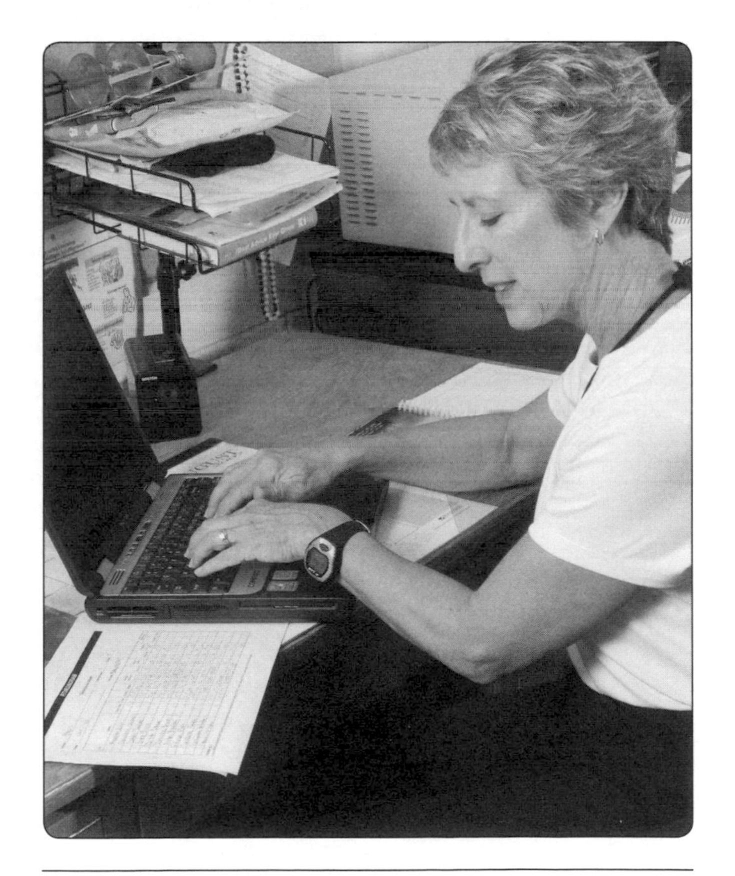

Scheduling blocks of time to write takes discipline, but will pay off in the long run.

- Title
- Abstract
- Background, introduction, or literature review
- Research aims, purpose, question, objective, intent, and hypothesis

- Methods
- Results
- Discussion
- Summary or conclusion
- References

Given that writing can begin well before the research has been completed, after determining a working title, it is worthwhile to focus initially on the areas of background, introduction, and literature review. This is because research planning requires that you will already have reviewed existing literature to determine the state of knowledge as it relates to your intended work. This review will be the basis of this early section. If you have not already done so, the first step could be to make notes of key points, findings, strengths, weaknesses, and the like on a blank sheet clipped to the front of each paper you will include in this section of your article.

Just as you need to plan the overall structure of the paper, you also need to plan the structure and flow of each section, particularly the introduction. Use subheadings to organize your thoughts, even though they may not appear as subheadings in the text. For example, in a paper focused on changes in self-efficacy experienced by patients with multiple sclerosis (MS) following MT, you might wish to include information on the following in your introduction:

- Definition and description of the disease
- Incidence and prevalence
- Classifications of disease
- Pathophysiology and medical treatment
- Commonly presented features, with those of greatest relevance to MT highlighted
- Theoretical basis for MT intervention
- Review of research related to the outcomes of MT in MS patients

Of course, the scope and depth of the review will be influenced by the type of paper you are submitting and the journal's requirements. Regardless of this, you should remember that this section sets the scene for how your own research will be presented in the sections that follow. The reader should be able to see how your research fits with previous studies and why it is important. The introduction should flow logically forward, so the reader appreciates the context, reason, and sense of what you will describe in the aims section.

Whether the aim or purpose is a section in its own right or appears at the end of the introduction or the beginning of the methods section, it should be a concise statement that captures the essence of what you set out to do. Although short, it is critical. It is what has guided your research, and it is what readers will refer back to in order to determine if your research aligns with your intent. When considering your aims, remember that research is about the search for facts or truth. An aim or intent should not posit a result or bias. For example, it would be inappropriate to declare that your aim is to prove that MT results in a certain effect. Clearly, this is not an unbiased position from which to start, since the conclusion has been reached before the data are in. More appropriately, the aim might be to determine if MT has a certain effect. Note that the latter reflects neutrality, where the former suggests bias.

Having stated the aims of the research, you will describe how you achieved those aims in the methods section. That is to say, what did you do? Menard (2009) indicates that this section should describe exactly how the study was carried out with enough detail to allow the study to be repeated by others (Rosenfeldt et al. 2000). While this is ideal, it must be remembered that journal requirements will influence how much detail can be included, such that authors must balance inclusion of detailed information while simultaneously adhering to a given journal's guidelines for length. Insufficient detail in this section is, of course, likely to be criticized by reviewers. As long as decisions about what to include and what to omit are logical and guided by the need to present the research truthfully, such criticism is the kind that researchers are prepared to address.

It is useful (and sometimes required) to break down the methods section into a number of subheadings, such as study design, participants, procedures, outcome measures, and data analysis. The study design should be described in a short statement that allows the reader to classify the research, such as "the research undertaken was a single-group pretest–posttest design with follow-up 8 to 12 weeks after the last treatment was delivered" (Finch 2007). Concerning participants, you should include quantities; sampling, selection, and allocation procedures; relevant demographic information; inclusion and exclusion criteria; procedures used to form experimental or control groups; and any other particularly important characteristics.

Under the heading of procedures, the goal is to present the details of what was done, from the selection and informed consent through the treatment, such that the study could be replicated by other researchers. An important caveat is that replicability pertains to another researcher familiar with the field, and certain assumptions have to be made about what that means. If it is stated that "grade-2 peripheral joint mobilization" was used as a part of treatment, you must assume that another researcher in the same field will know what peripheral joint mobilization is, and how to apply it in a general sense.

A summary of outcome measures tells your reader the tools or methods that you used to assess your dependent variables, those things that are being measured to determine if change has occurred. This can include self-report measures of pain or anxiety, or physiological measures of stress hormones, pedal plantar pressures, or HbA1c (a hemoglobin measurement test used in diabetes), to name just a few possibilities. You need to describe the measurement tools, how they were developed, and when possible, data on their reliability and validity. This worthwhile inclusion adds credibility to your results.

Under the heading of data analysis, you need to include a clear indication of the qualitative or quantitative approaches used to interpret the data. For example, this section of a quantitative paper might inform the reader that "the data were analyzed on an intention-to-treat basis, with a focus on the differences between mean values on the Multiple Sclerosis Self-Efficacy survey before and after treatment. Inferential testing was conducted using a paired *t*-test." Note that this section speaks to the management of the data; the research findings are not presented until the results section, which comes next.

The methods section answered the question "What did you do?" Similarly, the results section answers the question "What did you find?" The section must be straightforward. As Johnson (2008) notes, accuracy is of utmost importance. Duplication is to be avoided. Rather, any text, tables, and figures must complement each other. They must also be easily understood. Above all, do not clutter and distract the reader with background data that are not essential to the central findings. Resist the urge to discuss your findings in this section; save this for the aptly named discussion section that follows.

In the discussion section, you should not reiterate your findings. Rather, this is the place to evaluate the results of your study in the context of existing knowledge and theory and to note the implications of your findings. Your discussion should lead the reader logically toward the conclusion or summary. Sometimes, this is drawn out as a separate subsection, but at the very least, it should appear as a closing paragraph or two in the discussion. It is also important to address the limitations of your work and to suggest future studies that ought to be conducted, given what you found. Remember that knowledge evolves and is cumulative. Good research points the way to subsequent research that will further enhance the knowledge base.

Finally, there is the reference section. It might seem surprising, but this is often the first section reviewers will read. This is particularly so if the reviewers are very familiar with the area of research being presented, since they will be aware of the key studies that probably ought to be cited.

It is essential to present reference citations accurately and in accordance with the referencing system required by the target journal. Remember that readers may wish to follow up and obtain some of the studies you have referenced. You need to facilitate this by maintaining accuracy. Do not wait until the rest of the paper is finished before beginning to assemble the reference section. This task should begin at the point you start to search the literature, before you embark on your own research. Keep track of the references you come across and their key findings. Early attention to this will be time well spent that will make completing the reference section a lot less stressful.

WRITING STYLE

Experts generally agree that when writing a paper for publication, or indeed in any scientific writing, simplicity is desirable (Fahy 2008; Lee 2008). Additionally, an active voice should be used. Authors should strive for "accuracy, clarity, and brevity" (Johnson 2008). These tenets should inform careful choice of words, sentence structure, and paragraph structure, packaged such that the paper flows logically from introduction to conclusion. A useful strategy is for the writer to try to anticipate what questions readers might have as they read the paper, and to answer those questions in the paper as they arise. And, while it is important to acknowledge the limitations of your study, remember that it is also important to accentuate its positive aspects and the value of the work. When you submit a paper for publication you are, in essence, attempting to convince the editor and reviewers of its value.

As you move toward the first draft and beyond, colleagues with experience in scientific writing will be invaluable. Remember that the first draft of a paper represents the core text (Johnson 2008), but it is by no means a finished product. A manuscript may go through a dozen or more drafts before it is a completed, polished paper (Rosenfeldt et al. 2000). Do not be discouraged by this—it is a normal part of the publication process, and there is reward in seeing each version become progressively more refined. However, there comes a point when the document must be submitted. That point is when the edits that are generated result in wording changes, but do not substantially improve the paper. When this point has been reached, have a trusted colleague review the paper a final time and then put it aside for a while before revisiting it. If it passes muster, you can bask, at least for a moment, in a job well done.

SUMMARY

Writing journal articles relates to the adoption of an evidence-informed approach to MT practice in which conducting research, writing articles, reading articles, and applying findings to clinical problems becomes the rule rather than the exception.

If an evidence-informed, scholarly approach to MT is to thrive, then the norms of practice must shift. Practitioners must begin to see the time necessary to write and read articles, and to search the literature, as bona fide activities within the working day, and practice schedules must accommodate this. Practices must be planned such that access to electronic databases is easily accomplished on-site and relations with local library facilities are established and maintained. Subscriptions to key journals must be seen as legitimate and essential practice expenses. And, above all, a reflective approach to care must be adopted.

Evidence shows that two of the main barriers to evidence-informed practice in health care are time and access (Green and Ruff 2005). Additionally, energy and willingness to step into new and sometimes uncomfortable territory are essential components of developing new practice norms, which includes presenting the findings of our work in the form of journal articles. This is the challenge, and the opportunity, we face in continuing to advance our profession.

Critical Thinking Questions

1. What are the personal benefits to the author of publishing a journal article? What are the professional benefits to the author of publishing a journal article? How does the profession benefit when an author publishes an article? Provide at least two answers for each specific question.
2. List and describe at least three different types of journal articles.
3. What is *peer review,* and what purpose does it serve?
4. How should an author go about the process of selecting a journal for possible publication? Indicate at least three strategies and relevant considerations.
5. A general guideline in publishing research is that the author's methods should be described as completely and accurately as possible. Explain why this is important.

REFERENCES

Appleton, J.V., and D. Ratnaike. 2008. Sharing evidence: Community practitioners writing for publication. *Community Practitioner* 81(12): 22-25.

Fahy, K. 2008. Writing for publication: The basics. *Women and Birth* 21(2): 86-91.

Finch, P. 2007. Changes in the self-efficacy of multiple sclerosis clients following massage therapy. *J Bodyw Mov Ther* 11(3): 267-272.

Finch, P., and P. Becker. 2007. The evidence funnel: Highlighting the importance of research literacy in evidence based complementary health care. *J Bodyw Mov Ther* 11(1): 78-81.

Green, M.L., and T.R. Ruff. 2005. Why do residents fail to answer their clinical questions? A qualitative study of barriers to practicing evidence-based medicine. *Acad Med* 80(2): 176-182.

Johnson, T.M. 2008. Tips on how to write a paper. *J Am Acad Dermatol* 59(6): 1064-1069.

Keen, A. 2007. "Writing for publication: pressures, barriers and support strategies." *Nurse Educ Today* 27(5):382-388.

Lee, S.S. 2008. How to write a paper: An editor's tips. *Liver Int* 28(4): 421-422.

Menard, M.B. 2009. *Making sense of research.* 2nd ed. Toronto: Curties Overzet.

Rosenfeldt, F.L., J.T. Dowling, S. Pepe, and M.J. Fullerton. 2000. How to write a paper for publication. *Heart Lung Circ* 9(2): 82-87.

Rosenthal, R. 1998. Writing meta-analytic reviews. In *Methodological issues and strategies in clinical research,* 2nd ed., ed. A.E. Kazdin, 767-790. Washington, DC: American Psychological Association.

Sackett, D.L., S.E. Straits, W.S. Richardson, W. Rosenberg, and R.B. Haynes. 2000. *Evidence based medicine: How to practice and teach EBM.* 2nd ed. Toronto: Churchill-Livingston.

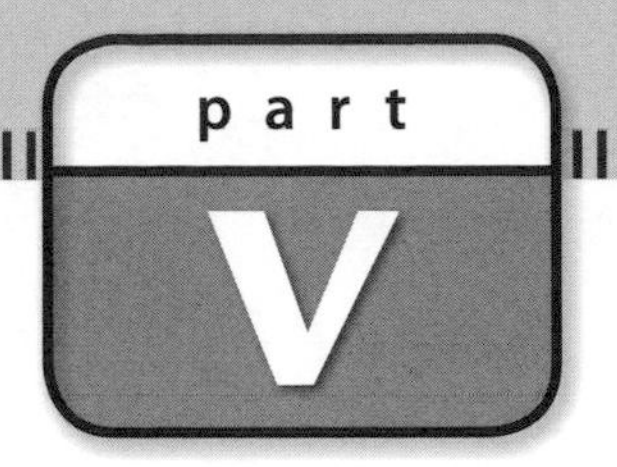

FUTURE DIRECTIONS

Where will the continued integration of research and practice lead the profession? Though this cannot be known for certain, the chapters presented here examine some of the most promising areas. In addition, the final chapter also identifies some of the dilemmas that have occasionally prevented massage therapy research from making the greatest possible progress, in the hope that they can be avoided or overcome heading forward.

chapter 22

Attitudes, Beliefs, and Expectations in Massage Therapy

Karen T. Boulanger, MS, CMT
Christopher A. Moyer, PhD

To best understand how massage therapy (MT) works and to optimize clients' subjective experiences and health benefits derived from this form of treatment, it is essential that the profession increase its scientific knowledge concerning the influence of attitudes, beliefs, and expectations. These factors undoubtedly affect a individual's decision to try new treatments, such that an increased understanding of their significance could improve the MT profession's ability to connect with and encourage people who have not yet experienced massage. In addition, evidence from the study of other therapeutic practices is increasingly demonstrating the importance of attitudes, beliefs, and expectations in affecting treatment outcomes (Finniss et al. 2010; Rothman and Salovey 1997; Apanovitch, McCarthy, and Salovey 2003; Thompson, Nanni, and Levine 1994; Scrimshaw, Engle, and Zambrana 1983). This chapter reviews the limited amount of research that has been conducted on attitudes, beliefs, and expectations about MT and recommends directions for subsequent research.

ATTITUDES, BELIEFS, AND EXPECTATIONS DEFINED AND DIFFERENTIATED

Though attitudes, beliefs, and expectations are concepts that can reasonably be considered to overlap, it is also true that they can be meaningfully differentiated. A *belief* is something that we think of as probable or true; for example, a person may believe that MT promotes relaxation. An *attitude* is an overall evaluation of our beliefs about something. People who believe that MT promotes relaxation might simultaneously see little value in relaxation, such that they believe MT is relaxing but have a generally neutral attitude about this. Alternately, and probably more likely, these people might see great value in relaxation, which would lead to a positive attitude toward MT for promoting relaxation. An *expectation* is a prediction about the outcome of an action or event; people might expect that a MT session will help them to relax.

belief
▸ Something that is thought of as probable or true.

attitude
▸ An overall evaluation of beliefs.

expectation
▸ A prediction about the outcome of an action or an event.

INFLUENTIAL MODELS NOT YET APPLIED TO MASSAGE THERAPY

health belief model

▸ A theory that attempts to explain health behaviors as a function of the person's belief that there is a threat to their health, combined with their belief that a specific health behavior may reduce that threat.

theory of planned behavior

▸ A theory that attempts to explain behavior as a function of a person's specific attitudes toward, and expectations of, that behavior.

self-efficacy

▸ The belief that one can perform a particular action or meet a particular goal.

Several general theoretical models make use of these concepts as they apply to health and wellness. Two of the most influential and widely applied are the *Health Belief Model* (Rosenstock 1966) and the *Theory of Planned Behavior* (Fishbein and Ajzen 1975; Fishbein and Ajzen 2010). Notably, neither of these has yet been used as a framework for research with MT.

As can be seen in figure 22.1, the health belief model focuses on a person's belief that their health is being threatened and that participating in a specific health intervention could reduce that threat. For a behavior to occur, people must perceive a threat from their current behavior and must expect that they are able to engage in a new behavior that has a valued outcome at a reasonable cost. For a long-term behavior change, perceived benefits must continue to outweigh costs. In addition to a graphical depiction of the health belief model, figure 22.1 includes a hypothetical example that illustrates how a person might evaluate MT as a possible treatment for depression according to this model.

Taylor (2009) notes that "interventions that draw on the health belief model have generally supported its predictions" for a variety of practices and conditions, but observes that the model has a weakness in that it "leaves out an important component of health behavior change: the perception that one will be able to engage in the health behavior" (57). The perception that one can do a particular thing, often referred to as *self-efficacy* (Bandura 1986), is particularly important in relation to many health behaviors, such as quitting smoking (Prochaska and DiClemente 1984) or changing eating habits (Schwarzer and Renner 2000). While an interesting study suggests that clients' self-efficacy in coping with a serious chronic illness may be improved by receiving MT (Finch and Becker 2007), the importance of self-efficacy in receiving and benefitting from MT has not been studied. Similarly, the well-validated beliefs represented in the health belief model have not been applied to MT, such that we can currently only speculate on the likely importance of beliefs in the pursuit of MT for treatment of particular conditions.

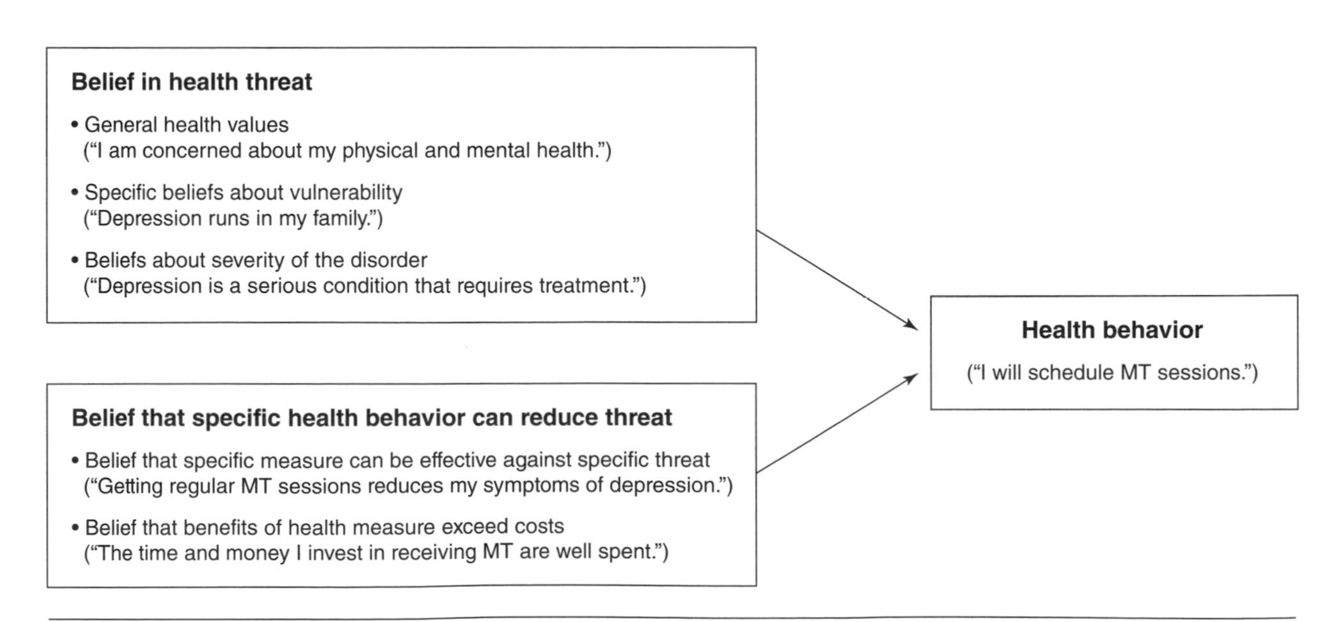

Figure 22.1 The health belief model, including a hypothetical example of how a a person might evaluate MT as a possible treatment for depression.

The theory of planned behavior acknowledges the importance of intentions and of the individual's actual control over a particular health behavior. Figure 22.2 illustrates this theory, including a hypothetical illustration of how it may apply to the use of MT for the treatment of anxiety.

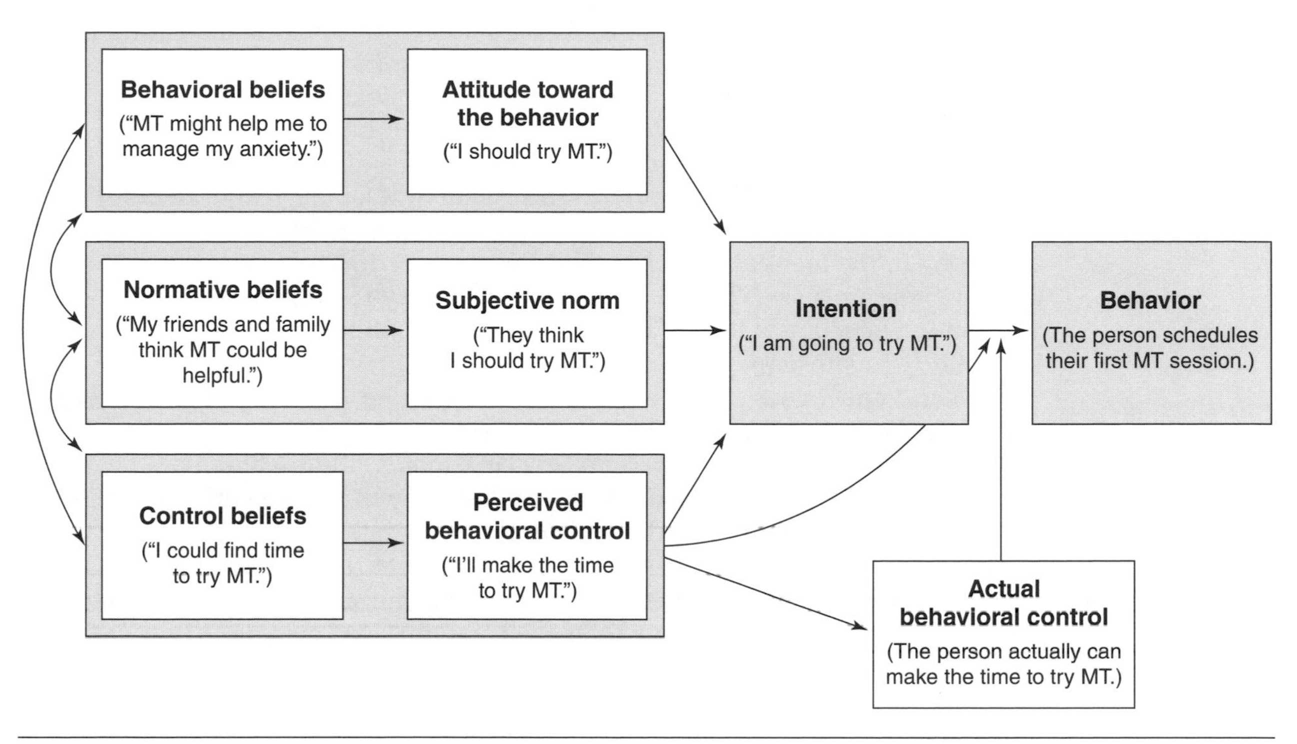

Figure 22.2 The theory of planned behavior, including a hypothetical example of how a person might evaluate MT as a possible treatment for anxiety.

This model has been shown to predict a wide range of important health behaviors, including testicular self-examination, reduction of soft-drink intake, use of sunscreen, and many others (Taylor 2009). An examination of its applicability to MT would undoubtedly be a valuable addition to the research literature.

EXISTING RESEARCH

Several studies have examined the role of attitudes, beliefs, and expectations within the context of massage therapy. These have included qualitative and quantitative approaches. They have examined these characteristics in massage recipients and massage therapists, as well as the interaction between recipients and therapists.

Clients' Attitudes and Expectations

Though the most influential theoretical models that attempt to integrate health attitudes, behaviors, and expectations have not been applied to MT, the relationship of these individual concepts to MT has been examined in a few studies. In a study that surveyed 285 respondents to develop a standardized instrument for the assessment of attitudes toward MT (Moyer and Rounds 2009), two distinct attitudes emerged. One is the degree to which a person sees MT as healthful and the other is the degree to which a person sees MT as pleasant. Respondents also completed standardized assessment of personality traits, which revealed that the traits most associated with vulnerability to anxiety and depression (neuroticism, and behavioral inhibition or anxiety) were predictive of less positive attitudes toward MT. Though these relationships were not surprising, they are unfortunate, given that MT shows great promise as a treatment for anxiety and depression (see chapter 13).

As such, it may be particularly important to explore strategies and informational materials that can help neurotic and anxious persons overcome their (possibly mistaken) attitude that MT is not or will not be pleasant. An additional set of questions administered in this study asked respondents about their preferences concerning the gender of their massage therapist and about any fear that they could become sexually aroused during a session of MT. Male respondents showed a strong average preference for female massage therapists, while in both men and women, the fear of becoming sexually aroused during a massage was correlated with neuroticism. The development of an easy-to-administer and validated assessment instrument for MT attitudes should permit further exploration of their importance in subsequent research.

Tsao and colleagues (2005) included MT with several other possible interventions in a study that assessed the expectations of 45 children who were chronic pain patients, as well as their parents' expectations. Children had more favorable expectations of medication and relaxation than they did for the other treatments, including MT. Their parents indicated similar expectations, though a comparison of the children's and parents' responses showed that the children's expectations of therapies nominally included in the category of complementary and alternative medicine were less positive than their parents'. In this study, that category included MT, hypnosis, acupuncture, yoga, and relaxation.

A recent qualitative study (Smith, Sullivan, and Baxter 2009) explored attributes of MT that were most valued by repeat clients. Focus groups conducted with a total of 19 MT clients, 17 of whom were female, resulted in the identification of six key elements (time for care and personal attention, an engaging and competent therapist, a trust partnership, holism and empowerment, effective touch, and enhancement of relaxation), all of which were considered to be grounded in effective communication. In addition, focus group members indicated that the expectation that their treatment goals would be met served as a strong motivation for returning to MT.

Bowerman (1989) completed a dissertation that assessed recipients' expectations of MT and how they were affected by brief empathic touch, which resulted in the creation of the massage expectation scale (MES). The MES consists of seven Likert-type items. The MES was administered individually to 81 female research participants at a Los Angeles MT clinic. Next, these participants were escorted into a MT room where they disrobed and lay in a prone position covered by a sheet. A massage therapist entered and performed an introductory session of empathic touch that lasted only 60 to 90 seconds, after which a research assistant entered the room and administered the MES a second time. The massage therapist then returned to perform either a 1-hour session of manual MT, or a time-matched alternate treatment administered with a handheld mechanical massage device.

Notably, MES scores were improved for all participants simply by the 60 to 90 seconds of empathic touch that began each session of therapy. This is evidence that even brief touch, performed skillfully, can be a powerful influence on the recipient. In addition, the MES scores were significantly more improved for the participants who were randomized to receive MT, even though the empathic touch session took place before research participants knew if they would receive the

MT or treatment with the mechanical massage device. Some massage therapists who participated in the research later informed Bowerman that they did not like administering the treatment using the device. They may have unintentionally influenced the expectations of the research participants as part of the empathic touch session.

Kalauokalani and colleagues (2001) examined expectations in a randomized clinical trial of acupuncture and MT for chronic low back pain. Before participants were randomly selected to receive one treatment or the other, their expectations of these treatments were assessed. Those with higher expectations had significantly greater pre- and postreduction of low back pain. Logistic regression, including adjustment for likely confounds, showed that those with high expectations were 5.3 times more likely to improve than those with low expectations. In addition, patients with different relative expectations for acupuncture or MT had significantly better improvements if they received their preferred treatment.

Massage Therapists' Expectations

A survey of 153 massage therapists currently being conducted by Boulanger asked the respondents to rate their agreement, using Likert-type scales (1 = strongly disagree, 7 = strongly agree), for 11 statements pertaining to MT. These respondents reported generally high expectations of MT, ranging from a mean score of 5.7 for the statement "Massage therapy will help my clients to concentrate better on a task" to 6.8 for the statement "Massage therapy will help my clients to relax." This is consistent with Kaptchuk's (2002) assertion that practitioners of complementary health modalities tend to be highly optimistic about the benefits of their respective interventions. In addition, it is likely that this optimism, when communicated to clients, can facilitate a healing response (Crow et al. 1999; DiBiasi et al. 2001).

Client–Therapist Interaction

In a clinical experiment to test the role of conversation during MT and the importance of a therapeutic bond between the massage therapist and client, Moyer and colleagues (2008) arranged for 30 persons with anxiety and depressive disorders to receive five weekly sessions of professionally administered MT. In addition, they were randomly assigned to either *talk-permissive MT* or *talk-restrictive MT* conditions. This group assignment was not revealed to them until after their participation was completed. All 30 MT recipients completed a modified version of the therapeutic bond scales (Saunders, Howard, and Orlinsky 1989), a standardized self-report instrument that is typically used to quantify the quality of the therapeutic bond in psychotherapy.

talk-permissive massage therapy

▸ A condition in which massage recipients may engage in conversation with their massage therapist, without limits, during treatment.

All MT recipients tended to improve in response to MT, but improvement was significantly better when subjects reported higher levels of therapeutic bond. Higher levels of therapeutic bond also predicted greater increases in MT attitudes across the treatment period. Further, though conversation during MT did not influence outcomes by itself, the interaction of conversation and therapeutic bond did have a significant effect, such that the symptom reduction was maximized when conversation was restricted and therapeutic bond was high. MT recipients who experienced these conditions achieved clinically significant symptom reductions after only three MT sessions, and they maintained these gains a month after the cessation of treatment.

talk-restrictive massage therapy

▸ A condition in which massage recipients are politely discouraged from engaging in unnecessary conversation with their massage therapist during treatment.

DIRECTIONS FOR FUTURE RESEARCH

As previously noted, the important role of attitudes, beliefs, and expectations in the broader fields of health and wellness has been firmly established. However, only a small amount of research has examined these factors in relation to MT. In some instances, the inclusion of these factors was only supplemental, rather than the main focus of study. New research that makes one or more of these factors the focus of study should be conducted. It is likely to be fruitful, given previous findings and the highly interpersonal nature of MT.

MT research should also make use of well-validated theories, such as the health belief model and the theory of planned behavior, that have been successfully applied to a range of other health practices and interventions. This has the potential to advance our understanding of MT, including the ways it is similar to or different from related treatments that have been more extensively researched.

Most importantly, an increased understanding of the perceptions of MT by clients and potential clients has the potential to influence the practice in ways that can maximize its effectiveness and to expand its reach to the greatest number of people who stand to benefit from it. The last point may be especially important; MT's most validated effect is its ability to reduce anxiety, and this effect likely underpins several of the more specific benefits that are associated with this form of treatment (Moyer 2008). However, for several reasons, anxious people are the ones most likely to let negative attitudes, beliefs, or expectations stand in the way of trying MT. Interventions and information aimed at reducing the fears associated with trying something new may deliver great benefit to a large and underserved population.

SUMMARY

Massage therapy is a physical treatment, but it is also an intervention in which the psychosocial context plays an important role. Attitudes, beliefs, and expectations are key elements of that context, and they must be acknowledged in research and in practice to further our understanding of massage therapy and to maximize its beneficial outcomes. Finally, researchers should apply well-validated models, such as the health belief model and the theory of planned behavior, to their studies. This will aid interpretation of results and help in connecting and relating massage therapy research to the broader fields of medicine and psychology.

Critical Thinking Questions

1. What are some of the ways that attitudes, beliefs, and expectations affect treatment outcomes? Give specific and detailed examples.
2. Apply the *health belief model* to a hypothetical case of a person considering massage therapy for a specific condition.
3. Apply the *theory of planned behavior* to a hypothetical case of a person considering massage therapy for a specific condition.
4. What is *self-efficacy*, and how might it play a role in massage therapy? Give specific and detailed examples.
5. What are some of the specific attitudes about massage therapy that have been identified in research studies? Why is it important for the profession to recognize them? How do you think they should be dealt with in practice?

6. As noted in the chapter, health researcher Ted Kaptchuk asserts that practitioners of complementary health modalities tend to be highly optimistic about the benefits of their respective interventions. Discuss the pros and the cons of such optimism on the part of practitioners.
7. In your own training and practice, have you tended to emphasize a *talk-permissive* or *talk-restrictive* approach to treatment? How and why did you arrive at this style? What are the likely pros and cons of each style?

REFERENCES

Apanovitch, A.M., D. McCarthy, and P. Salovey. 2003. Using message framing to motivate HIV testing among low-income, ethnic minority women. *Health Psychol* 22(1): 60-67.

Bandura, A.J. 1986. *Social foundations of thought and action: A social cognitive theory.* Englewood Cliffs: Prentice Hall.

Bowerman, S.B. 1989. The effect of empathic touch and expectations on mood change during a therapeutic massage treatment. *Dissertation Abstracts International* 50 (10).

Crow, R., H. Gage, S. Hampson, J. Hart, A. Kimber, and H. Thomas. 1999. The role of expectancies in the placebo effect and their use in the delivery of health care: A systematic review. *Health Technol Asses* 3(3): 1-96.

DiBiasi, Z., E. Harkness, E. Ernst, A. Georgiou, and J. Kleijnen. 2001. Influence of context effects on health outcomes: A systematic review. *Lancet* 357: 757-762.

Finch, P., and P. Becker. 2007. Changes in the self-efficacy of multiple sclerosis clients following massage therapy. *J Bodyw Mov Ther* 11(3): 267-272.

Finniss, D.G., T.J. Kaptchuk, F. Miller, and F. Benedetti. 2010. Biological, clinical, and ethical advances of placebo effects. *Lancet* 375(9715): 686-695.

Fishbein, M., and I. Ajzen. 1975. *Belief, attitude, intention, and behavior: An introduction to theory and research.* Reading, MA: Addison-Wesley.

———. 2010. *Predicting and changing behavior: The reasoned action approach.* New York: Psychology Press.

Kalauokalani, D., D.C. Cherkin, K.J. Sherman, T.D. Koepsell, and R.A. Deyo. 2001. Lessons from a trial of acupuncture and massage for low back pain: Patient expectations and treatment effects. *Spine* 26(13): 1418-1424.

Kaptchuk, T.J. 2002. The placebo effect in alternative medicine: Can the performance of a healing ritual have clinical significance? *Ann Intern Med* 136: 817-825.

Moyer, C.A. 2008. Affective massage therapy. *Int J Ther Massage Bodywork* 1(2): 3-5.

Moyer, C.A., and J. Rounds. 2009. The attitudes toward massage (ATOM) scale: Reliability, validity, and associated findings. *J Bodyw Mov Ther* 13(1): 22-33.

Moyer, C.A., J. Rounds, and J. Hannum. 2008. The non-talking cure: Massage therapy's psychotherapeutic effects are associated with therapeutic bond. Poster presented at the 20th annual convention of the Association for Psychological Science. Chicago, IL. May 22-25, 2008.

Prochaska , J.O., and C.C. DiClemente. 1984. *The transtheoretical approach: Crossing traditional boundaries of therapy.* Chicago: Dow Jones/Irwin.

Rosenstock, I.M. 1966. Why people use health services. *Milbank Meml Fund Q* 44(3): S94-S127.

Rothman, A.J., and P. Salovey. 1997. Shaping perceptions to motivate healthy behavior: The role of message framing. *Psychol Bull* 121(1): 3-19.

Saunders, S.M., K.I. Howard, and D.E. Orlinsky. 1989. The therapeutic bond scales: Psychometric characteristics and relationship to treatment effectiveness. *Psychol Assessment* 1(4): 323-330.

Schwarzer, R., and B. Renner. 2000. Social-cognitive predictors of health behavior: Action self-efficacy and coping self-efficacy. *Health Psychol* 19(5): 487-495.

Scrimshaw, S.M., P.L. Engle, and R.E. Zambrana. 1983. Prenatal anxiety and birth outcome in U.S. Latinas: implications for psychosocial interventions. Paper presented at the annual meeting of the American Psychological Association, Anaheim, California, August 26-30.

Smith, J.M., S.J. Sullivan, and G.D. Baxter. 2009. The culture of massage therapy: Valued elements and the role of comfort, contact, connection, and caring. *Complement Ther Med* 17(4): 181-189.

Taylor, S.E. 2009. *Health psychology.* 7th ed. New York: McGraw-Hill.

Thompson, S.C., C. Nanni, and A. Levine. 1994. Primary versus secondary and central versus consequence-related control in HIV-positive men. *J Pers Soc Psychol* 67(3): 540-547.

Tsao, J.C.I., M. Meldrum, B. Bursch, M.C. Jacob, S.C. Kim, and L.K. Zeltzer. 2005. Treatment expectations for cam interventions in pediatric chronic pain patients and their parents. *Evid-Based Complement Alternat Med* 2(4): 521-527.

Directions and Dilemmas in Massage Therapy Research

A Workshop Report From the 2009 North American Research Conference on Complementary and Integrative Medicine[1]

Christopher A. Moyer, PhD
Trish Dryden, MEd, RMT
Stacey Shipwright, BA, RMT

While we were working on this book, we also collaborated to conduct a workshop at the 2009 North American Research Conference on Complementary and Integrative Medicine. We were lucky that our workshop was well attended by some of the most knowledgeable, experienced, and enthusiastic persons connected with massage therapy and related health modalities. We were also grateful that they helped us to take stock of the state of massage therapy research, which we published as an article in the *International Journal of Therapeutic Massage and Bodywork*. Though we hadn't planned it, we later realized that this timely article makes all of the points that we needed to emphasize in our final chapter.

Though the practice of massage therapy (MT) is very old, it is only in the last 20 years or so that scientific research on it has begun to accumulate. And, while this growing body of research has certainly refined our understanding of MT and its effects, it is also true that it has serious shortcomings that hamper the field's progress. To best ensure that the next 20 years of MT research will be of maximum value, we endeavored to take stock of established findings, determine what new research is most needed, and identify consistent weaknesses that need to be

[1]Reprinted from C.A. Moyer, T. Dryden, and S. Shipwright, 2009, "Directions and dilemmas in massage therapy research: A workshop report from the 2009 North American Research Conference on Complementary and Integrative Medicine," *International Journal of Therapeutic Massage & Bodywork: Research, Education, & Practice* 2(2): 15-27.

The authors thank the participants in our workshop at the 2009 North American Research Conference on Complementary and Integrative Medicine Conference. We also thank Glenn M. Hymel and Karen T. Boulanger for their helpful feedback in response to a draft of this report.

addressed in this field. Logically, discussion of these topics should also lead to the identification of other issues that have the potential to inform the next two decades of MT research.

The 2009 North American Conference on Complementary and Integrative Medicine was a rare opportunity to assemble MT researchers, educators, and practitioners, and other health care practitioners who work interprofessionally with MT. We seized this opportunity by conducting an interactive, participatory workshop to identify needed directions and current dilemmas in MT research. This report presents the results of that workshop.

METHOD

On Wednesday, May 13th, 2009, the authors of the present report facilitated a 90-minute workshop titled *Directions and Dilemmas in Massage Therapy Research* at the 2009 North American Research Conference on Complementary and Integrative Medicine in Minneapolis, MN. Thirty-seven workshop participants (see appendix) were asked to form subgroups of three to six people and to take approximately 5 minutes to introduce themselves to each other and to record their names, institutional affiliations, and e-mail addresses on a provided handout. Next, the facilitators spent approximately 15 minutes presenting a general overview of MT research progress covering the 20-year time period from 1988 to 2008. Finally, the remainder of the scheduled time was conducted by means of a modified Delphi method (Dalkey 1969), in which the subgroups generated responses to topics provided by the facilitators; subsequently, after each individual topic was addressed in the subgroups, the entire group reconvened to hear the subgroups' responses, recognize consensus (or lack thereof) among subgroup responses, and engage in brief discussion.

The facilitators prepared five topics with corresponding instructions for the subgroups:

1. *Established MT research findings.* Indicate MT effects, mechanisms, processes, or other details that are already relatively well understood as a result of research.
2. *Needed MT research.* Indicate MT effects, mechanisms, processes, or other details that are most in need of research.
3. *Methodological strengths in MT research.* Indicate ways in which MT research, as a field, has made good use of scientific methods, tools, and approaches to optimally increase our knowledge of MT.
4. *Methodological weaknesses and limitations in MT research.* Indicate ways in which MT research, as a field, has failed to use scientific methods, tools, and approaches to optimally increase our knowledge of MT.
5. *Conclusions.* After considering what MT has and has not accomplished in the previous 20 years, what, as a field, is most important for us to consider as we go forward in the next 20 years?

During the workshop, the decision was made to skip topic number three, on methodological strengths, due to time limitations. The remaining topics were addressed in the order presented, with approximately an equal amount of time devoted to each.

Three techniques were used during the full-group portions of the workshop to ensure clear and accurate communication and recording of information. First, when subgroups were reporting their contributions to the larger group, we attempted to verbally reiterate these, and provided the subgroups with the opportunity to refine or restate their contributions in response to these reiterations. Second, we used an easel pad to visually organize and summarize the contributions of the subgroups. Third, after informing participants that we would do so, we used a shareware digital recording program (Audacity 1.2.6) running on a personal computer, attached to an outboard boundary microphone, to make an audio recording of the entire 90-minute workshop.

MT Research Overview, 1988 to 2008

Prior to the participatory portion of the workshop, the information in this section was presented to provide an overview of and context for the previous 20 years of MT research. This helped ensure that a diverse group of participants would begin the workshop with a common knowledge base. Approximately 15 minutes total were devoted to covering the four topics that follow.

Quantity of MT Research

There has been a rapid increase in MT research during the 20-year period from 1988 to 2008. Proof of this can be demonstrated by a year-to-year search in any one of a number of scholarly or scientific databases, such as PubMed, PsycInfo, or CINAHL. However, for present purposes, we selected the publicly accessible and wide-ranging Google Scholar database (http://scholar.google.com), which allows anyone with basic Internet access to replicate our procedure.

As shown in figure 23.1, the quantity of documents retrieved with the keyword "massage therapy" in the three most relevant Google Scholar subcategories increases dramatically during this time period. Note, however, that these raw

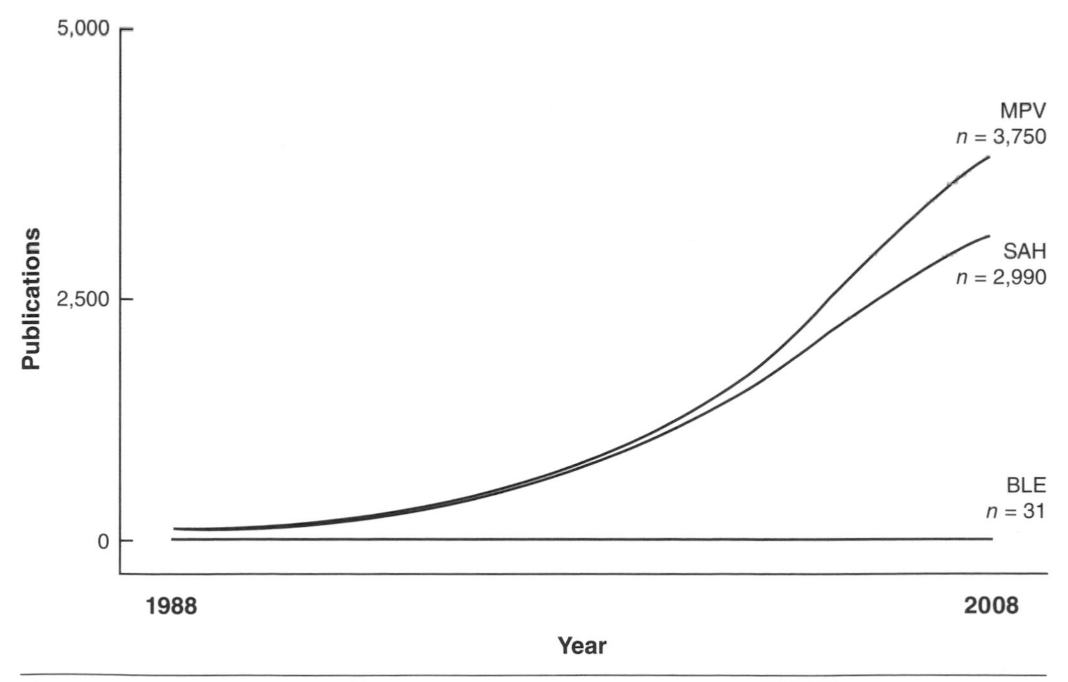

Figure 23.1 Number of Documents Retrieved, in a Year-by-Year Search With the Key Phrase "Massage Therapy," From Three Google Scholar database categories. BLE = Biology, Life sciences, and Environmental science; MPV = Medicine, Pharmacology, and Veterinary science; SAH = Social sciences, Arts, and Humanities.

numbers can be misleading; only a small portion of these retrieved documents are original research, and only a portion of those will be research of high quality. For example, a 2004 study identified only 37 MT studies of sufficient quality for inclusion in a meta-analysis (Moyer, Rounds, and Hannum et al. 2004). However, even with this in mind, the overall trend is still evident; the quantity of scholarly and scientific writing on MT has increased rapidly during the previous 20 years.

At first glance, this appears to be remarkable progress; there are now several thousand MT documents when, just 20 years ago, there were essentially none. But before we can be certain that our field is entitled to a self-congratulatory pat on the back for such amazing progress and impressive present-day totals, a comparison that puts these results in context would be useful. Is this pattern of results unique to MT, or would we find this general pattern for any number of related searches we might conduct? Similarly, we might question whether the remarkably low numbers in the earliest years are an accurate representation of the state of MT research during that time period, given that they could just as easily be an artifact rooted in the idiosyncrasies and relative newness of this particular database.

Though many comparisons are possible (and we encourage interested readers to make them), we believe that psychotherapy is a logical choice due to the many parallels that exist between these forms of therapy. For instance, both forms of treatment share the following characteristics:

1. They have existed for considerable time.
2. They have scientifically documented effects.
3. No clear scientific consensus exists on the mechanisms that underlie their effects.
4. They have numerous schools and approaches in which therapists are trained that guide their assumptions and selection of specific techniques.
5. They have numerous structural similarities, including typical session length, number of sessions that make up a course of treatment, and the likelihood of repeated, private interpersonal contact between therapist and patient (Moyer, Rounds, and Hannum 2004).

As can be seen in figure 23.2, the same search procedures conducted with the keyword "psychotherapy" yields a very different result; there are so many more documents that it is necessary to change the scale of the vertical axis so that results can be displayed in the tens of thousands, instead of just thousands. For these results, it makes sense to display linear regression lines rather than the raw data, which serves to smooth out minor retrieval anomalies that can result when the search yield is large. Clearly, there has been much more scholarly writing and scientific research on psychotherapy than there has been on massage therapy, such that the result of this comparison is humbling.

In sum, it is undeniably true that MT research progressed dramatically in these 20 years. At the same time, though, it is also true that our field is probably far behind where it could be, and that it has a long way to go. It is important for us to recognize that MT research is still in its infancy.

MT Research Reviews

A number of MT research reviews were published during this time period. While a detailed account of them is beyond the scope of the current report, it is worth noting that the results of narrative MT research reviews (in which review authors rely heavily on the written conclusions of the original studies) and those of quantitative MT research reviews (in which review authors measure treatment effects by apply-

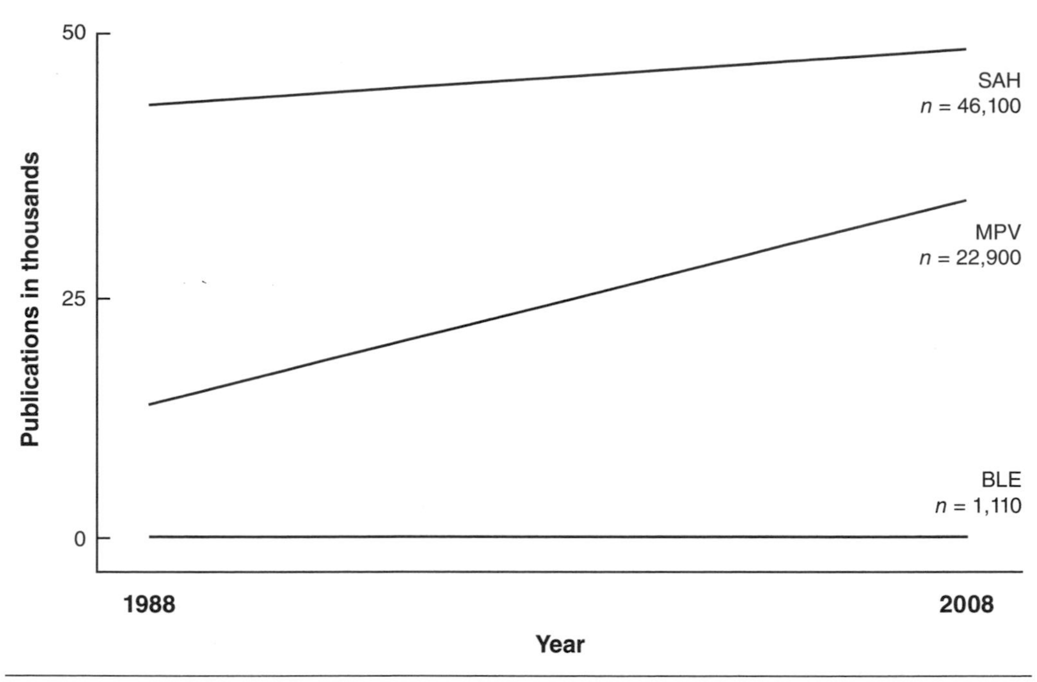

Figure 23.2 Linear Regression Lines Corresponding to Documents Retrieved, in a Year-by-Year Search with the Keyword "Psychotherapy," from Three Google Scholar database categories.

ing statistical procedures to the actual data reported in the original studies) often diverge in their basic findings. Table 23.1 highlights some of these discrepancies.

Meetings to Determine Directions for MT Research

There have been at least two important meetings that have attempted to chart the direction for research on MT and related therapies. In 2002, the American Massage Therapy Foundation (now known as the Massage Therapy Foundation) reported the conclusions of its Massage Therapy Research Agenda Workgroup (Kahn 2002),

Table 23.1 Comparison of Basic Conclusions Reached by Narrative and Quantitative Massage Therapy Research Reviews

Narrative MT research reviews	Quantitative MT research reviews
MT facilitates growth in newborns.[2,3,4]	"Evidence that massage for preterm infants is of benefit for developmental outcomes is weak and does not warrant wider use of preterm infant massage."[5]
MT reduces pain.[2,4]	MT produces generally small reductions of pain in adult recipients,[1] but appears to have a large specific effect on arthritis pain in children.[6]
MT increases alertness.[2,4]	This effect is unexamined in quantitative reviews.
MT reduces anxiety and depression.[2,4]	MT consistently produces moderate to large reductions of anxiety and depression in children[6] and adults.[1]
MT enhances immune function.[2,4]	MT shows no effect on immunity in children;[6] in adults, this effect is unexamined in quantitative reviews.
MT reduces cortisol levels.[2,4]	MT shows little to no effect on cortisol levels in children[6] or adults.[1]

[1](Moyer, Rounds, and Hannum 2004); [2](Field 1998); [3](Field 1992); [4](Field, Diego, and Hernandez-Reif 2007); [5](Vickers et al. 2004); [6](Beider and Moyer 2007)

which emphasized five main recommendations for the field. Specifically, it was recommended that the field do the following:

1. Build a research infrastructure within the massage therapy profession.
2. Fund research into the safety and efficacy of massage therapy.
3. Fund studies of physiological or other mechanisms by which massage therapy achieves its effects (including the dubious recommendation that this include exploration of so-called "subtle energy").
4. Fund studies stemming from a wellness paradigm.
5. Fund studies of the profession of therapeutic massage, including what makes a good or great massage therapist and what contributes to a positive therapeutic encounter.

In general, these recommendations do seem to have driven meaningful progress in MT research, including the establishment of several Massage Therapy Foundation initiatives, such as their research grant program, separate student and practitioner case report contests, the *International Journal of Therapeutic Massage and Bodywork,* and the MT-specific research conference detailed later in this report.

In 2005, the National Center for Complementary and Alternative Medicine (NCCAM) sponsored the Conference on the Biology of Manual Therapies to bring together U.S. and Canadian health experts and members of academic, patient advocacy, and professional organizations to assess current knowledge and identify opportunities for further research in manual therapies, such as massage therapy and chiropractic and osteopathic manipulation. Numerous directions for research were organized under three main headings corresponding to (1) general questions pertaining to mechanisms of action for massage therapy (e.g., Does paraspinal tissue have any unique physiology compared to appendicular tissues?), (2) questions relating to peripheral mechanisms of action for manual therapy (e.g., How do various manual therapies affect peripheral nerve biomechanics?), and (3) questions relating to central mechanisms of action for manual therapy (e.g., Do different types of manual therapies evoke different patterns of neural activity in the central nervous system or autonomic nervous system?). Apart from its intended influence on NCCAM's research agenda and funding priorities for manual therapies, the impact of this fairly recent and more broadly focused conference is difficult to assess. It should be noted, though, that the broader focus of this conference may have been its most valuable element, given that it required attendees "to step out of [their] individual disciplines and look together at what [they] collectively know about the effects of manual therapeutic techniques" (Kahn 2005).

MT-Specific Research Conferences

While there have been scientific conferences concerned with the broader field of touch-based therapies (most notably, the outstanding 2002 and 2004 International Symposiums on the Science of Touch), the first MT-specific research conference was not held until 2005 in Albuquerque, New Mexico. The *Highlighting Massage Therapy Research in Complementary and Alternative Medicine* conference (Massage Therapy Foundation 2005) combined terrific networking opportunities with a healthy amount of quality research presentations, and demonstrated that there is sufficient interest and activity in MT research to support a dedicated conference. The recent announcement of a second such conference to be held in 2010 in Seattle, Washington, is an exciting development (Massage Therapy Foundation 2010).

In sum, MT research progressed rapidly between 1988 and 2008, and there is now sufficient interest and productivity to support the first conferences and journals dedicated to research in the field. At the same time, it must be acknowledged that, where research is concerned, the field is still in its earliest stages. In a comparative sense, MT is significantly behind fields that have their own research infrastructure. This perspective, presented to workshop participants, set the stage for the discussion of subsequent topics.

RESULTS

Established Effects

Directed to "indicate MT effects, mechanisms, processes, or other details that are already relatively well understood as a result of research," workshop subgroups chose the following conclusions as their most important ones to report to the full group. The order in which they were discussed in the workshop is preserved in this section of the report. However, the format and time limitations of the workshop did not allow for the provision of specific references; these were researched and added when this report was written.

Effect on Mood

MT's effect on mood was nominated as an established effect. Note, however, that workshop time limitations did not allow detailed discussion of the fact that MT's effect on negative mood does not attain statistical significance when quantitatively reviewed in adult (Moyer, Rounds, and Hannum 2004) or child (Beider and Moyer 2007) populations.

Reduction of Musculoskeletal Pain, Including Low Back Pain

MT is known to reduce some forms of musculoskeletal pain. It was noted that assessment of MT's effect on pain more generally can be problematic, because averaging or otherwise combining the results of MT for different painful conditions may not be justifiable if it means that a robust effect on one condition may be washed out when combined with MT's lack of effect on another condition. For instance, a Cochrane review of MT for low back pain indicates that this form of treatment "might be beneficial for patients with subacute and chronic nonspecific low back pain" (Furlan et al. 2008), while another Cochrane review of MT for mechanical neck disorders concludes that "no recommendations for practice can be made at this time because the effectiveness of massage for neck pain remains uncertain" (Haraldsson et al. 2006). A very recent study of MT for chronic neck pain, which has not yet been incorporated to the continually updated Cochrane reviews, finds that "therapeutic massage is safe and may have benefits for treating chronic neck pain, at least in the short term" (Sherman et al. 2009).

Reduction of Anxiety

MT's effect on anxiety was noted as one of its most well-established effects (Moyer, Rounds, and Hannum 2004; Beider and Moyer 2007). Further, one of the subgroups echoed a point made in a recent IJTMB editorial, which noted that it may be especially important because it may be a main effect that is the basis for a host of other, secondary effects associated with MT (Moyer 2008b).

Arthritis

MT's beneficial effects for arthritis were nominated as an established effect, and there is evidence to support this. However, it is remarkable how little research is actually available on MT for arthritis, given the prevalence of the condition (Hootman and Helmick 2006; Hootman et al. 2006) and the promising results for MT in two studies. In a 1997 study of children suffering from mild to moderate juvenile rheumatoid arthritis (Field et al. 1997), MT greatly outperformed relaxation therapy for reducing the pain associated with this condition. Similarly, a more recent study of adults with osteoarthritis of the knee (Perlman et al. 2006) found that MT significantly outperformed a wait-list control condition for reducing pain and improving physical functioning.

Lymphedema

Reduction of lymphedema, the swelling of a limb due to a blockage of the lymphatic system, was offered as an established MT effect. A large-scale (n = 299) prospective study of multimodal treatment for lymphedema concluded that lymphatic MT in combination with other treatments, such as compression bandaging, remedial exercises, and skin care, was highly effective (Dicken et al. 1998). In addition, MT is endorsed by the Mayo Clinic as a treatment for lymphedema (Mayo Clinic 2007).

Amelioration of the Effects of Cancer Treatment

The diagnosis of cancer and its associated treatments are stressful to the patient (Spiegel 1997; Hobbie et al. 2000). MT, while not a treatment for cancer itself, can be effective in combating the stressful effects of the diagnosis and treatment. A number of studies (Wilkie et al. 2000; Weinrich and Weinrich 1990; Cassileth and Vickers 2004; Grealish, Lomansey, and Whiteman 2000; Kutner et al. 2008; Myers, Walton, and Small 2008; Billhult, Bergbom, and Stener-Victorin 2007; Post-White et al. 2009) suggest there may be specific effects of particular benefit to cancer patients, including reductions of anxiety, nausea, and pain, and improvements in appetite and sleep.

Stress Reduction

MT's ability to reduce stress was nominated as an established effect. Taken at face value, this seems obvious, but in scientific practice, the concept of stress reduction has been operationally defined in so many ways that it may be difficult to say precisely what it is (Ong, Linden, and Young 2004). In a recent review, the stress-reducing effects of MT were examined by means of treatment-induced changes in physiological parameters, such as cortisol level, heart rate, and blood pressure. Findings were mixed, and the researchers observed that the primary studies generally lack "the necessary scientific rigor to provide a definitive understanding of the effect massage therapy has on many physiological variables associated with stress" (Moraska et al. 2008). Based on currently available evidence, it may be pragmatic to consider MT to be a form of emotion-focused coping (Folkman et al. 1986) that works by improving a recipient's affective state (Moyer 2008b), which, in turn, reduces the perceived effect of negative stressors.

Increased Oxytocin

Oxytocin is a neuropeptide that plays a key role in mammalian social attachment and affiliation (Kosfeld et al. 2005). MT may, under certain conditions, lead to an increase of oxytocin that would be consistent with feelings of well-being, prosocial behavior, and the promotion of health. In a fascinating study that examined the interactions of physical contact and trust, Morhenn and colleagues (2008) found that 15-minute doses of moderate-pressure MT increased oxytocin levels if they were followed by an intentional act of trust performed during an experimental procedure known as the "trust game." Further, these MT recipients who participated in the trust game made larger altruistic sacrifices of money during the game than persons who played without first receiving MT. Increased oxytocin was not observed in a group of participants who only received MT, nor in the group that played the trust game without first receiving MT.

How Should We Define "Well Understood?"

After briefly discussing these well-understood effects, workshop participants raised the question: How, exactly, should we define *well understood?* While there is no simple answer, the question is an important one for our field to consider. MT's effect on anxiety is probably the one that is best supported by scientific evidence, and that effect has only been examined in a few dozen high-quality studies, while some other effects nominated as well understood have only been studied a handful of times. The concept of *well understood* can probably only be applied in a relative way. For example, within our field, it would be accurate to say that MT's effect on anxiety is better understood than MT's effect on arthritis, based simply on the number of studies that have examined each of these effects. And, while comparisons across fields are conceptually harder to make, it would almost certainly be accurate to say that MT is not as well understood as psychotherapy, which is also a conclusion that is based on the number of studies that have examined each of these forms of treatment. In either case, it should be clear that further research is needed, even on these well-understood effects.

Needed Research

Next, subgroups reconvened and worked together to indicate MT effects, mechanisms, processes, or other details that are most in need of research. The following are those they considered important enough to report to the entire group, and are presented here in the same order as discussed in the workshop, with the exception of a topic that the present authors have moved to the conclusions section for organizational purposes.

Multidimensional Studies

Workshop participants believed that individual MT studies have too often been limited to one type of outcome, where examples of such types might be self-report, or behavior, or biochemistry, among others. Individual MT studies that assess multiple outcome types would be preferable in many, if not all, cases, because they would make greater use of the resources committed to a study, and would permit examination of the degree to which different types of MT outcomes converge.

What Is MT?

MT is an umbrella term that can include all manner of theoretical assumptions, levels of training, specific strokes, variations in pressure, special techniques, and anatomical sites to which treatment is being applied. Despite this—or, possibly, because of it—researchers often include only the most basic information on what constituted MT in a particular study. To improve matters, researchers can and should take care to indicate, in detail, what they mean when they report having examined massage therapy. This would facilitate experimental replication and increase the potential of research to inform practice.

Neuroimaging Studies

Modern technology makes it possible to see what happens in the brain and the extended nervous system in response to treatment, and a few studies have examined the effect of MT on brain activity (e.g., Diego et al. 2004). Still, more studies that examine the effects of MT using the range of neuroimaging methods are certainly needed, since an increased understanding of the effect of MT on central and peripheral nervous system activity is likely to be especially valuable (Sagar, Dryden, and Wong 2007).

Studies That Define the Profession

Just as it can be hard to say precisely what MT is, the same could be said of the field's practitioners. Levels and types of training can differ widely among states, regions, territories, and countries. In some cases, health care practitioners who are not specifically or traditionally trained as massage therapists may still provide MT as part of health care delivery (e.g., nurses, chiropractors, physical therapists, and so on). This raises the question of who, exactly, is a massage therapist? Studies that examine the relationship between amount and type of training, the tasks and techniques that such training makes possible, and the outcomes that a practitioner is able to achieve could be valuable additions to MT research. Similarly, it is important for all MT research studies to provide detail on the background, training, and specialties of the massage therapists who provide treatment. This has been absent from many study reports.

Body Awareness as a Mechanism of Action, and as an Outcome

Some MT effects may result from the treatment's potential to improve recipients' sense of their own bodies. This could take several forms, such as enhanced proprioception, improved body image, or the reduction of dissociation. In some cases, these may be desired outcomes by themselves. While a few studies have examined these interesting possibilities (Bredin 1999; Price 2007; Price 2005), more research is necessary.[2]

Examinations of Dosage

An examination of dosage is fundamental to understanding a treatment, and relatively little is known about optimal dosing in MT. For a given condition, what constitutes an effective and efficient treatment dose? What constitutes an effective and efficient maintenance dose?

Determine MT Effect on Medication Uptake

It is possible that, for certain conditions, MT benefits patients by improving how, or triggering when, the body utilizes medications (Trubetskoy et al. 1998). This interesting application of MT is certainly worth scientific investigation.

What Takes Place in the Therapist During MT?

Though we know some of what takes place in the recipient during MT, we know hardly anything about what takes place in the therapist. Examination of intra-

[2]See chapter 14 for additional information.

therapist processes, both physiological and psychological, that take place during treatment could serve to improve MT training, identify optimal treatment and working conditions, and promote career satisfaction, to name just a few interesting possibilities.

Examine the Nature of the Therapeutic Encounter

Undoubtedly, effective MT depends on more than the application of manual manipulation of soft tissue. Therapists and recipients are thinking, feeling persons who communicate and form impressions of each other, and all of this takes place within an environmental context that inevitably shapes the encounter. Research that examines the nature of these therapeutic encounters to identify factors in the therapist, recipient, environmental context, and their interactions that contribute to desired outcomes has great potential to inform the field.

Education and Training Research

Training and education are critical to the success of a profession. What knowledge content is essential to good practice? How much training is necessary to consistently yield competency? Which methods for teaching and training MT students work best? Does the amount or type of training that a MT student receives predict career satisfaction, success, or tenure? These and other questions pertaining to MT education and training are all worthy of study.

Methodological Weaknesses and Limitations in MT Research

Workshop subgroups convened once more to indicate ways in which MT research, as a field, has failed to use scientific methods, tools, and approaches to optimally increase our knowledge of MT. Subsequently, the following seven topics, in the order reported here, were presented by the subgroups to the larger group.

Lack of Standards in the Profession

As noted previously, the training, education, knowledge of research, and clinical experience of massage therapists varies widely, so much so that it can be difficult to precisely define what a massage therapist is. The resulting lack of commonly held knowledge across the profession limits the contribution that massage therapists are able to make to MT research.

What is a Good Comparison or Control in MT Research?

Most often, it is desirable for MT research studies to compare the effects of MT to another form of treatment (or, in some cases, to no treatment at all). This controls for confounds, such as attention, expectation, spontaneous improvement, the passage of time, and statistical regression, so that we can most accurately determine the amount of improvement that is directly attributable to MT. But to what, exactly, should the control group be subjected? In most medical research, the choice is straightforward: Control-group participants should receive a *placebo* that is identical to the real treatment in all ways but one—the placebo does not deliver the active ingredient being examined in the study. Ideally, placebo-controlled studies must be *double blind,* which means that neither the participants in the study nor the researchers know who is receiving the active treatment and who is receiving the placebo until the results have been generated. This design feature ensures

placebo

▸ A treatment that cannot logically be expected to have a unique therapeutic effect beyond that produced by the recipients' expectation that they have received a true treatment. As such, placebo treatments are frequently used in research to control for the expectation of benefit and related psychological mechanisms, so that they may be compared with and separated from a treatment's unique effects.

double blind

▸ A condition imposed in some research studies in which neither participants nor researchers know, until the conclusion of the study, who is receiving the treatment under examination and who is receiving a placebo. This is often the best way to control for expectation effects.

that both the active-treatment and placebo control groups will be equally affected by the previously mentioned confounds, such that any additional improvement observed in the active-treatment group must be attributable to the active ingredient that only those participants have received.

It would be ideal if the logic of double-blind, placebo-controlled studies could be easily extended to MT research, but, in most cases, it cannot. The reason for this is not because any so-called alternative medicine treatments are somehow antithetical to scientific examination, as is sometimes claimed (Tonelli and Callahan 2001). Rather, it is for a very simple reason: There is no way to blind the massage therapists participating in a research study. Obviously, they must know whether or not they are administering a real treatment, and this knowledge and the resulting expectations can always, even inadvertently, be communicated to the treatment recipients. (Note that the exact same problem arises in psychotherapy research [Seligman 1995].)

To what, then, should we compare MT? A related question we must also ask ourselves is how does our eventual selection of a particular comparison or control condition affect the interpretation of a study's results? There are no simple answers to these questions. Rather, it is incumbent on MT researchers to make thoughtful choices and to clearly communicate the logic behind them. It is also necessary that we make many different comparisons, such that the idiosyncratic strengths and weaknesses of individual studies can complement each other and their results can be considered together, to best address the questions that MT research asks.

Restriction in the Range of Outcomes That Have Been Assessed

Some workshop participants felt that the field has inadequately assessed both the physiological outcomes of MT and the patient- or recipient-centered outcomes that motivate persons to receive this form of treatment.

An Overemphasis on Reductionism at the Expense of Ecological Validity and the Whole System

As is evident from a recent exchange in this journal (Moyer 2008; Lott 2009; Moyer 2009), the value of, need for, and even the proper definition of reductionism as it applies to MT research can be vociferously debated. Reductive methods in clinical research are sometimes criticized because they may remove a treatment from its context in a way that harms its effectiveness, or because they may not allow for the customization and individualization on which a major portion of a treatment's effectiveness may depend (Verhoef et al. 2005). A solution is to design and conduct research that maximizes *ecological validity*, such that study details maintain or closely resemble the way a treatment is conducted in the real world (Schmuckler 2001). Some complementary, alternative, and integrative medicine researchers emphasize ecological validity in whole-systems research (Ritenbaugh et al. 2003). Regardless of the terminology our field adopts, it is certainly true that we must complement standardized and laboratory-based MT research with studies that more accurately reflect how this form of treatment is delivered in the real world. Further, if the results of these approaches to MT research do not converge, it is essential to conduct further research that can uncover the source of the discrepancies.

ecological validity

▸ The extent to which the details of a research study resemble the way an intervention is conducted in real life.

Lack of Research Literacy Among Massage Therapists

As has previously been noted, the field of MT does not have a research tradition or infrastructure. The result is that most massage therapists are not accustomed to reading, participating in, or benefitting from research. Increasing research literacy is likely to benefit the practice and profession of MT.

When Research Questions are Driven by Methodology

A field's progress can be limited by dependence on a narrow set of research methods. If we are only familiar or comfortable with, say, the randomized controlled trial, we may never even ask important questions that can be answered by a qualitative approach, survey method, case study, or naturalistic observation. Workshop participants noted that careful consideration of research questions should precede the selection of a research method. This is sound advice that all researchers need to be reminded of occasionally.

Confusion of Within-Group and Between-Groups Effects

Many between-groups MT studies (that is, studies that compare the effects of MT against another treatment or no treatment) carelessly emphasize within-group effects (the before-and-after changes that take place in just the MT group) in their analyses and results (Moyer 2009b). This misleading practice could be problematic in any treatment field because it fails to separate treatment effects from placebo effects and other confounds, which has the effect of distorting and obscuring the true effects of the treatment under examination. The problem is made worse when it occurs in a field, such as MT, that does not have a strong research tradition, because the majority of the research consumers will not be in a position to critically evaluate methodologies and analytical strategies, and must instead depend on the narrative description of the results provided by the researchers. The solution is, in essence, a simple one: MT researchers need to specify and conduct the correct analyses for their research design, and journal reviewers and editors must ensure that this has been done before agreeing to publish a study.

Conclusions

Finally, it was determined that there was insufficient time for subgroups to reconvene to discuss the final prepared topic. Instead, the larger group was asked to give their thoughts in response to this question: After considering what MT has, and has not, accomplished in the previous 20 years, what, as a field, is most important for us to consider as we go forward in the next 20 years? The following issues and topics were raised. In this section, we have omitted the repetition of a point which has already been covered in detail in another section. We also slightly reordered the points for better organization and emphasis in this section of the written report.

Bridge the Disconnect That Can Arise Between Researchers and Clinicians

The point was made that, because the MT researchers are rarely practicing MT clinicians, they may be disconnected from some of the most important issues and questions that are arising from practice. As MT research moves forward, researchers should endeavor to stay in close contact with clinicians to build collaborative interprofessional research teams and to ask clinicians for their perspective on needed research.

Issues Pertaining to MT Protocols and Reporting Must Be Carefully Considered

Several problems surrounding the area of MT research protocols must be addressed. One is that protocols are often poorly described in research studies. Future studies need to improve on vague descriptions in the form of "15 minutes of Swedish massage were performed on the upper body." Protocols need to be reported in sufficient detail and with clearly defined terminology to permit precise replication and to aid in the eventual examination of the differential effectiveness of particular MT techniques, modalities, and dosages.

Progress can also be maximized by ensuring that research protocols reflect how MT is performed in practice. Addressing this important detail by means of close collaboration with working therapists helps to maximize the ecological validity of studies and increases the value of research to the field.

Additionally, there is a need for greater standardization of MT protocols in MT research. At first, this may seem to contradict the point just made—that MT research protocols must reflect practice in the real world—but in actuality, these are not mutually exclusive. Both are needed. Standardization of techniques, procedures, and guidelines for clinical decision making, when accompanied by accurate and detailed description in research reports, permits meaningful comparisons that eventually lead to progress in clinical settings.

It is insufficient for researchers to specify a protocol and then assume that it unfolded in the study exactly as planned. High-quality MT research should also evaluate the clinical processes that emerge in the course of research and report on the fidelity with which protocols were carried out. Logically, one hopes that research proceeds as planned and that fidelity to specified protocols is high, but it is always better to check. And, even when research does not proceed as planned, unexpected events and details, and instances where the treatment diverges from that which was planned, have great potential to inform future research and practice.

Finally, the quality of MT research could probably benefit from agreeing on a set of reporting standards. It was pointed out that, all too often, some important detail about a research study gets omitted from the report. Adoption of formalized reporting standards for MT research, possibly based on the CONSORT guidelines (Moher, Schulz, and Altman 2001), could guide researchers and help to prevent such oversights.

Progress Will Accelerate as Funding Agencies Learn More About MT Research

It is terrific if one can come up with an innovative, large-scale research design to address an important question, but the question will never get answered if one cannot obtain funding to actually conduct the study. And in some cases, a strong and innovative proposal may fail to impress reviewers because they are unacquainted with how a proposal addresses some of the issues presented in this report, or because they dogmatically apply a rule of thumb that is frequently correct (e.g., clinical research must have a placebo control group), but is not applicable to a particular MT study proposal. This may be a difficult problem to solve, but there are at least two things our field can do. The first is to write clear research proposals that anticipate the blind spots some reviewers may have related to MT research. The second is that those of us with MT research expertise should, when opportunities arise, devote time to serving on research grant review boards and to educating our colleagues in other clinical fields to some of the challenges presented by conducting MT research.

MT's Role in Integrative Health Should Be Examined

It was pointed out that there is value in expanding the research focus to examine how MT integrates with health and health care more broadly. When, where, and how is MT being used in health care settings and as a complement to other treatments, and what effect does MT have on the delivery and effects of other treatments? How should we evaluate the contribution MT makes to wellness and health maintenance, as opposed to limiting our examination to its benefit for certain conditions and symptoms? Does MT have a professional identity crisis that results from the fact that it is performed alongside medical treatments in some settings and as a personal service in other settings? Clearly, many interesting questions arise from considering the broader role of MT in integrative health, and these need to be researched.

Cost-Effectiveness Studies Should Be Conducted

Results in the form of degrees added to range of motion, lowered scores on an anxiety measure, and statistically significant p-values are fine, but in the end, money may be the best outcome metric of all, and it is one that our field has tended to ignore. Studies that assess the cost-effectiveness of MT have the potential to make a big effect, and can lead to health insurance reimbursement in cases where the treatment is demonstrated to be economically viable.

There Is a Need for Longitudinal MT Research

All of the MT research that we are aware of has been limited to treatment periods of days or weeks. The result is that nothing scientific is known about the effects of MT when it is applied across months or years. Longitudinal research that follows research participants for extended time periods is definitely needed, and it is likely to yield valuable and surprising results.

Innovative Ways to Assess the Therapeutic Encounter Must Be Developed

Probably all of us agree that MT provides benefit not simply by means of the manual manipulation of the recipient's body. This is part of it, of course, but surrounding this is a complex interplay between how the therapist and recipient think and feel about each other, their expectations of and attitudes toward MT, and their prior experiences, to name just a few factors that are probably important. Scientific examination of the complex interaction of multiple intangible variables is daunting, but, in this case, it is also too important to ignore. We must develop innovative ways to assess the therapeutic encounter if we are going to improve our scientific understanding of MT.

These Issues Are Not Unique to MT Research

The process of conducting our workshop and of writing this report identified many issues pertaining to MT research, and it may seem logical to assume that many are unique to the field. However, this is almost certainly not the case. In fact, it is likely that each of these issues has already been encountered, and attempts have been made to address them in related fields belonging to the wider world of applied and clinical research. Presently, MT research has so many issues to address, not because it is unique, but because it is so young. As it matures, MT research will undoubtedly contribute some innovations to the wider world of clinical research, but our own progress will be maximized if we first acquaint ourselves with how other clinical fields have addressed issues identical to or parallel to our own.

SUMMARY

MT research has made considerable progress in the 20-year period from 1988 to 2008, but that time period can also be seen as the infancy of systematic MT research, which places us far behind many other health modalities, especially those with a research tradition and infrastructure. While time lost can never be recovered, our field's late start need not be a demoralizing handicap to progress. Indeed, it may even present certain opportunities and benefits; consider how much more rapidly medical research could have progressed and how many mistakes and dead ends would have been avoided if it had begun with the methods and technologies of the late 20th and early 21st centuries. This is precisely the situation that MT as a field finds itself in today. The technologies available in the Information Age ensure that we can communicate rapidly, collaborate efficiently, and maximally leverage the depth and breadth of modern scientific knowledge as we address the fundamental issues arising at this early stage of MT research. The progress that MT research makes in the next 20 years should be impressive.

Critical Thinking Questions

1. How much scientific research has there been on the topic of massage therapy? There could be more than one correct answer, but make sure your own answer puts the amount in context by comparing it with other fields of research.
2. What, if anything, is well understood about massage therapy as a result of research? Explain your answer.
3. This chapter identifies massage therapy effects, mechanisms, processes, and other details that workshop participants considered to be most in need of research. Indicate which one you think is most important and explain your reasoning.
4. The case is made that massage therapy does not easily lend itself to double-blind, placebo-controlled trials. Explain why this is so, and then generate some possible control-group conditions that would be well suited to future massage therapy research. Be sure to provide the reasoning for your choices.
5. A major issue in massage therapy research has been the confusion of within-group and between-groups effects. Why is the distinction important? How can the confusion between the two distort an understanding of massage therapy effects? (Refer to chapter 3 for a detailed treatment of this issue, if necessary.)

REFERENCES

Beider, S., and C.A. Moyer. 2007. Randomized controlled trials of pediatric massage: A review. *Evid Based Complement Alternat Med* 4(1): 23-34.

Billhult, A., I. Bergbom, and E. Stener-Victorin. 2007. Massage relieves nausea in women with breast cancer who are undergoing chemotherapy. *J Altern Complement Med* 13(1): 53-57.

Bredin, M. 1999. Mastectomy, body image and therapeutic massage: A qualitative study of women's experience. *J Adv Nurs* 29(5): 1113-1120.

Cassileth, B., and A. Vickers. 2004. Massage therapy for symptom control: Outcomes study at a major cancer center. *J Pain Symptom Manag* 28(3): 244-249.

Conference on the Biology of Manual Therapies. 2005. National Center for Complementary and Alternative Medicine. http://nccam.nih.gov/news/events/Manual-Therapy/manual-conference.htm.

Dalkey, N.C. 1969. *The Delphi method: An experimental study of group opinion*. Santa Monica, CA: Rand Corporation. www.rand.org/pubs/research_memoranda/RM5888/RM5888.pdf.

Dicken, S.C., R. Lerner, G. Klose, and A.B. Cosimi. 1998. Effective treatment of lymphedema of the extremities. *Arch Surg* 133(4): 452-458.

Diego, M.A., T. Field, C. Sanders, and M. Hernandez-Reif. 2004. Massage therapy of moderate and light pressure and vibrator effects on EEG and heart rate. *Intern J Neuroscience* 114(1): 31-45.

Field, T. 1992. Interventions in early infancy. *Inf Mental Hlth J* 13(4): 329-336.

———. 1998. Massage therapy effects. *Am Psychol* 53(12): 1270-1281.

Field, T., M. Hernandez-Reif, S. Seligman, J. Krasgenor, W. Sunshine, R. Rivas-Chacon, S. Schanberg, and C. Kuhn. 1997. Juvenile rheumatoid arthritis: Benefits from massage therapy. *J Pediatr Psychol* 22(5): 607-617.

Field, T., M. Diego, and M. Hernandez-Reif. 2007. Massage therapy research. *Dev Rev* 27(1): 75-89.

Folkman, S., R.S. Lazarus, C. Dunkel-Schetter, A. DeLongis, and R.J. Gruen. 1986. Dynamics of a stressful encounter: Cognitive appraisal, coping, and encounter outcomes. *J Pers Soc Psychol* 50(5): 992-1003.

Furlan, A.D., M. Imamura, T. Dryden, and E. Irvin. 2008. Massage for low-back pain. *Cochrane Db Syst Rev* 4: CD001929. DOI: 10.1002/14651858.CD001929.pub2.

Grealish, L., A. Lomansey, and B. Whiteman. 2000. Foot massage: A nursing intervention to modify the distressing symptoms of pain and nausea in patients hospitalized with cancer. *Cancer Nurs* 23(3): 237-243.

Haraldsson, B., A. Gross, C.D. Myers, J. Ezzo, A. Morien, C.H. Goldsmith, P.M.J. Peloso, and G. Brønfort. 2006. Cervical Overview Group. Massage for mechanical neck disorders. *Cochrane Db Syst Rev* 3: CD004871. DOI: 10.1002/14651858.CD004871.pub3.

Hobbie, W.L., M. Stuber, K. Meeske, K. Wissler, M.T. Rourke, K. Ruccione, A. Hinkle, and A.E. Kazak. 2000. Symptoms of posttraumatic stress in young adult survivors of childhood cancer. *J Clin Oncol* 18(24): 4060-4066.

Hootman, J.M., and C.G. Helmick. 2006. Projections of U.S. prevalence of arthritis and associated activity limitations. *Arthritis Rheum* 54(1): 226-229.

Hootman J.M., J. Bolen, C.G. Helmick, and G. Langmaid. 2006. Centers for Disease Control and Prevention. Prevalence of doctor-diagnosed arthritis and arthritis-attributable activity limitation: United States 2003-2005. *Morbidity and Mortality Weekly Report* 55(40): 1089-1092. www.cdc.gov/mmwr/PDF/wk/mm5540.pdf.

Kahn, J. 2002. Massage therapy research agenda. American Massage Therapy Association Foundation. www.massagetherapyfoundation.org/pdf/MRAW-3-02.pdf.

———. 2005. Research matters. *Massage Magazine,* Sept/Oct. www.massagemag.com/Magazine/2005/issue118/Research118.1.php.

Kosfeld, M., M. Heinrichs, P.J. Zak, U. Fischbacher, and E. Fehr. 2005. Oxytocin increases trust in humans. *Nature* 435(June 2): 673-676.

Kutner, J.S., M.C. Smith, L. Corbin, L. Hemphill, K. Benton, B.K. Mellis, B. Beaty, S. Felton, T.E. Yamashita, L.L. Bryant, and D.L. Fairclough. 2008. Massage therapy versus simple touch to improve pain and mood in patients with advanced cancer: A randomized trial. *Ann Intern Med* 149(6): 369-379.

Lott, D.T. 2009. Letter to the editor. *Int J Ther Massage Bodywork* 2(1): 17-18. www.ijtmb.org/index.php/ijtmb/article/view/31/43.

Massage Therapy Foundation. 2005. Highlighting massage therapy in CAM research. www.massagetherapyfoundation.org/pdf/Highlighting%20Program.pdf.

———. 2010. Highlighting massage therapy in CIM research 2010. www.massagetherapyfoundation.org/researchconference2010.html.

Mayo Clinic. 2007. Lymphedema. www.mayoclinic.com/health/lymphedema/DS00609.

Moher, D., K.F. Schulz, and D.G. Altman. 2001. The CONSORT statement: Revised recommendations for improving the quality of reports of parallel group randomized trials. *BMC Med Res Methodol* 1(2). www.biomedcentral.com/content/pdf/1471-2288-1-2.pdf.

Moraska, A., R.A. Pollini, K. Boulanger, M.Z. Brooks, and L. Teitlebaum. 2008. Physiological adjustments to stress measures following massage therapy: A review of the literature. *Evid-Based Compl Alt.* http://ecam.oxfordjournals.org/cgi/reprint/nen029.

Morhenn, V.B., J.W. Park, E. Piper, and P.J. Zak. 2008. Monetary sacrifice among strangers is mediated by endogenous oxytocin release after physical contact. *Evol Hum Behav* 29(6): 375-383.

Moyer, C.A. 2008. From the research section editor's perspective. *Int J Ther Massage Bodywork* 1(1): 7-9. www.ijtmb.org/index.php/ijtmb/article/view/11/16.

———. 2008b. Research section editorial: Affective massage therapy. *Int J Ther Massage Bodywork* 1(2): 3-5. www.ijtmb.org/index.php/ijtmb/article/view/30/31.

———. 2009. Response to Dylan Thomas Lott. *Int J Ther Massage Bodywork* 2(1): 19-20. www.ijtmb.org/index.php/ijtmb/article/view/38/44.

———. 2009b. Between-groups study designs demand between-groups analyses: A response to Hernandez-Reif, Shor-Posner, Baez, Soto, Mendoza, Castillo, Quintero, Perez, and Zhang. *Evid-Based Compl Alt* 6(1): 49-50. http://ecam.oxfordjournals.org/cgi/reprint/6/1/49.

Moyer, C.A., J. Rounds, and J.W. Hannum. 2004. A meta-analysis of massage therapy research. *Psychol Bull* 130(1): 3-18.

Myers, C.D., T. Walton, and B.J. Small. 2008. The value of massage therapy in cancer care. *Hematol Oncol Clin North Am* 22(4): 649-660.

Ong, L., W. Linden, and S. Young. 2004. Stress management: What is it? *J Psychosom Res* 56(1): 133-137.

Perlman, A.I., A. Sabina, A. Williams, V.Y. Njike, and D.L. Katz. 2006. Massage therapy for osteoarthritis of the knee. A randomized controlled trial. *Arch Intern Med* 166(22): 2533-2538.

Post-White, J., M. Fitzgerald, K. Savik, M.C. Hooke, A.B. Hannahan, and S.F. Sencer. 2009. Massage therapy for children with cancer. *J Pediatr Oncol Nurs* 26(1): 16-28.

Price, C. 2005. Body-oriented therapy in recovery from child sexual abuse: An efficacy study. *Altern Ther Health Med* 11(5): 46-57.

———. 2007. Dissociation reduction in body therapy during sexual abuse recovery. *Complement Ther Clin Pract* 13(2): 116-128.

Ritenbaugh, C., M. Verhoef, S. Fleishman, H. Boon, and A. Leis. 2003. Whole systems research: A discipline for studying complementary and alternative medicine. *Altern Ther Health Med* 9(4): 32-36.

Sagar, S.M., T. Dryden, and R.K. Wong. 2007. Massage therapy for cancer patients: A reciprocal relationship between body and mind. *Curr Oncol* 14(2): 45-56.

Schmuckler, M.A. 2001. What is ecological validity? A dimensional analysis. *Infancy* 2(4): 419-436.

Seligman, M.E.P. 1995. The effectiveness of psychotherapy. *Am Psychol* 50(12): 965-974.

Sherman, K.J., D.C. Cherkin, R.J. Hawkes, D.L. Miglioretti, and R.A. Devo. 2009. Randomized trial of therapeutic massage for chronic neck pain. *Clin J Pain*. 25(3): 233-238.

Spiegel, D. 1997. Psychosocial aspects of breast cancer treatment. *Semin Oncol* 24(1): S1-36-S1-47.

Tonelli, M.R., and T.C. Callahan. 2001. Why alternative medicine cannot be evidence-based. *Acad Med* 76(12): 1213-1220.

Trubetskoy, V.S., K.R. Whiteman, V.P. Torchilin, and G.L. Wolf. 1998. Massage-induced release of subcutaneously injected liposome-encapsulated drugs to the blood. *J Control Release* 50(1-3): 13-19.

Verhoef, M.J., G. Lewith, C. Ritenbaugh, H. Boon, S. Fleishman, and A. Leis. 2005. Complementary and alternative medicine whole systems research: Beyond identification of inadequacies of the RCT. *Complement Ther Med* 13(3): 206-212.

Vickers, A., A. Ohlsson, J.B. Lacy, and A. Horsley. 2004. Massage for promoting growth and development of preterm and/or low birth-weight infants. *Cochrane Db Syst Rev* CD000390. DOI: 10.1002/14651858.CD000390.pub.

Weinrich, S.P., and M.C. Weinrich. 1990. The effect of massage on pain in cancer patients. *Appl Nurs Res* 3(4): 140-145.

Wilkie, D.J., J. Kampbell, S. Cutshall, H. Halabisky, H. Harmon, L.P. Johnson, L. Weinacht, and M. Rake-Marona. 2000. Effects of massage on pain intensity, analgesics and quality of life in patients with cancer pain. *Hospice J* 15(3): 31-53.

APPENDIX

Participants	Affiliation
Lois Bogenschultz	Cincinnati Children's Hospital Medical Center
Karen Boulanger	Massage Therapy Foundation and University of Iowa
M.K. Brennan	American Massage Therapy Association
Marissa Brooks	Massage Therapy Foundation
Dongyuan Cao	Palmer College of Chiropractic
Dan Cherkin	Group Health Center for Health Studies
Lisa Corbin	University of Colorado Denver
Susanne Cutshall	Mayo Clinic
Elaine Danelesko	Mount Royal College
Bernadette Della Bitta Nicholson	Commission on Massage Therapy Accreditation
Kinga Dziembowski	
Kathleen Farah	Children's Clinic of Minnesota and Red Cedar Medical Center
Maura Fitzgerald	Children's Hospital of Minnesota
Michael Hamm	Cortiva Institute-Seattle
Nancy Jallo	Virginia Commonwealth University
Anna C. Jensen	Northwestern Health Sciences University
Ania Kania	IN-CAM and University of Calgary
Hollis King	A.T. Still University School of Osteopathic Medicine
Romy Lauche	
Wolf Mehling	University of California, San Francisco
Martha Menard	University of Virginia School of Medicine
Jeremy E. Miller	Abbott Northwestern Hospital-Penny George Institute for Health and Healing
Adam Perlman	University of Medicine and Dentistry of New Jersey
Joel Pickar	Palmer College of Chiropractic
Katherine Pohlman	Palmer College of Chiropractic
Antony Porcino	University of British Columbia and University of Calgary
Cynthia Price	University of Washington
William Reed	Palmer College of Chiropractic
Beatrix Roemheld-Hamm	University of Medicine and Dentistry of New Jersey
Jo Smith	Southern Institute of Technology

Participants	Affiliation
Kiyoshi Suzuki	MOA Health Science Foundation
Ann Gill Taylor	University of Virginia
Lesley Teitelbaum	Crouse Irving Hospital
Barb Thomley	Mayo Clinic
Diana Thompson	Massage Therapy Foundation
John Toews	University of Calgary
Ruth Werner	Massage Therapy Foundation

Index

Note: The italicized *f* and *t* following page numbers refer to figures and tables, respectively.

D

About the Editors

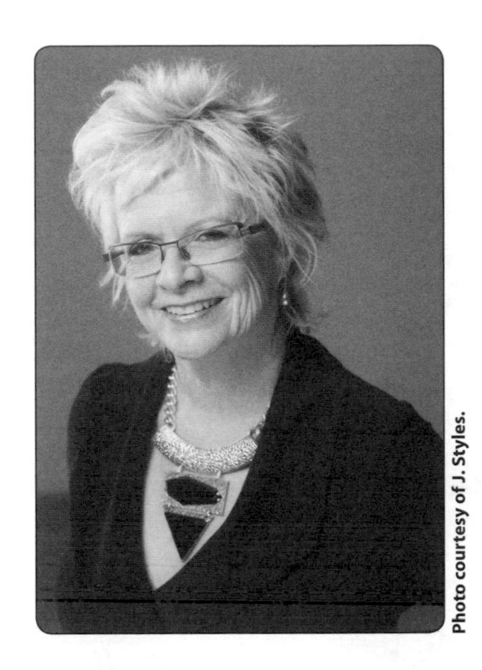
Photo courtesy of J. Styles.

Trish Dryden, MEd, RMT, is the associate vice president of research and corporate planning at Centennial College in Toronto, Ontario, Canada. In addition, she is a registered massage therapist with over thirty years of clinical, education, and research experience. As a massage therapist, Trish specializes in working with individuals recovering from the experience of trauma. A trailblazer and catalyst for change, she is instrumental to the professionalization of massage therapy and the development of integrative and interprofessional research and health care in Canada and internationally. Her work is an extension of her lifelong commitment to equity and social justice, and excellence in public policy, education, and health care. She is the recipient of the President's Award, Centennial College (2010), the President's Award: American Massage Therapy Association (2008), Outstanding Achievement Award, Canadian Massage Therapist Alliance (2005), and the President's Award, Ontario Massage Therapist Association (2003). Trish lives with her husband Lee and sister Diane in the lovely village of Port Hope, Ontario, where she is an avid gardener in summer and intrepid snowshoer in winter. She has two grown children, Bryn and Jesse, and revels in their life adventures with their partners and friends.

Christopher A. Moyer, PhD, is an Assistant Professor of Psychology at University of Wisconsin-Stout. He has been publishing massage therapy research since 2004, and has recently extended his research focus to also examine meditation. He is the Research Section Editor of the *International Journal of Therapeutic Massage and Bodywork: Research, Education, and Practice*, is on the editorial board of the *Journal of Bodywork and Movement Therapies*, and has presented his research findings at international conferences. He and his wife, a professor in the field of Information Studies, reside in Wisconsin with their dog Stewart and their cats Cleo, Tiggy, Smokey, and Charles.

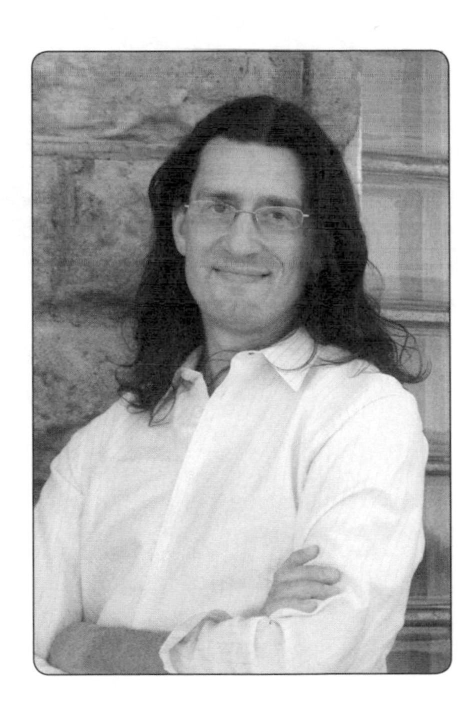

191998
UCB